RICHARD R. LINGEMAN

DRUGS FROM A TO Z

REVISED & UPDATED
SECOND EDITION

A DICTIONARY

McGraw-Hill Book Company

New York • St. Louis • San Francisco • London • Paris • Düsseldorf
Tokyo • Kuala Lumpur • Mexico • Montreal • Panama • São Paulo
Sydney • Toronto • Johannesburg • New Delhi • Singapore

3456789 MUMU 798765

Library of Congress Cataloging in Publication Data

Lingeman, Richard R
   Drugs from A to Z.

1. Drug abuse—Dictionaries. 2. Drugs—Diction-
aries. I. Title. [DNLM: 1. Drug abuse. 2. Hallu-
cinogens—Dictionaries. 3. Narcotics—Dictionaries.
QV13 L755d]
HV5804.L54 1974   613.8'3'03   74-13363
ISBN 0-07-037913-0
ISBN 0-07-037912-2 (pbk.)

Grateful acknowledgment is hereby made to the authors and publishers for permission to quote from the following (which are also cited within this text):

Tom Alexander, "Drugs and the Law." Reproduced from *The Drug Takers.* Copyright
1965, Time Inc., New York.

Jack Altman and Marvin Ziporyn, M.D., *Born to Raise Hell: The Untold Story of Richard
Speck.* Reprinted by permission of Grove Press, Inc. Copyright © 1967 by Jack
Altman and Marvin Ziporyn, M.D.

Charles Baudelaire, *Les Paradis Artificiels* (translated by Norman Cameron), Weiden-
feld and Nicolson Ltd., London, 1860.

Claude Brown, *Manchild in the Promised Land.* Reprinted by permission of The
Macmillan Company, New York, 1965, and Jonathan Cape, Ltd., London.

Tom Buckley, "The LSD Trigger," *The New Republic,* © 1966, Harrison-Blaine of
New Jersey, Inc.

William Burroughs, *Junkie,* Ace Books, New York, 1953.

William Burroughs, *Naked Lunch.* Copyright © 1959 by William Burroughs. Reprinted by permission of Grove Press, Inc., and Calder and Boyars, Ltd.

John Cashman, *The LSD Story,* Fawcett Publications, Inc., Greenwich, Connecticut,
1966.

"The Cheapest Turn-On in Town", *"World Journal Tribune,* November 6, 1966.

Desoxyn (Manufacturer's Statement), Abbott Laboratories, Chicago, 1967.

Havelock Ellis, "Mescal: A New Artificial Paradise," *The Contemporary Review,* January, 1898, by permission of Leonard Scott Publication Co.

"Everybody's Turning On," *Look,* August 8, 1967.

Seymour Fiddle, *Portraits from a Shooting Gallery,* Harper & Row, Publishers, Incorporated, New York, 1967.

Paul J. Fink, Morris J. Goldman, and Irwin Lyons, "Morning Glory Seed Psychosis," *Archives of General Psychiatry,* Vol. 15, August, 1966.

Théophile Gautier, *Revue des Deux Mondes,* 1846. Translation by Polly Kraft for David Ebin (ed.), *The Drug Experience,* The Orion Press, New York, 1961.

Allen Ginsberg, *Kaddish and Other Poems.* Copyright © 1961 by Allen Ginsberg. Reprinted by permission of City Lights Books.

Louis S. Goodman and A. Z. Gilman (eds.), *The Pharmacological Basis of Therapeutics,* The Macmillan Company, New York, 1965.

Richard Goldstein, *One in Seven: Drugs on Campus.* Reprinted by permission of Walker and Company. Copyright © 1966 by Richard Goldstein.

Albert Hofmann, in H. J. DeShon, M. Rinkel and H. C. Solomon, "Mental Changes Experimentally Produced by LSD," *Psychiatric Quarterly,* Vol. 57, 1952.

M. Hoffman, *Comprehensive Psychology,* Vol. 5, 1964.

Helen MacGill Hughes (ed.), *The Fantastic Lodge,* Houghton Mifflin Company, Boston, 1961.

Aldous Huxley, *The Doors of Perception,* Harper & Row, Publishers, Incorporated, New York, 1954.

"Iceberg Slim," *Pimp. The Story of My Life,* Holloway House Publishing Company, Los Angeles, 1967.

Alexander King, *Mine Enemy Grows Older.* Copyright © 1958 by Alexander King. Reprinted by permission of Margie King.

Heinz Kusel, "Ayahuasca Drinkers among the Chama Indians," *Psychedelic Review,* No. 6, 1964.

Jeremy Larner and Ralph Tefferteller, *The Addict in the Street.* Copyright © 1964 by Grove Press, Inc. Reprinted by permission of Grove Press, Inc.

Peter Laurie, *Drugs,* Penguin Books, Ltd., Harmondsworth, England, 1967.

Louis Lewin, *Phantastica: Narcotic and Stimulating Drugs.* Translated by P. H. A. Wirth. Copyright, ©, 1964 by Routledge & Kegan Paul, Ltd. Reprinted by permission of Routledge & Kegan Paul, Ltd.

Dr. Donald Louria, *Nightmare Drugs.* Copyright, ©, 1966 by Mel Sokolow Associates. Reprinted by permission of Simon & Schuster, Inc.

Don McNeill, "Green Grows the Grass on the Lower East Side," *Village Voice,* December 1, 1966.

Don McNeill, "Is Acid Obsolete? The New Initials Are STP," *Village Voice,* April 13, 1967.

B. Manzini and Saraval, in *Delysid (LSD-25), Annotated Bibliography Addendum No. 3,* Sandoz Pharmaceuticals, Hanover, New Jersey, 1961.

The Marihuana Problem in the City of New York, by The Mayor's Committee on Marihuana, Copyright 1944, The Ronald Press Company. Copyright renewed © 1972 by The Ronald Press Company, New York.

The Marijuana Newsletter, Peace Eye Press (Ed Sanders, Publisher), 1965. Reprinted by permission of William Beckman.

Milton Mezzrow and Bernard Wolfe, *Really the Blues.* Copyright 1956 by Milton Mezzrow and Bernard Wolfe. Reprinted by permission of The Harold Matson Company, Inc.

James Mills, "Karen and John: Two Young Lives Lost to Heroin." Reproduced from *The Drug Takers.* Copyright 1965, Time Inc., New York

James Mills, *The Panic in Needle Park.* Copyright © 1965, 1966 by James Mills. Reprinted by permission of Farrar, Straus & Giroux, Inc., and Marvin Josephson Associates, Inc.

Claudio Naranjo, *The Healing Journey.* Copyright © 1973 by Claudio Naranjo. Reprinted by permission of Pantheon Books, a Division of Random House, Inc.

The New York Post, August 17, 1972.

Ed Sanders, *Coming Down,* United International Copyright Representatives, Ltd., New York © 1966.

Richard E. Schultes, "Botanical Sources of the New World Narcotics," *Psychedelic Review,* No. 2, 1964.

Hubert Selby, Jr., *Last Exit to Brooklyn.* Copyright © 1957, 1960, 1961, 1964, by Hubert Selby, Jr. Reprinted by permission of Grove Press, Inc., and Calder and Boyars, Ltd.

J. S. Slotkin, "Menomini Peyotism," *Transactions of the American Philosophical Society,* Vol. 42, Part 4, 1952.

Howard Smith, "Scenes" (Column), *Village Voice,* 1966.

Richard B. Stolley, "Synanon: The Open Door and the Blunt Truth." Reproduced from *The Drug Takers.* Copyright 1965, Time, Inc.

Piri Thomas, *Down These Mean Streets.* Copyright © 1967 by Piri Thomas. Reprinted by permission of Alfred A. Knopf, Inc., and International Famous Agency, Inc.

Hunter S. Thompson, *Hell's Angels.* Copyright © 1966, 1967 by Hunter S. Thompson. Reprinted by permission of Random House, Inc., and Ballantine Books, Inc., a Division of Random House, Inc.

Alexander Trocchi, *Cain's Book.* Copyright © 1960 by Grove Press, Inc. Reprinted by permission of Grove Press, Inc., and Calder and Boyars, Ltd.

R. Gordon Wasson, "Rite of the Magic Mushroom." Reproduced from *The Drug Takers.* Copyright 1965, Time Inc., New York.

Abraham Wikler, *Opiate Addiction. Psychological and Neurophysiological Aspects in Relation to Clinical Practice,* Charles C. Thomas, Publisher, Springfield, Ill., 1953.

Warren R. Young and Joseph R. Hixon (eds.), *LSD on Campus,* Dell Publishing Co., Inc., New York, 1966.

To Anthea

Preface to
the Second Edition

Back when I began the first edition of this book, I mentioned it to Allen Ginsberg, the poet, whom I'd interviewed for an article on the drug culture. Impossible to do, he said, the slang terms change too fast. Well, the existence of the first edition of *Drugs from A to Z* was testimony that such a project was not impossible, while the appearance of the second edition affirms the ever-changing nature of the drug culture, its language and its chemicals. As I pointed out in the preface to the first edition, drug terminology is frequently quite conservative, with some words in use for over half a century; yet obviously new terms arise along with new drugs and now, five years after the first edition appeared, it is time to focus on the *plus ça change* of the French equation that is completed by *plus c'est la même chose*.

Dr. Sidney Cohen of the University of California, a leading authority on drugs, outlined the changing fads in drug usage the country has undergone since the 1960s, when drug use first broke out from the socially erected enclosure of the demimonde. 1966, Dr. Cohen said, was The Year of Acid; 1968, The Year of Speed; 1970, The Year of Smack; and 1972, The Year of the Downer. One might add that 1973 was The Year of Coke—not to mention the most popular drug of all, alcohol, which has spread from what Dr. Timothy Leary once called the "whiskey-drinking establishment" to the current younger generation in a kind of reverse migration.

Dr. Leary is one of the many names from the past a rereading of the first edition summons up; once the high priest of the chemical road to Nirvana, he is back in the California prison from which he escaped, serving a harshly long term for marijuana possession—a last casualty of the once-raging war to stamp out the weed, a war that now rests in an uneasy truce. LSD and the rest of the hallucinogens he once sanctified are still around (or at least their names are applied to the bizarre pharmacopoeia of chemicals now being sold on the street) but the benign furor of the love generation, which in its heyday prompted a cover story by *Time* magazine and an LSD trip by its publisher, Henry R. Luce (a good trip, incidentally; Luce, formerly tone-deaf, "heard" music for the first time), has now faded into memory. As the pop culture sociologists never used to tire of saying, Woodstock gave way to Altamont, and in Haight-Ashbury the paranoia of speed ousted whatever love the flower children had brought there. The hippies have largely fled the cities for the countryside and natural, often drug-free trips. Love turned to protest and the object of protest, the Vietnam war, imported another agony to these shores in the form of heroin addiction among veterans. And all this time drugs continued their steady transmigration across socioeconomic boundaries, out of the ghettos, on to the campuses, and into the suburbs. Heroin, the ultimate downer, was being shot up in Scarsdale as well as on the corner of Seventh Avenue and 128th Street in Harlem.

In the inner city, the methadone clinics were popping up everywhere—157 of them in New York City alone—as the front line of a now-mobilized society's attack on hard drugs. For the first time, law enforcement agencies were getting a handle on the heroin traffic, and it was only recently announced that the "French connection"—the Corsican smugglers in Marseille—has been severed. Under pressure from the United States government, Turkey stopped growing poppies, but in 1974 that opium connection was resumed. The Mexican border, traditional egress for most United States marijuana, has also been stoppered, it is claimed, with the assistance of the once-indifferent Mexican police. Domestically, manufacturing quotas were imposed upon commercially made amphetamines in 1971 (cutting what might be dubbed the Smith, Kline & French connection), and this has reduced amphetamine usage. Similar quotas were imposed on certain barbiturates in 1973.

Yet the drugs were still there, or substitutes were found. The profit margin was sky high; the need remained: *Plus ça change. . . .* Methadone became a street drug and in 1973 passed heroin as the leading cause of opiate-type drug deaths in New York City. Other downers came into vogue—notably methaqualone. Cocaine became an "in" drug, replacing amphetamines although it is more expensive. New hallucinogens were —or could be—synthesized; apparently the number of possible chemical permutations was almost infinite. And there were always new frontiers remaining to be crossed: tranquilizers, stimulant-barbiturate combinations, and the numerous synthetic opiates listed in somewhat tedious detail in this very book. Marijuana and hashish continue to flow in, imported by daring ex-hippie smugglers from Jamaica and Colombia or by returning travelers on the golden road from Samarkand. Like the snakes on Hydra's head, lop off one source and another would appear.

At the same time, the country's attitudes toward drugs was undergoing a rapid change. Marijuana, once the devil's weed of the thirties, had become so common that numerous establishment figures were urging its "decriminalization"; something which, in 1966, when I happened to do an article on the subject, was the rallying cry of a small band of deviants in the underground. A presidential commission on marijuana, appointed by Lyndon B. Johnson, recommended a drastic revision of legal sanctions on private use of the drug; President Nixon, his antennae attuned to *his* silent majority, rejected its conclusions, but many states quietly went about holding referenda on liberalization of their marijuana laws. At least one, Oregon, placed marijuana possession in a legal category lower than a misdemeanor. Texas and Maine loosened their laws, and other states will probably follow their lead, though glacially.

At the same time, New York State experimented with new drug laws of drastic severity for hard drugs. Despite some dire predictions by liberals, the law did seem to reduce trafficking although the final returns are not yet in. Yet the liberals' question—does the end justify the means?—remains as we hear of small-time student coke sellers facing life sentences.

The yawning generational schism between the predominately young, who wanted some liberalization of the marijuana laws, and the predominately old, who didn't, still gaped; yet the intervening years since the first edition of this book appeared have seen numerous bridges thrown across the chasm and a steadily increasing flow of traffic toward the liberalization side. Young and old are now talking to each other; the newspapers are no longer hypnotized by the gaudy freaks of psychedelia; old hardline attitudes pinioning drug use as criminal behavior are loosening, so far as the compulsive user of the more destructive drugs is concerned. So, on the one hand, we see the drug mystique dissipating and drug usage, especially of hard drugs, achieving a plateau, rather than ascending a steadily climbing curve. On the other hand, the need for drugs—for anodynes to assuage the pain of living—seems to be as present as ever. "One must seek drunkenness," Baudelaire said, "in wine or poetry or virtue." What each individual must continue to search out are the age-old alternatives to the kind of ecstasy found in chemicals—the quiet private ecstasies of daily living, as well as the profounder spiritual answers each man seeks for himself along the troublous passage of his life. Drugs were invented by man, almost as inevitably as fire, to ease his body when pain became too much, to strum the chords of his senses, or even to open his mind to wider varieties of consciousness; nonetheless, we must keep them in their place, as servants, for human experience has shown again and again what tyrannical, destructive masters drugs can become.

R.R.L.
New York City

Preface

When I was in college, drugs were things you bought at the drugstore. Oh, there was a small benzedrine scene on campus around exam time, and one read about marijuana in Jack Kerouac, who was then in vogue, but an offer of marijuana probably would have been turned down without the slightest compunction. In those benighted days, in the early fifties, our "trip," if we indeed had one, was Ortlieb's beer. LSD had been discovered, but if someone had mentioned it, we would probably have thought he meant an honorary degree.

The fact that in recent years drug use, or more correctly abuse, has radically changed is, of course, the *raison d'être* of this book. My maiden entry into the new drug scene came a couple of years ago, when I wrote an article for the *New York Times Sunday Magazine* on the then infant subculture of hallucinogenic-drug users. For an innocent user of nicotine, caffeine, and alcohol, it was a case of what the anthropologists call "cultural shock." New York's "East Village" (known to Harry Golden fans as the lower East Side) was just opening itself up to a new wave of immigrants—young people who were knowledgeable about "trips"; who talked of "burn artists," "narcs," and "fuzz"; who patronized "head shops" and had Timothy Leary as their idol and LSD as their sacrament. In the course of the article I did considerable research in the excellent New York County Medical Society Library and interviewed such students of the field as Dr. Jerome Jaffe and Mr. Leon Brill, of Albert Einstein Medical College; Dr. Donald B. Louria, of Belleuve Hospital; and Mr. George Belk, District Supervisor of the Federal Bureau of Narcotics.

So when the opportunity arose to do a book about drugs in dictionary format, I was immediately intrigued—not only because, as a thrifty writer, I would have an opportunity to employ some of the research which was necessarily omitted from *The Times* article—but because the subject itself had become a fascinating one to me.

I must express my gratitude to Dr. Herbert Berger for reading the manuscript and pointing out the inevitable errors of a layman and for writing an introduction to the book. The views expressed and any present errors are, of course, the author's responsibility. Dr. Berger has a distinguished record of public service in the drug-addiction field and in the treatment of drug addicts—an act of courage for a physician in view of our rigid narcotics laws, which have transformed narcotics abuse from a medical into a penal problem. (In his comments on the manuscript, Dr. Berger remarked *en passant:* "Note—addict is really self-destructive. He is consciously committing suicide slowly! One once described drugs as 'Having all the advantages of death without its permanence.' ") Because of the high relapse rate and the low economic level of the typical addict, it is also rather unrewarding both emotionally and financially.

A word about the purpose and format of this book. It is primarily intended for laymen, especially those who through occupation or association have become concerned about drugs. The approach is two-pronged. Drugs are discussed from both a pharmacological and sociological point of view. It might be appropriate here to define what we mean by a "drug" in the context of this book. Generally speaking, a drug is any substance, synthetic or naturally occurring, with a more or less predictable effect on the human physiology. We here are concerned with the so-called "mind" drugs, that is, drugs which alter consciousness, mood, affect, and emotions, which intoxicate and induce pleasurable sensations, and which have been used for extramedical purposes by persons seeking these effects. A "drug" really has five facets: *(1)* its chemistry or molecular structure; *(2)* its pharmacological action, that is, its effects upon mind and body; *(3)* its clinical use, that is, the selective employment of these effects in medical therapy; *(4)* its sociopsychological context, that is, who takes it and by what methods, their motives, the subcultures they form, and so on; and finally, *(5)* its implications to society, that is, how it is used in medicine (if it is used) and with what implications, how society regards its extramedical use, what the moral attitude toward it is, what legal controls exist for it, and how society defines its "abuse," in other words, what uses the culture sanctions and what uses it considers abnormal.

Tying in with the last two categories, since language is a social gesture, is the slang, argot, or cant employed by drug users. It is part of the mystique of drugs to give them special names, different from their common or medical names. It provides a kind of code for the drug subculture in carrying out illegal transactions, and it serves to forge loose fraternal bonds among them and keep the "square" world on the outside. There are probably deeper, more primitive motives at work, too, as well as the desire to be "hip," "in," or easily colloquial. Cocaine is called "coke," and it is easy to understand the abbreviating process. But why is it also called "girl"? And why is heroin called "junk" or "shit" or "crap"? I have attempted, whenever possible, to go into these origins, both psychological and etymological. In doing so, I have found Eric Partridge's work in the field of slang a great help. Two of his books which were of particular assistance are *A Dictionary of Slang and Unconventional English, 6th ed.* (The Macmillan Company, New York, 1967) and *A Dictionary of the Underworld, rev. ed.* (The Macmillan Company, New York, 1961).

Drug slang changes, and some words pass out of vogue as others come along. New drugs demand new words, and there is even a form of technological change at work in that new drugs sometimes replace other drugs in favor, making the slang that grew up around them obsolete. The discovery of heroin, a highly potent narcotic easily trafficked, meant that the use of opium declined, at least in the United States. Nevertheless, as Partridge points out, much underworld argot is conservative in its development. For example, "junk" for narcotics has been with us since at least the turn of the century. New classes of drug users (college students, for example) also adopt many of the old words from the addict underworld, sometimes altering their meanings, sometimes taking them over intact. Some of the words in this book are admittedly what Partridge calls "cliquisms and ephemerides"; they are included, nevertheless, because of the light they cast upon the drug user's world. Similarly, some words which are probably obsolete (so indicated, whenever possible) are also included for the same reason and because they may be lineal relatives of current terms.

A word on the form of this dictionary. Slang and drug names are intermixed. All entries are in alphabetical order, dictionary style; that is, *AMT* follows *amphetamines.* A word is often followed by brackets enclosing the derivation; the chemical composition, or the chemical, generic, and manufacturer's names of a drug; or the meaning of foreign words. There are two abbreviations used to credit source for derivations of entries, i.e., EP for Eric Partridge, and MM for Mezz Mezzrow. The other less frequently appearing sources are not abbreviated. Cross references are indicated by SMALL CAPITALS. In the body of an entry on a drug the cross reference generally refers to specific kinds of drugs, such as particular brands of amphetamines, e.g., BENZEDRINE, or, conversely, to a more general discussion of a specific drug; that is, in the entry for Seconal, a brand name of a barbiturate, the reader is referred to the general discussion of BARBITURATES or else to a term, such as WITHDRAWAL SYMPTOMS, discussed at greater length as a separate entry. With some slang words, related terms are referred to for purposes of comparison. An entry is cross-referenced only once in a given article. Words are generally not marked for cross reference if they are merely synonyms. With *compare,* however, small capitals are used for such entries. When an entry is followed by a word or words in small capitals, it is a synonym for that main entry. When such a cross reference is preceded by *see,* the second term is not a synonym but an entry where more information can be found.

Quotations that follow the definitions are intended to illustrate how a slang term is used or its implications or to provide a subjective description of the effects of a drug. Such accounts, it should be noted, represent one man's experience, and thus are not necessarily typical.

A final caveat: this book is not intended to be a guide to drug taking. As practically all the drugs in this book should be taken only under the directions of a physician (if at all), only his advice, and not the amounts set down herein, should be heeded.

R.R.L.
New York City

Contents

Preface to the Second Edition   *vii*

Preface   *xi*

Introduction by Herbert Berger, M.D.   *xvii*

Addenda   *xxi*

Drugs from A to Z   *1*

Appendix I   Nonsynthetic derivatives of opium, morphine, and cocaine   *258*

Appendix II   Generic names of synthetic opiates   *258*

Appendix III   Schedule I drugs under the Controlled Substances Act of 1970   *260*

Appendix IV   Schedule II drugs under the Controlled Substances Act of 1970, as revised in 1973   *260*

Appendix V   Schedules III, IV, and V drugs under the Controlled Substances Act of 1970, as revised in 1973   *274*

Introduction

It is now five years since the first edition of *Drugs from A to Z* appeared; a period when many aspects of the multifaceted drug syndrome have changed materially. The drug culture has spread from the ghettos to all segments of society, all over the world.

During my recent tour of duty as visiting professor of medicine at Ghaga Mada University in Indonesia, I was surprised to be greeted with a request for information on drug addiction—even before I could begin my lectures on medicine to the students.

The number of new drugs is limited only by the ingenuity of our pharmaceutical chemists. Always the more recent chemicals integrate poorly or disastrously with older ones. The addict buys what the pusher has; not what he believes he is purchasing. There continue to be far too many deaths from overdose among young people whose whole lives should be before them; often because the drug they buy is not one to which they have developed a tolerance.

Mr. Lingeman's book and the efforts of all of us who struggle against drug abuse need no excuse. A physician thinks nothing of working five hours in an intensive care unit to save the life of a 75-year-old cardiac patient. But what has been accomplished? The preservation of life for another year or two. A young addict who is salvaged can have 50 years of life to live. This is what drives us all to attempt to understand, prevent, and treat addiction.

There is some reason to believe that drugs may no longer be the "in" thing and that addiction is falling off. This is, of course, fine—but there are no addictive drugs, there are only addictive personalities. Thus the person who leaves the scylla of opiates finds himself swallowed by the charybdis of alcohol.

Methadone maintenance has caused methadone to be legalized under strict control. In this way the addict can be weaned away from a life of crime to a place in our society. All hospitals must admit addicts; all physicians who wish to, should be permitted to treat them; all insurance companies must cover the costs of their care.

Causes of addiction must be determined. We treat the addict with only a modicum of success—we must therefore bend our efforts toward prevention. All of these problems will move toward solution as many disciplines work together. Should we succeed, the data obtained can be extrapolated for use in the management of alcoholism and obesity. The numerous disciplines must cooperate if this legal, social, and medical problem of addiction is to be managed and prevented. To this end, Mr. Lingeman's contribution in fostering better communication is exemplary.

When Richard Lingeman's pioneer and monumental effort to compile a lexicon of terms from the world of drug abuse first came to my attention in 1968, I greeted it with ambivalence—first, with enthusiasm, for it was long overdue; second with remorse, for why didn't I think of doing this myself?

Over the past years, I have taken part in many symposia in which experts representing various disciplines explored the problems of narcotic addiction. Here were police officials, pharmacologists, public prosecutors, judges, teachers, guidance counsellors, clergymen, and physicians. A good part of our time had to be spent in defining terms to everyone's satisfaction.

Since our efforts would help various legislatives bodies draft laws to combat drug addiction, we were acutely aware of the need for precise definitions: ambiguity in the meaning of the law would result in confusion and even chaos in its enforcement. We therefore compiled a glossary of terms. But our definitions were necessarily arbitrary because there was no standard reference work that adequately covered the subject. Most of the terms used by addicts are slang, and they increase and change too rapidly for most dictionaries to cope with them.

Not too many years ago the students of addiction were concerned only with the opiates—tinctures and infusions prepared from powdered opium. Some addicts smoke the product of the poppy directly. Then the various alkaloids, the active principles, of opium were isolated, and we were faced with addiction to much more potent materials, such as morphine. Still later, heroin was introduced as a nonaddictive substitute for morphine. Unfortunately heroin did indeed replace its predecessor, only to produce the much more complicated addiction problem which faces us today.

As time went on, many new synthetic drugs appeared—demerol, methadone, and laterine, to name a few—whose formulas were very different from those of morphine, heroin, and the other alkaloids of opium. But their effects were almost identical with those of the opium derivatives. These new drugs, too, were looked upon as panaceas which one day would cure addictions, but they proved to be as dangerous and as habit-forming as their precursors.

Then came the barbiturates—the sleeping pills and sedatives. Still more recently, the tranquilizers have appeared on the scene, and at the other end of the spectrum stimulants like the amphetamines have been introduced.

A drug group now receiving wide publicity is the psychedelics, or hallucinogens. New hallucinogens are being synthesized almost daily. Others, such as marijuana, have been in use for centuries. Chemicals like psilocybin and fly agaric have been used by primitive peoples to produce trances as a part of religious rituals. There seems never to have been a single race of man that has not felt the need to escape from reality through the medium of drugs!

We cannot help but reflect on this truth as we blame our present preoccupation with drugs on the pressures of modern society. It is quite probable that the contemporary American is less subject to stress than was any predecessor. At no time in history were people's basic needs met so adequately. Yet modern men and women, like their neanderthal forebears, are beset by frustration. Sometimes they respond by running away from problems. Physical flight is the often-attempted means of escape; drug-taking is another.

As pharmaceutical chemists continue to synthesize new drugs, many of which find their way onto the market both licitly and illicitly, the narcotics problem multiplies exponentially. Until recently most addicts used heroin or barbiturates or stimulants such as amphetamine. Today multiple addictions are the rule rather than the exception. A variety of materials is used because one drug or the other is not obtainable at the time or because the addict hopes to overcome different kinds of discomfort with different kinds of drugs. Several years ago a cartoon appeared in the *New Yorker* magazine which depicted a man standing before a vending machine. Across the top was the legend "Start the Day Right." The machine buttons had such labels as "Tired—Benzedrine"; "Nervous–Phenobarbital." It was difficult for me to smile at this piece of humor; too many of my patients could have posed as the bewildered man reaching for a coin to insert in the machine. For it is all too true that the multiple addict often starts his day with amphetamine and keeps using it all day long in order to be "the life of the party." However, when night time approaches, he is still hopped up and thus unable to sleep. He then turns to a barbiturate sedative for relief. In the morning he has such a hangover from the massive dose of barbiturate he needed to bring on sleep that he must have still larger amounts of his stimulant.

Multiple addictions are also found in the world of sports. Some boxers, for example, take a combination of heroin and amphetamine in the hope that the former will keep them from suffering too much from the blows while the latter will keep them from tiring. This is often specious reasoning in the extreme, but it tends to further complicate the study of addictions.

How many addicts are there? No one knows. Laws which drive these people underground obscure the answer, but some figures are available. Over thirty thousand narcotic addicts were registered in New York City in a two-year period. Names are obtained primarily from police records; some addicts voluntarily come to physicians' offices or clinics. Most impoverished addicts must eventually come to the attention of the authorities because the cost of narcotics usually exceeds their earning capacity. Addicts are often unemployable. They are not dependable, often steal from their employers, and are narcotized—largely incapacitated—much of the time, so they usually lose their jobs. Most become addicted too young to acquire a salable skill, so they must steal to support the enormous cost of their habits. The district attorney of New York County tells me that fences pay only about one-fifth the retail price for stolen goods. Thus, a $50-a-day addict must steal about $250 worth of merchandise daily. Most addicts cannot maintain this scale of theft without getting caught eventually. Thus, for this class of addict, the police figures are fairly accurate.

The wealthy addict, however, doesn't have to break laws to buy drugs and therefore rarely becomes a police statistic. The public has become aware of something which physicians have known for some time: There are as many addicts on Fifth Avenue as there are on First. Addiction is no longer a disease afflicting just the subcultures of our great cities. It has become an urgent problem for all segments of society.

To these addicts must be added the 6 million homeless alcoholics. This is not the total figure, for only some 5 percent of such addicts are female. Females are just as prone to addiction as males, but they are hidden and protected by their families—often sequestered in upstairs bedrooms with "sick headaches," "female troubles," and the like.

How much does addiction cost? Some years ago I was commissioned with some others by Mayor Robert F. Wagner to find the cost of drug addiction in New York City. The figure we arrived at—$5 billion—seemed so large that we reviewed it by various accounting methods. All yielded similar answers—narcotic addiction costs $625 per person per year. This included the cost of apprehending, trying, and jailing addicts and pushers; the cost of welfare for addicts and their dependents; and—the largest sum of all—the value of the stolen goods. Yet neither the number of registered addicts nor the material cost of addiction tells the whole story. The real immeasurable price is paid in threatened lives, wasted potential, broken homes, and misery. Is narcotic addiction increasing? This, too, is hard to evaluate. There are many more arrests today—but this may indicate more police activity rather than more addiction. For whatever this figure is worth, arrests have increased over 1,000 percent in the past ten years. Significantly, such distressing figures are found not only in a known addiction center like New York City but also in a prosperous suburban area like Westchester County. Such data certainly suggest that addiction is increasing.

It is no secret that drugs are a problem on college campuses. A Harvard survey suggested that over 25 percent of the student body has experimented with drugs and that over half of the experimenters continue to use them. Although these figures are obtained through questionnaires with guaranteed anonymity, they are inaccurate, as are all estimates of the incidence of drug abuse.

Addiction is no respecter of class, race, education, or geography. It has become imperative that our ignorance of its causes and consequences be dispelled as rapidly as possible. Richard Lingeman's *Drugs from A to Z* is a signal contribution to the understanding of this problem.

Herbert Berger, M.D.
New York Medical College

Addenda

banker. one who puts up the capital to finance a marijuana-buying expedition, assuming none of the risk of arrest.

blanco. [Spanish, white] HEROIN.

boogie. a trip to buy drugs for smuggling, as in, "I'm going to do a boogie to Mexico."

cocaine. As usage of cocaine spread during the early 1970s drug experts began to study cocaine users and, as a result, traditional medical notions about the drug came into question. For example, a number of experts submitting affidavits at a trial in the Federal District Court in Newark, N.J., in 1974 generally agreed upon the following: (1) cocaine use does not lead to criminal activity in obtaining the drug or violent behavior; (2) death by overdosage is almost nonexistent, certainly rare; (3) in amounts taken by most users cocaine has no adverse effect on the health; (4) cocaine has less abuse potential than heroin, alcohol, tobacco, barbiturates, or amphetamines; (5) most cocaine users take it infrequently, intermittently, as a special treat; (6) cocaine is less harmful organically than amphetamines; (7) cocaine users did not disrupt their lives or their work; (8) intermittent users felt no depression after cocaine use that would compel them to take more; (9) the drug did not engender psychotic reactions; (10) users could stop without psychological discomfort; (11) the effect of the drug is subtle and the "high" must be learned as is the case with marijuana; (12) in the United States the drug is usually taken in a diluted state—50 to 90 percent pure—though sometimes it is cut with amphetamines by dealers. These observations of cocaine users suggest that some of the adverse reactions attributed to the drug in the main entry are actually associated with extreme abuse. Since the preponderance of users sniff the drug in a diluted form, they do not receive its full effects, just as the sniffer of heroin (or the opium smoker) receives less potent doses of the drug. Further, cocaine use is by custom analogous to joy-popping among heroin users. Injecting cocaine, however, especially intravenously, would no doubt increase the danger of lethal reaction, when taken in amounts equal to the generally given lethal dose (1,200 milligrams).

colas. [Spanish, tails] the flowering tops of the MARIJUANA plant.

cold bust. an arrest made when the person stopped is, by coincidence, concealing drugs. Compare HOT BUST.

domestic. MARIJUANA grown in the United States. Compare HOMEGROWN.

doobie. a MARIJUANA cigarette.

dope run. a trip to buy drugs for oneself or someone else.

gold. also, any high-potency MARIJUANA.

grower. a MARIJUANA cultivator, uninvolved in smuggling.

homegrown. MARIJUANA grown in the United States. Compare DOMESTIC.

hot bust. an arrest resulting from a trip by an informant or other police action. Compare COLD BUST.

incentive. COCAINE.

Johnson grass. [from Lyndon B. Johnson, a Texan] low-potency MARIJUANA—strictly for Texans.

load. also STASH.

lumber. MARIJUANA waste. Compare STICKS.

move. to traffic in MARIJUANA.

number. a MARIJUANA cigarette.

pop. also, arrest.

primo. number-one quality.

Purple. see ZACATECAS PURPLE.

sniff. COCAINE.

snort. also, COCAINE.

stepped on. cut; diluted.

sticks. MARIJUANA twigs; waste.

weight. also, a large quantity of a drug, as in, "Can you bring me weight?"

Zacatecas Purple. MARIJUANA grown in Zacatecas, a central Mexican state; the seeds turn purple when dried; supposedly very potent.

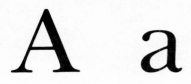

A a

A. AMPHETAMINES.

A-bomb. [since the 1940s—*EP*] a mixture of MARIJUANA and HEROIN smoked in a cigarette. *Obsolete.* See DUSTER, DUSTING, PALL MALL AND PAREGORIC.

Acapulco gold. [from the golden brown color] also called gold and golden leaf. A variety of MARIJUANA considered especially potent by users, grown near Acapulco, Mexico (potency of marijuana varies with its origin; see CANNABIS SATIVA). It is priced from 15 to 60 percent higher than the lowest "grades." Compare MEXICAN GREEN, PANAMA RED.

> This is a special grade of pot growing only in the vicinity of Acapulco. The color is either brownish gold or a mixture of gold and green. This grade has a potency surpassed by few of the green varieties and usually comes at slightly higher prices or in short weights.
> –*The Marijuana Newsletter No. 1* (Jan. 30, 1965)

ace. [from *ace*, highest card in the deck; unparalleled, number one; since the 1940s] a MARIJUANA cigarette. *Obsolete.*

l-acetyl-*d*-lysergic acid diethylamide. a chemical congener of LSD-25.

acid. [from a shortening of *d*-lysergic *acid* diethylamide; since around 1960] LSD-25.

acid freak. [from *acid*, LSD-25, and FREAK, suggested by bizarre behavior and states of consciousness induced by a HALLUCINOGEN, and *to freak*, to be under the influence of LSD-25] *1.* a user of LSD-25. *2.* one who exhibits the dress, behavior patterns, etc., of the LSD cult and whose behavior is bizarre.

acid head. [compare HEAD] frequent, habitual, heavy user of LSD-25; similar to ACID FREAK, except that the term connotes a subjective state of choice as much as a characteristic pattern of behavior.

acid rock. a kind of rock and roll music emphasizing electronically produced sounds, songs with surrealist imagery and loud, monotonous, sometimes atonal sound, the use of Indian instruments such as the sitar, or a primitive pounding, coarse blues sound, considered to be inspired by, and compatible with, LSD-induced states of consciousness. The music originated in San Francisco and was performed by groups such as Jefferson Airplane, Dow-Jones and the Industrials, and The Grateful Dead. The music was initially played at ACID TESTS and associated with the use of HALLUCINOGENS, and many of its composers and performers were users of hallucinogenic drugs.

acid test. [from *acid*, LSD-25, and *test* in the sense of a psychic trial by fire] parties held in the mid-sixties at which the guests wore bizarre, colorful costumes and clown makeup and danced randomly to the accompaniment of raga music or ACID ROCK, while slides and stroboscopic lights were flashed on the walls, the intention being to mimic and enhance the LSD experience. A punch containing LSD, called ELECTRIC KOOL-ADE, was often served, sometimes causing BAD TRIPS among those who drank it unwittingly.

action. [in the sense of an illegal activity, such as gambling] selling of narcotics, as in "There's no action around here."

active principle. the chemical substance in a plant which produces mind-altering and toxic effects, e.g., the active principle in PEYOTE is MESCALINE, in MARIJUANA is TETRAHYDROCANNABINOL, in OPIUM is MORPHINE.

addiction. an overwhelming involvement with, and craving for, a substance, often accompanied by PHYSICAL DEPENDENCE (although one can be physically dependent without being addicted and vice versa), which motivates continuing usage, resulting in TOLERANCE to a drug's effects and a syndrome of identifiable symptoms appearing when it is suddenly withdrawn. The addicts' use of the substance becomes compulsive so that they feel they cannot function without it, orient their lives around acquiring it (unless they have an unlimited source), at whatever the personal social cost, and are subjectively preoccupied with repeating their intake in quantities that are excessive for their culture, often to their physical detriment. Addiction is also characterized by a high rate of relapse among those who attempt or are compelled to stop using the substance addicted to. Although in common parlance addiction refers to such compulsive, excessive use of narcotic and other physical dependence-producing drugs, the term properly encompasses any substance so used. As the World Health Organization says:

> There is scarcely any agent which can be taken into the body to which some individuals will not get a reaction satisfactory or pleasurable to them, persuading them to continue its use even to the point of abuse— that is, to excessive or persistent use beyond medical need.

Of course some drugs, because of their pharmacological effects and the severe disapproval with which a culture regards their use, wreak greater harm than other drugs. The opium user in nineteenth-century China was regarded with the same tolerance as that extended by many Americans to heavy social drinking as long as it does not result in violent behavior, or smoking, while a narcotic addict in this country generally must resort to desperate criminality to support addiction. Because the social and medical problems of addiction often vary with the type of drug, the WHO has recommended that the use of the term be abandoned in favor of the formula "drug DEPENDENCE of the [name of drug] type," further differentiating between PHYSICAL DEPENDENCE and PSYCHIC DEPENDENCE, the latter referring to a compulsive need for the drug's mental effects such that users feel their well-being depends upon continuing to use the drug.

The three main approaches to treatment of addiction are (1) treating the specific drug dependence by addicting the patient to another drug (see METHADONE, CYCLAZOCINE); (2) treating the character structure through intensive group or individual therapy directed by professionals in mental health or by cured addicts who serve as discussion leaders and authority figures (see SYNANON); and (3) incarceration and compulsory withdrawal.

adrenochrome. one of the components of "pink adrenaline," a derivative of the epinephrine produced in the body. It has an indole nucleus identical to the HALLUCINOGENS and for this reason was thought to be the chemical cause of schizophrenia, since some of the effects of that disease are similar to those produced by the hallucinogens (see SEROTONIN). This theory has all but been discarded, however. When injected, adrenochrome will cause immediate physical pain unless it is mixed with the subject's own blood. Mixed or not, it produces certain abnormal and unpredictable mental effects, including changes in color and texture of the environment, distorted visual patterns, vague paranoia, and irritability with those not participating in the experience.

A-head. [from A, AMPHETAMINES, HEAD, a frequent drug user] a frequent, habitual, often exclusive user of amphetamines.

a la canona. [Puerto Rican addicts' slang] abruptly stopping HEROIN and undergoing WITHDRAWAL SYMPTOMS without medication. COLD TURKEY.

> He was gonna let me make it—cold turkey—*a la canona.*
> —Piri Thomas, *Down These Mean Streets* (1967)

alcohol. also called ethanol, ethyl alcohol. A primary and continuous depressant of the central nervous system. The effect is analogous to a general anesthetic, though usually less profound and longer lasting since the alcohol is slowly metabolized in the liver, at the average rate of 10 milliliters per hour (the equivalent of 0.6 ounce of 100-proof whiskey). The amount necessary to produce anesthesia is dangerously close to the lethal dose. The body can metabolize at the very maximum 400 to 500 milliliters in a day, the equivalent of about a fifth of 100-proof whiskey. It takes the average adult five or six hours to metabolize the alcohol in 4 ounces of whiskey or 1.25 quarts of beer, however, which means that roughly a pint of 100-proof whiskey or 5 quarts of beer would be metabolized in a day.

Alcohol acts on the primitive part of the brain, the reticular activating system, releasing it from the integrative control of the cortex, with the result that thoughts occur in a disorganized, jumbled fashion and bodily coordination is disrupted. Though basically a depressant, alcohol can foster a pseudo-stimulant effect which results from the hyperactivity of various primitive parts of the brain suddenly freed from the inhibitory control of the cortex. This activity is short-lived and gives way to the depressant effects, with resultant coma if consumption is continued.

The degree of alcoholic intoxication is fairly accurately reflected by the percentage of alcohol in the bloodstream. Various "drunkometer" or "breathalyzer" tests to establish this percentage have been devised and are employed by legal authorities to determine whether a person was criminally under the influence of alcohol when he committed a crime, i.e., certain crimes such as negligent homicide while driving a motor vehicle in which the key element is whether the driver was drunk or not. The following percentage concentrations of milligrams of alcohol in proportion to milliliters of the blood are commonly accepted as causing corresponding states of alcoholic intoxication:

0.05%	no intoxication (but the American Medical Association says that this concentration can impair driving ability in some individuals)
0.05–0.15%	some intoxication, but not in itself legal proof of intoxication
0.15%	legal presumption of intoxication according to the criterion established by the National Safety Council (which later recommended it be lowered to 0.10%)
0.25%	mild to moderate intoxication
0.3%	severe intoxication

0.4%   extremely severe intoxication, at the threshold of coma and even death

0.5–0.8%   fatal concentration of alcohol in the blood

It is estimated that the ingestion of 4 ounces of whiskey or 5.5 ounces of a martini cocktail on an empty stomach results in a blood concentration of 0.06 to 0.09 percent, or 0.03 to 0.05 percent on a full stomach. The same amount of alcohol taken as beer (1.25 quart) results in a maximum blood concentration of 0.041 to 0.049 percent on an empty stomach and 0.020 to 0.023 percent on a full one. Thus four average-sized highballs or martinis will produce a concentration in the blood of 0.134 to 0.184 percent, the legally defined state of intoxication.

PSYCHIC DEPENDENCE upon alcohol, where users drink in ways and amounts that are abnormal for their culture, may be mild, i.e., they miss the presence of alcohol at social functions; moderate, i.e., they feel compelled to drink in order to work or function socially and make determined action to see that alcohol is available for those purposes; or strong, i.e., they use amounts far in excess of the norm, drink more or less steadily and on occasions not customary in their culture, and are so obsessed with obtaining alcohol that they will go to any lengths to do so and will drink whatever is available, even poisonous mixtures. Motivations for psychic dependence range from (1) socially acceptable half rationalizations (he "needs" it to relax, to stimulate appetite, relieve boredom, or to sleep) to (2) subconscious compulsions (anxiety, latent aggression that he can express only when inhibitory controls are removed, or inhibited masculininity or feminity) to (3) a desire to withdraw from a world perceived as threatening.

TOLERANCE to the action of alcohol develops, but imperfectly; during sustained drinking the amount of alcohol necessary to maintain an intoxicatory percentage in the blood must be increased, and an alcoholic's performance while intoxicated may be slightly less impaired than that of a nonalcoholic. But this tolerance is nothing like that seen with MORPHINE. The symptoms of chronic alcoholic intoxication, too well-known to be described here, resemble chronic BARBITURATE intoxication. PHYSICAL DEPENDENCE on alcohol definitely occurs (an estimated 10 percent of the 60 million users of alcohol in the United States are alcoholics), with WITHDRAWAL SYMPTOMS ranging in severity from the morning-after hangover (although this is not really a withdrawal symptom since a first-time drinker can have a hangover) to convulsions and delirium, including confusion, disorientation, delusions, and vivid visual hallucinations.

Delirium tremens, when severe, has an 8 percent fatality rate. There is a degree of CROSS-TOLERANCE between the barbiturates and alcohol; hence, barbiturates will relieve the alcoholic withdrawal syndrome, as will certain nonbarbiturate hypnotics, especially the frequently used PARALDEHYDE. TRANQUILIZERS are also effective in alleviating the rigors of the withdrawal state.

Prolonged use of alcohol, especially in conjunction with the inadequate diet often associated with it, also has a debilitating effect on the body (cirrhosis of the liver, lowered resistance to disease, stomach trouble, heart disease); the barbiturates do not have these effects. Even if the heavy drinker gets an adequate diet, alcohol's toxic effects will damage the liver, eventually causing death. The usual long-term progression is fatty liver (which can be reversed by abstinence), alcoholic hepatitis, and fatal cirrhosis of the liver. Liver damage represents the chief health hazard of alcohol, and cirrhosis of the liver ranks as the third leading cause of death, after heart trouble and cancer, in New York City.

Because of its action in releasing aggressive drives from inhibitory controls, alcohol is a significant factor in over half the crimes of violence in this country and over half the automobile fatalities. And because of its ability to POTENTIATE many drugs, alcohol is often an important factor in drug fatalities, especially when large doses are not involved.

alley. inmate's name for a dormitory corridor at the U.S. Public Health Service (Narcotics) Hospital, Lexington, Kentucky.

alphaprodine. a synthetic compound similar in its effects to MORPHINE, though a larger dosage (40 to 60 milligrams) is necessary to produce the ANALGESIC (pain-relieving) effect of the standard 10-milligram dose of morphine. Its duration is one to two hours, somewhat less than that of morphine. Prolonged use of the drug results in PHYSICAL DEPENDENCE. WITHDRAWAL SYMPTOMS are not so severe as those associated with morphine. Alphaprodine is sold commercially as Nisentil, Nisintil, and Prisiliden. A Schedule II drug under the CONTROLLED SUBSTANCES ACT. Compare MEPERIDINE, DEMEROL.

amanita muscaria. FLY AGARIC.

amobarbital. AMYTAL.

amphetamines. synthetic amines which act with a pronounced stimulant effect on the central nervous system. They are thought to POTENTIATE the effects of norepinephrine, a neurohormone which activates parts of the sympathetic nervous system. Chemically there are three types; salts of racemic amphetamines, dextro amphetamines, and methamphetamines, which vary in the degree of side effects and in potency (methamphetamine—SPEED—being the most potent). The dextro amphetamines have the least peripheral activity and in general use produce fewer side effects, e.g., decrease in saliva and mucus, alteration in blood pressure, tremors, enlargement of the nasal and bronchial passages, and faster heartbeat, while continuing to stimulate the brain.

Amphetamine was first discovered in 1887, but its medical effects were not known until 1927. The first amphetamine preparation on the market was BENZEDRINE, used in an inhaler to reduce nasal congestion (see B-BOMB). The amphetamines were found useful in narcolepsy (involuntary sleep), in controlling hyperactive children (in whom they have the paradoxical effect of calming down), in psychological depression, and as an aid to dieting (since they seem to depress the appetite center). Since amphetamines provide a feeling of euphoria—considerably enhanced when they are injected—and dull the sense of taste and smell, they are useful in dieting up to a point, but are more likely to be abused for their pleasurable effects. Their appetite-depressant effects are also short-lived (unless the dosage is markedly increased). As a result, their use in dieting is no longer recommended and their chief medical use now is in narcolepsy, hyperkinesis, and sometimes depression (controversial).

Although many medical users of amphetamines have continued at the same dose level for a long period of time, TOLERANCE does develop to the drug's euphoriant, energizing effect, necessitating an increased dosage to achieve the same pleasure experienced from the initial dose. Injection of amphetamines in soluble form (METHEDRINE and DESOXYN are the main commercial preparations) probably became popular among HEROIN users in the 1950s (amphetamines potentiate heroin's analgesic effects, while the heroin counters excitation). The combination of the two drugs was known as a SPEEDBALL. Knowledge of the intensified pleasure to be gotten from injecting spread in the early sixties and such usage became widespread among the HIPPIES in the HAIGHT-ASHBURY section of San Francisco.

Amphetamines are not effective in treating deep-seated or psychotic depressions (heavy usage may produce paranoid psychoses, see below); if used in mild depression, the depression may be intensified after the drug is stopped. Psychotherapists have employed them to make a repressed patient more talkative. They are also used to combat overdosages of central nervous system depressants, depending upon the drug used, because of their stimulant effects on the central nervous system. This treatment is controversial, however. Usual prescribed dosages range from 15 to 30 milligrams per day up to (by gradually increasing the daily dose) 50 milligrams in narcolepsy. If tolerance to the stimulant's effects develops and if users increase their daily dosage beyond recommended limits, they suffer loss of appetite, chronic insomnia, marked restlessness, depression, fatigue, acute paranoia, delusions, irritability, and combativeness. A single dose of 50 milligrams (ten 5-milligram Benzedrine tablets) when there is no tolerance to the drug may produce in some persons a toxic psychosis, with hallucinations and paranoid delusions. More prevalent are the paranoid delusions that inevitably follow prolonged, heavy injection of the methamphetamines (speed). These heavy users also report the delusion that bugs are crawling on their skin (CRANK BUGS) and suffer from malnutrition.

Fatalities due to an overdose of amphetamines are fairly rare but have occurred. The symptoms are convulsions, coma, and cerebral hemorrhage. The lethal dose is not known and varies among individuals. A dose of 120 milligrams was fatal in one case, whereas a dose of 500 milligrams was survived in another. Based on experiments with monkeys, the lethal dose in human adults would be around 20 to 25 milligrams per kilogram (2.2 pounds) of body weight (or 780 to 890 milligrams in a 150-pound man), and for children, about one-fourth to one-fifth of this amount. In certain sensitive individuals the lethal dose may be much lower. If prolonged use has produced tolerance to the drug, larger amounts can be consumed; a habitual user probably ingests anywhere from 200 to 1,000 milligrams a day, although not all at one time. A case was reported of a heavy user injecting 15,000 milligrams and surviving!

Amphetamines raise the blood pressure and stimulate the heartbeat and are thus hazardous to people with high blood pressure or heart trouble. Overdosages may also be followed by chills, collapse, and loss of consciousness. Prolonged heavy users may view the resultant paranoia with some detachment, but at length their delusions become real and they sometimes slip over into full-blown psychosis. In most cases, though, users will return to a normal state within six months to a year if the drug is given up completely, the only long-term effect being some loss of memory. Prolonged use of amphetamines to counter fatigue is a form of PSYCHIC DEPENDENCE. The truck drivers who take amphetamines to stay awake risk severely impaired judgment, psychoses, and accompanying hallucinations, which have been the proximate cause of serious accidents. Deaths from heart failure have occurred among athletes, another common group of abusers, who use them to increase energy, alertness, and endurance—most prominently long-distance bicycle racers. In Japan, where amphetamine abuse was widespread, medical authorities contended the drug caused brain damage. Babies with defective hearts have been born to amphetamine-using mothers.

Although psychic dependence upon amphetamines does occur, PHYSICAL DEPENDENCE does not, and there are no specific WITHDRAWAL SYMPTONS. Still the hyperexcitability and masking of fatigue resulting from their use will take their toll: upon withdrawal the heavy user will experience massively accumulated fatigue and suffer from general depression, weakness, tremors, gastrointestinal disturbances, and a long, exhausted sleep, sometimes lasting days (CRASHING). Amphetamines can be detected in the blood and the urine by laboratory tests. The amphetamine user often has dilated pupils, dry mouth and nasal passages; exhibits excited, aggressive behavior; and talks incessantly. The community of SPEED FREAKS which grew up around San Francisco was extremely antisocial, even violent, given to stealing from other users, and did not exhibit the talent for HUSTLING that heroin users often display.

Amphetamines are often used by students and persons engaged in intellectual work to "get them started," stimulate their mental processes and promote alertness, retention, and wakefulness. Such users commonly take one or two tablets and use the drug only when they need added mental energy to cope with a difficult task, or simply to stay awake in order to complete a large amount of work. Apparently amphetamines do not improve performance (errors may be increased); they do stimulate the initiative to undertake and keep on with a task. Correspondingly, persons undertaking unusual physical stress employ amphetamines to mask fatigue and keep them going. Thus they were issued to soldiers by both sides in World War II, a practice which continued through the Vietnam war. The danger, of course, is that prolonged use will produce a relapse, impaired judgment, and perhaps mental disturbance.

As several writers have noted, the sustained use of amphetamines to mask fatigue and produce a continuous state of stimulation is overdrawing one's account at one's energy bank, and one may have to pay up later in the form of an unpleasant mental state. Unlike foods, amphetamines do not create energy; they mobilize adrenalin, which is the neurohormone that activates the bodily system. Further, amphetamines, when used in large amounts, can have bizarre effects upon the operation of the mind and indeed be inimical to systematic intellectual work. The speed freak often compulsively engages in some grotesque parody of a mechanical task; he will start to repair something, then find himself staring for hours at the object to be repaired before taking the simplest step; he may repeat an operation, or a form of physical activity, such as flipping a coin or dancing, over and over and over—an action known as hypomania; and though his mind may be full of brilliant ideas and verbal energy, he may be unable to apply these in any way other than dissipating them in a talking jag or singing the same song repeatedly.

A common character structure among heavy amphetamine users—especially the young—is a low sense of self-esteem and recurring depression; by producing euphoria, an enhanced sense of power, and excessive energy, the amphetamines alleviate this feeling of worthlessness. Others use them simply to feel "HIGH" over a long period of time, to stay awake, or to savor the illusion of increased intellectual activity unleashed by the drug.

Specific commercial preparations most commonly taken by drug abusers include Benzedrine, DEXEDRINE, Methedrine, DESBUTAL, Desoxyn, DEXAMYL, and DAPRISAL (a combination of amphetamine and BARBITURATE; compare TEDRAL). The federal government's tighter regulations of commercial amphetamine production resulted in increased black market activity with amphetamines being smuggled in from Mexico, the growth of clandestine laboratories manufacturing injectable speed, and finally the increased use of COCAINE, which is quite similar in its effects to amphetamines, although it is not effective if taken orally and does not last as long. Production controls under the CONTROLLED SUBSTANCES ACT, however, have substantially decreased the amount of legally produced amphetamines in the illicit market, where they once constituted 80 percent of the supply. Amphetamine substitutes, usually marketed as diet drugs such as PRELUDIN or RITALIN, are also used. Amphetamine and amphetamine-barbiturate preparations are Schedule II drugs under the Controlled Substances Act. Compare MAO INHIBITORS. Slang names: A, cranks, splash, rhythms, chalk, ups, thrusters, forwards, crystal, water, whites, speed, bennies, dexies, benz, cartwheels, fives, tens, lid poppers, peaches, roses, sparkle plenties.

> Georgette twisted her face with pain, not too much though, and they wondered and thrilled. Goldie handed her half a dozen bennie and she swallowed them, gulped hot coffee and sat silent . . . trying to think the bennie into her mind . . . not wanting to wait for it to dissolve and be absorbed by the blood and pumped through her body; wanting her heart to pound *now;* wanting the chills *now;* wanting the lie *now;* Now!!! . . . Goldie sent Rosie, a demented female who acted as sortofa

housemaid, for gin, cigarettes and another gross of bennie. They made a small pot of bouillon and danced around it dropping tablets in and chanting *ben*nie in the *bouil*lon, *ben*nie in the *bouil*lon, whirling away the fear and boredom, gibbling, popping bennie, drinking gin, toasting Georgette. . . .

But the boys were having a ball, not too sure what they were laughing about, but really digging the bennie scene, enjoying the cold chills and the strange feeling in their jaws as they clenched and ground their teeth. . . .

Goldie opened the box of bennie slowly and proffered it to Georgette. She took two, just two thank you, smiled and laid them on her tongue and sipped her gin. They spoke quietly, smiling, sipping their drinks, at peace with all and Georgette leaned back in her chair speaking softly with Vinnie, and the others when addressed; all her movements, smoking, drinking, nodding, soft and regal; feeling extremely human; looking upon her world (kingdom) with kindness, softness; waiting, excitedly yet not nervously, for the time, soon for her to nod to her lover. . . . Goldie kept glancing at her watch and listening to hear Sheila and her john leaving, wanting to get out of this ugly room and upstairs with the boys before the light brought them down and they lost what Georgette had given them; afraid if a bennie depression set in that the boys would simply become rough and not trade. . . .

—Hubert Selby, Jr., *Last Exit to Brooklyn* (1964)

AMT. [perhaps a play on the HALLUCINOGEN DMT] AMPHETAMINES.

amyl nitrite. an inhalant dilator of the small blood vessels, which also acts to lower high blood pressure; the drug relaxes the smooth (involuntary) muscles of the body.

Amyl nitrite was discovered by Sobrero in 1857; its first medical use was in the treatment of angina pectoris. The drug is active only when inhaled; hence, it is sold as a clear, yellow, volatile liquid in glass ampuls, which are called *pearls* in the medical profession; a slang name is *snapper*. Each contains 2/10 milliliter.

Amyl nitrite is still used to relieve the pain of angina pectoris and to prevent seizures, which it does by dilating the blood vessels leading to the heart. Amyl nitrite is very quick acting, taking effect within thirty seconds, hence its value in such seizures. The effects last only two to three minutes. Sometimes unpleasant side effects, such as headaches, nausea, vomiting, and flushing of the face, are experienced; the drug may also cause temporary visual disorders, e.g., halos of yellow or blue surrounding dark objects seen against a light background.

Among illicit users, the drug is prized for its alleged sexual stimulation or intensification of orgasm as well as the perceptual and consciousness distortions it produces. In most states it is sold without prescription. TOLERANCE develops to the effects of drugs of the nitrite family. Deaths from nitrite poisoning are rare.

amys. small glass vials containing AMYL NITRITE.

Amytal. [amobarbital, Eli Lilly and Company] an intermediate-acting BARBITURATE hypnotic and sedative, which acts in fifteen to thirty minutes and lasts three to six hours. The sedative dose is 20 to 50 milligrams, two to three times daily. The hypnotic (sleep-inducing) dose is 100 to 200 milligrams. Amytal comes in capsule-shaped scored tablets inscribed "Lilly," in different colors, depending on the amount of the drug:

color	milligrams	grains
light green	15	1/4
yellow	30	1/2
orange	50	3/4
pink	100	1-1/2

Amytal is a Schedule II drug under the CONTROLLED SUBSTANCES ACT.

Amytal Sodium. more frequently the choice of drug abusers than AMYTAL, this form comes in pale blue capsules, with a darker band of blue where the upper and lower parts join, in 60- and 180-milligram (1- and 3-grain) sizes. Prolonged heavy use, i.e., 600 milligrams per day, will result in PHYSICAL DEPENDENCE and severe WITHDRAWAL SYMPTOMS and convulsions if abruptly stopped. A Schedule II drug under the CONTROLLED SUBSTANCES ACT. Slang names: blue heavens, bluebirds, blues.

analgesic. [from the Greek *an-,* without, and *algesia,* pain] a drug producing relief from pain without loss of consciousness (although the more potent narcotics, such as MORPHINE, in large doses will produce sedation).

angel dust. PHENCYCLIDINE (Sernylan) which is mixed in powdered form with MARIJUANA or other HALLUCINOGENS and smoked, inhaled, or swallowed. Compare HOG, ELEPHANT.

angel off. [police term; from (?) *angel,* a person easily victimized, like a theatrical angel, who puts up money for a show, or one who puts up the money for a criminal venture—*EP*] to arrest the customers of a drug peddler who is under surveillance.

. . . but we figure we'll go up and *angel off* some of his customers. Angeling off is when you know someone's dealing and you lay back some place and bust the customers coming out. Sometimes you do it to get information on exactly where the dealer is and sometimes you do it, like this time, just to make business rough for him.

—narcotics detective in James Mills,
The Panic in Needle Park (1966)

anileridine. a synthetic compound similar in effects to MORPHINE, anileridine is also very similar to MEPERIDINE, another SYNTHETIC OPIATE, in chemical structure and pharmacological actions. It is not so constipating as morphine but otherwise has similar side reactions, e.g., vomiting, nausea, feelings of warmth, faintness, and dizziness. Injections of 30 to 40 milligrams will produce analgesia equal to that of 10 milligrams of morphine with a shorter duration (two to three hours) than morphine. As with morphine, overdosage can cause respiratory depression and death. PHYSICAL DEPENDENCE results from long-term usage, with WITHDRAWAL SYMPTOMS similar to those of morphine in severity. Commercial preparations are Lerinol and LERITINE. Compare DEMEROL. A Schedule II drug under the CONTROLLED SUBSTANCES ACT.

antihistamines. drugs which block the action of histamine on effector cells in the nerves. A large number of commercial preparations are marketed but there is little difference among them, except in potency. The drugs are most effective in alleviating various allergies and mitigating symptoms, such as sneezing, runny nose, itching of the eyes and throat, and skin conditions. Some are also useful in preventing motion sickness, and because of the drugs' sedative effects, they are used in certain nonprescription sleeping tablets. Drug abusers mainly use them either mixed with CODEINE and terpin hydrate elixir (BLUE VELVET) or as found in commercial cough syrups such as Robitussin A-C, which contains codeine, pheniramine maleate (the antihistamine), and glyceryl guaiacolate (a muscle relaxant). The effects sought are probably sedation and some euphoria. Alcohol (of which there is a high percentage in terpin hydrate elixir) acts synergistically with antihistamines, thus magnifying the sedative effects of both and possibly lowering the toxic dose of the antihistamine. Toxic doses engender excitation, restlessness, and convulsions followed by central nervous system depression; death, if it occurs, is a result of respiratory arrest. In these effects, the antihistamines resemble ATROPINE and SCOPOLAMINE. Antihistamines can also generate various unpleasant side effects among approximately 20 percent of the population. Abuse of antihistamine combinations is a fairly recent (1968) phenomenon.

anywhere. possessing drugs, as in "are you *anywhere?*" meaning "do you have any drugs?" Compare HOLDING.

army disease. MORPHINE addiction among soldiers. During the Civil War the hypodermic needle was first employed to inject the drug and was used widely and indiscriminately. Because only soldiers were so widely affected, the addiction became known as the army disease. After the war, the number of addicts in the United States was estimated at 400,000, or 1 percent of the population.

artillery. equipment for injecting narcotics. Compare WORKS.

Asthmador. an obsolete asthma cigarette containing 50.4 percent STRAMONIUM and 4.5 percent BELLADONNA, both of which are toxic in large amounts and produce hallucinations. Three cases of experiments with this drug by teen-agers with resultant hallucinations have been reported, and use is becoming more widespread.

ataraxic drug. [from Greek, *ataraxia,* perfect peace of mind] also called ataractic drug. A drug that acts as a TRANQUILIZER.

atropine. [from *Atropos,* one of the three Fates; so named because BELLADONNA was used in the Middle Ages as a poison] an alkaloid found in deadly nightshade, *Atropa belladonna,* henbane, *Hyoscyamus niger,* and other plants of the potato family (*Solanaceae*). It is also synthesized.

The drug is used mainly as an antispasmodic (in parkinsonism, gastrointestinal upset, peptic ulcer, vomiting, etc.) because it acts to block the action of acetylcholine, a neural activator, on the parasympathetic nerves, thus tranquilizing the smooth muscles and glands. It is also used to reduce nasal congestion, for parkinsonism and, in heavy doses, as shock therapy for schizophrenia. The average dose of atropine is 0.5 milligram. Such small doses do not depress the central nervous system or inhibit normal bodily activity.

Since it does not depress the central nervous system or cause sedation to the extent that SCOPOLAMINE, a related alkaloid, does, atropine is preferred as an antispasmodic. In massive doses, atropine can cause death through medullary paralysis and respiratory failure. The lethal dose is not known, and fatalities in adults are rare. Dosages of 1,000 milligrams have been survived; however, toxic reactions usually occur in doses of 10 milligrams or more. Atropine is considered less toxic than scopolamine. Fatalities among children from atropine poisoning (mainly due to eating the plants containing it) are much more common, in doses as small as 10 milligrams. Doses above 1 milligram will result in stimulation; those above 10 milligrams will be toxic, producing in adults rapid weak pulse; enlargement of the pupil so that the iris is almost obliterated (thus it may induce or aggravate glaucoma); blurred vision; flushed hot dry skin; loss of motor control; restlessness, excitement, wakefulness, hallucinations, and delirium (the "belladonna jag"); followed by paralysis and coma.

Atropine acts as an antidote to the deadly poison MUSCARINE, found in the mushrooms *Amanita muscaria,* FLY AGARIC, and *A. pantherina.* It is also an antidote to certain poisons used as insecticides and in chemical warfare.

ayahuasca. [Peruvian Indian word] also called CAAPI, NATÉMA, and YAGE. A hallucinogenic beverage brewed from various species of the tropical liana *Banisteriopsis,* especially BANISTERIOPSIS CAAPI, by the Chama Indians of northeastern Peru. Sometimes the beverage is prepared with the vine alone, and sometimes in conjunction with other leaves, especially *Haemadictyon amazonica,* a member of the family *Apocynaceae.*

When ill, the Indians take the beverage in the belief that the plants they see in their hallucinations are those which will cure them. They also take it before an important enterprise, in the hope that their visions will foretell the future, and for pleasure and escape from the harsh reality of their life. The drug is little known among North Americans, though there is evidence that it is appearing now on college campuses. Slang name: jungle drug.

> The first visual experience was like fireworks. . . . There were patterns that consisted of twining repeats, and others geometrically organized with rectangles or squares that were like Maya designs or those decorations which the Chamas paint on their thin, ringing pottery. . . . At times snake-like stems of plants were growing profusely in the depths, at others these were covered with arrangements of myriads of lights that like dewdrops or gems adorned them. . . . A big ship with many flags appeared in one of these flashes, a merry-go-round with people dressed in highly colored garments in another. . . . The color scheme became a harmony of dark browns and greens. . . . Naked dancers appeared turning slowly in spiral movements. Spots of brassy lights played on their bodies which gave them the texture of polished stones. . . .
>
> —Heinz Kusel, *Psychedelic Review* (1964)

B b

baby. *1.* MARIJUANA. *2.* a small, irregular HEROIN habit.

backwards. [certain TRANQUILIZERS will calm an LSD panic reaction; thus they reverse the drug's action] *1.* tranquilizers or BARBITURATES. *2.* a reacquired drug habit.

back up. *1.* to inject part of a shot of HEROIN into a vein, then withdraw blood back into the syringe or eyedropper. Compare BOOTING, JERK OFF. *2.* to back out of a narcotics sale at the last moment.

bador. [Aztec, little children] Aztec name for the hallucinogenic seeds of *Rivea corymbea.* See MORNING GLORY SEEDS.

bad. very good, potent, as in "That's *bad* dope."

bad seed. [probably a pun based upon the appearance of the cactus buds and the common phrase meaning ill-fated offspring] PEYOTE.

bad trip. a panic reaction or temporary or chronic psychosis after taking a HALLUCINOGEN, especially LSD, or other drugs.

bag. *1.* a measure of HEROIN diluted with MILK SUGAR or quinine and packed in folded paper or the small glassine envelopes used by stamp collectors. The proportion of heroin ranges from 1 to 80 percent, and the addict is never certain of the strength of the dose he is taking. The usual bag contains about 5 grains of diluted substance, of which about 1 to 5 percent is pure heroin. This is the equivalent of 3 to 15 milligrams (average bag contains 5 milligrams) of heroin with the analgesic potency of 9 to 45 milligrams of MORPHINE, the latter amount being used medically for severe pain. Often referred to as a FIVE-DOLLAR BAG. *2.* a measure of MARIJUANA, usually called a NICKEL ($5) BAG, containing 1/7 to 1/5 ounce of marijuana. *3.* something one is interested in, occupied with, obsessed with; a drug one is using exclusively at the time, as in "He is in a *speed* bag."

bagman. [from BAG; since the 1950s] a narcotics peddler, though usually one who holds the money in an illegal transaction.

bale. a pound of MARIJUANA.

balloons. drugs, usually HEROIN, sold in rubber balloons; in case of pending arrest they can be swallowed in this form and later excreted and the contents used.

bam. [from *bombita*] amphetamine pill, or amphetamine for injection.

Bambu. a kind of cigarette paper used in rolling a MARIJUANA cigarette.

banana smoking. a hoax perpetrated in 1966 and instigated by Marvin Garson. It was alleged that the inside of a banana peel scraped off and dried in the oven would, if smoked, produce a HIGH. Prohibition of bananas would, of course, be impossible. After due investigation, federal authorities pronounced the claims a hoax. The purpose of the jest—to twit narcotics authorities—thus may be said to have been accomplished.

bang. [from a pun on *shoot* or *shot*] *1.* an injection of narcotics, as in "I had a *bang.*" *2.* to inject narcotics, as in "I was *banging* heroin."

Banisteriopsis caapi. a species of jungle liana belonging to the family *Malpighiaceae* and known to the Chama Indians of northeastern Peru as the "vine of death." The entire vine or the more tender inner part is used by South American Indians to prepare a beverage with hallucinogenic effects under the names YAGE, AYAHUASCA, NATÉMA, or CAAPI.

The Indians used it simply as an intoxicant, to get in touch with the spirits of their ancestors, for divination, in religious ritual, and for anesthesia during painful initiation ceremonies. In small doses it reportedly produces vomiting, and it is a powerful stimulant of the genital organs, causing erection in the male and engorgement of the clitoris accompanied by vaginal spasm in the female. Enhancement of the visual powers so that the user sees lights too dim for ordinary vision and enhanced auditory acuity so that the user hears sounds too faint for normal hearing have also been reported. Other effects include blue flashes before the eyes; sensations of heat alternating with sensations of cold; wild bravado alternating with fear; vertigo; intensification of colors; and hallucinations of ornamental objects and animals.

The drug has a fast onset, taking effect within five minutes; a profound sleep, accompanied by dreams full of forms fluctuating between the microscopic and the megascopic, is said to complete the hallucinatory cycle. The drug is thought to act as an excitant upon the central nervous system. The lethal dose for human beings is not known, but the lethal dose for dogs has been experimentally determined as 200 milligrams per kilogram of body weight. Death results from respiratory paralysis, while toxic doses produce muscle incoordination and convulsions. The active alkaloid extracted from the vine is HARMALINE, which contains the same indole nucleus as SEROTONIN (also present in LSD-25).

bank bandit pills. BARBITURATES or other sedative pills.

bar. a solid block of MARIJUANA, bound together with honey or sugar water. Compare BRICK, SUGAR WEED.

barbiturates. central nervous-system depressant drugs derived from barbituric acid (malonylurea), which in itself does not have these effects. The first hypnotic (sleep-producing) barbiturate was issued in 1903 under the trade name Veronal. Its basis was barbital (diethylbarbituric acid), and it is still used today. In 1912 came LUMINAL, a phenobarbital, and since its appearance over 2,500 barbituric acid derivatives have been synthesized; some fifty commercial brands are presently on the market although, according to the American Medical Association, five or six types are sufficient for most clinical purposes. Barbiturate production rose from 3.1 billion 300 mg. dosage-units in 1967 to 5 billion in 1971—an increase of 30 percent; the Food and Drug Administration (FDA) estimates that 20 percent of these find their way into the illicit market.

The barbiturate derivatives act to depress the central nervous system, which is profoundly sensitive to their action. Their first medical usage was to induce sleep, replacing alcohol, bromides, the opiates, and such drugs as CHLORAL HYDRATE and PARALDEHYDE. They do not have to be ingested in large quantities in order to induce sleep as do alcohol and opiates; and chloral hydrate and paraldehyde have an unpleasant taste and smell. In small doses ("daytime sedation") they are effective in relieving tension and anxiety and, like TRANQUILIZERS, do not cause excessive drowsiness. In larger doses their selective activity is lost, while their depressant actions spread to all parts of the central nervous system and the spinal cord, causing drowsiness, loginess, and sleep under normal circumstances. A barbiturate-induced sleep resembles natural sleep, except that a disturbance of the random eye movement (REM) factor has been noted, indicating that dreaming is impaired, which could have as yet unexplored psychological consequences.

In addition to producing sedation or sleep, certain of the barbiturate derivatives are useful as anticonvulsants (e.g., in epilepsy) and as analgesics when minor pain is preventing sleep (though in severe pain they have no analgesic effect and may produce excitation); the ultra-fast-acting barbiturates are used to induce anesthesia or as anesthetics for minor surgery.

The various barbiturates are metabolized and eliminated through the liver and kidneys at varying rates of speed. Hence, they are classified according to three categories: *long-acting barbiturates,* which move slowly through the blood to the brain and hence are slow in taking effect but which produce a more profound and prolonged sleep because they are slow in passing through the kidneys; *short- to intermediate-acting* or *fast-acting barbiturates,* which have a faster onset and do not last so long because they are more rapidly metabolized, thus tending to eliminate "barbiturate hangover," the morning-after drowsiness caused by barbiturates remaining in the system, and making them preferable for persons who have difficulty in falling alseep but, once asleep, tend not to wake up; and *very fast-acting barbiturates,* which take effect in approximately ten minutes when taken intravenously, producing hypnosis for about fifteen minutes, and are thus useful in inducing a rapid onset of vapor anesthetics such as NITROUS OXIDE.

Because they seek the drug's effects quickly, barbiturate abusers almost uniformly choose the fast-acting drugs. The Drug Enforcement Agency says that the most widely abused barbiturates are AMYTAL (amobarbital), TUINAL (amobarbital and secobarbital), NEMBUTAL (pentobarbital), and SECONAL (secobarbital). These have been classified as Schedule II drugs under the CONTROLLED SUBSTANCES ACT. The fast-acting barbiturates are also considered more likely to produce PHYSICAL DEPENDENCE.

In the presence of severe pain or psychological disturbance, the barbiturates in clinical doses may produce delirium, rashes, nausea, diarrhea, anxiety, nervousness, and other undesirable side effects in some persons. If for some reason ingestion of a hypnotic dose is not followed by sleep, the patient may show signs of mental confusion and euphoria, even stimulation, closely resembling alcohol intoxication, with slurred speech, excessive drowsiness, loss of motor coordination, staggering gait, and eventual unconsciousness. Anxious persons with low self-esteem find the drug an excellent palliative for their symptoms, and of course it is also used for a sense of HIGH, relaxation, and intoxication.

TOLERANCE to the sedative effects of the drug will develop after prolonged heavy use because the rate of its elimination from the system increases (the drug seems to stimulate the enzymes in the liver, where it is metabolized). This necessitates more frequent doses to preserve the high, or higher initial doses to achieve the initial euphoria previously produced by a lower dose. Tolerance does not significantly increase the lethal dose, varying widely among individuals, beyond which the barbiturate user, no matter how tolerant to the drug, cannot go and live. Since tolerance to the drug's desired effects builds up, users may continue to increase their dose until they reach the lethal level. Since the long-acting barbiturates achieve their effects more slowly, yet more profoundly over a longer time, an overdose would seem more likely to be fatal, because there is less chance that it will be discovered in time for medical attention. In practice, however, the barbiturates most frequently used in suicides or overdoses are undoubtedly the four short-acting barbiturates mentioned above as being most widely abused. They tend to be available, and the chance of accidental overdosage is higher since they take effect before the user can seek help.

The lethal dose is assumed by a rough rule of thumb to be something more—varying with the individual—than ten times the hypnotic dose, or 1,000 to 2,000 milligrams. With such a dosage severe central respiratory depression will occur, producing deep coma, respiratory and kidney failure, complications, and death. A person who has taken an overdose develops a typical shock syndrome, including a weak, rapid pulse, cold sweaty skin, and breathing that is either slow or rapid and shallow. The large medical armamentarium available is usually effective if hospital treatment is undertaken in time, barring complications.

Nevertheless, barbiturates are a leading mode of suicide. Detailed studies, in Santa Clara County, California, showed, between the period January 1, 1971 and May 1, 1972, there were 1,771 barbiturate suicides and 3,475 overdoses; in Los Angeles County in 1971 the Coroner's Office reported 54 barbiturate-related suicides and 259 accidental deaths. Another study showed that about 42 percent of the barbiturate overdoses were related to the intention to commit suicide, while the remainder were accidental overdoses. Thus, the drug provides an easy way of suicide and is also dangerous because of accidental overdose. Since the insomnia states for which they are prescribed are often symptomatic of an underlying depression that may be in itself suicidal, they tend to be available to the suicide-prone individual, thus becoming a self-fulfilling prophecy. Further, since oblivion may be the effect sought, the temptation to overdose is often present. Use of barbiturates with alcohol, which

POTENTIATES their effects (meaning that a small dose may be fatal), is another cause of death. DRUG AUTOMATISM, the state of mental confusion in which the barbiturate user forgets how many doses he has taken, is another potential cause of overdose. On the other hand, overdosage is usually deliberate. The person who, out of impatience because his usual dose has not brought sleep, repeats the dose several times usually falls asleep before he can take a sufficient amount to cause death. Used under proper medical supervision, the barbiturates have proved to be useful hypnotics, sedatives, and anticonvulsants.

At the usual therapeutic dose (100 to 200 milligrams a day) physical dependence is unlikely to develop. However, if taken in amounts exceeding 800 milligrams per day for at least sixty days, physical dependence, with WITHDRAWAL SYMPTOMS following cessation, will occur. In the matter of barbiturate dependence among those who do not use large amounts or seek frequent, chronic barbiturate intoxication, Dr. Henry L. Price and Dr. Robert D. Dripps say:

> The danger of *severe* physical dependence and addiction is overemphasized; more pertinent is the question whether regular use of barbiturates and other hypnotics may not tend to obscure or exacerbate the condition underlying the insomnia, thus establishing a vicious cycle in which the patient becomes psychologically dependent on, or habituated to the drug.
> —In L.S. Goodman and A.Z. Gilman (eds.),
> *The Pharmacological Basis of Therapeutics* (1965)

Barbiturate withdrawal symptoms are severe—in fact, more severe than HEROIN withdrawal symptoms, especially since the heroin addict often has a milder physical dependence due to the diluted nature of the heroin he has been taking. (The use of barbiturates among heroin addicts and those on METHADONE maintenance programs is on the upswing; the former often use them when they cannot get heroin, while the latter, unable to achieve a heroin high, simply substitute another drug). Withdrawal symptoms closely resemble the delirium tremens of the alcoholic and include weakness, violent tremors, anxiety, rise in temperature, rapid pulse, and violent epileptic-like seizures, which are sometimes fatal (in 5 to 7 percent of the cases where withdrawal is not eased by medication). By the third day psychoses resembling schizophrenia with paranoid delusions and vivid hallucinations may occur; sometimes patients die of exhaustion during this psychotic stage, which lasts up to two weeks. The treatment for withdrawal symptoms is gradually decreased doses of barbiturates. Alcohol also helps and barbiturate users show a CROSS-TOLERANCE for alcohol, and vice versa.

Barbiturates are also used in combination with other drugs, in addition to heroin and methadone. The combination with alcohol is common (compare GERONIMO) and potentially lethal, since the drugs potentiate each other, with the result that a dosage of barbiturates that might normally not be fatal *is* when combined with alcohol.

Barbiturates tend to enhance the euphoric effects of the AMPHETAMINES while calming the overwrought nervous state they produce. Hence, the two were sometimes combined commercially in capsules, e.g., DEXAMYL, which was used in dieting. The FDA has banned such combinations, but drug manufacturers have appealed this ruling. Amphetamine users also take barbiturates after a prolonged JAG in order to sleep. Persons taking barbiturates in large amounts in order to sleep often fall into the habit of taking amphetamines in the morning to wake up and combat barbiturate hangover. As their barbiturate dosage increases, their amphetamine dosage does also; this results in worse insomnia and necessitates even more barbiturates, and so on in a vicious cycle. See MULTI-HABITUATION.

Barbiturates are also used to combat alcoholic hangover and medically to alleviate delirium tremens. This is another illustration of the chemical affinity of the two drugs. Predictably, heavy barbiturate users resemble alcoholics. Experiments at the United States Public Health Service Hospital, Lexington, Kentucky, demonstrated that subjects given regular daily doses of barbiturates soon deteriorated in their behavior patterns so that they markedly resembled skid row alcoholics.

The abuse of barbiturates among young people has shown a marked increase, as has that of other sedatives such as METHAQUALONE and DORIDEN (which are not barbiturates). Unlike amphetamines and the HALLUCINOGENS, the black market trade in barbiturates does not originate in clandestine laboratories; rather, they are siphoned out of legitimate channels or smuggled in from Mexico. Barbiturates are rarely injected (if barbiturate preparations containing soluble salts are injected subcutaneously they cause skin irritation); the onset of the fast-acting barbiturates is so rapid that most users achieve the desired high by swallowing them.

The barbiturate addict exhibits marked social and emotional deterioration and resembles the chronic alcoholic. He neglects his appearance, loses his job, and is rejected by friends and family. Addicts undergo wild swings in moods from elation to deep depression or hostility. Barbiturate users are prone to violence, and in New York City they have the highest percentage of aggravated assault charges among all drug users. Some users may develop dangerous paranoid delusions; a tendency to suicidal depression will be intensified by chronic intoxication. Barbiturate users are also dangerous drivers; 100 milligrams will impair driving performance to the same extent that the legal minimum of alcohol does. The presence of barbiturates in the blood or urine can be determined by laboratory tests. Barbiturates penetrate the placental walls, thus affecting the fetus, so that babies of addicted mothers are born addicted. For descriptions of specific commercial preparations see Amytal, Dexamyl, Luminal, Tuinal, Nembutal, Seconal. Slang names: reds, blues, yellows, nemmies, seggies, barbs, sleepers, downs, blockbusters, bluebirds, blue heavens, courage pills, gangster pills, G.B., goofballs, goofers, gorilla pills, idiot pills, King Kong pills, nebbie, nemish, yellow jackets, yellows, pinks, seccy, sleepers, stumblers, tooies, rainbows, red and blues, red birds.

CATEGORIES OF BARBITURATES

long-acting	aprobarbital, e.g., Alurate
	barbital, e.g., Veronal
	diallybarbituric acid, e.g., Dial
	phenobarbital, e.g., LUMINAL
short- to intermediate-acting	amobarbital, e.g., AMYTAL
	butabarbital, e.g., BUTISOL SODIUM
	cyclobarbital, e.g., Phanodorn
	heptabarbital, e.g., Medomin
	hexethal, e.g., Ortal
	pentobarbital, e.g., NEMBUTAL
	probarbital, e.g., Ipral
	secobarbital, e.g., SECONAL
	talbutal, e.g., Lotusate
	vinbarbital, e.g., Delvinal
very short-acting	thiopental, e.g., PENTOTHAL SODIUM

The barbiturate addict presents a shocking spectacle. He cannot coordinate, he staggers, falls off bar stools, goes to sleep in the middle of a sentence, drops food out of his mouth. He is confused, quarrelsome and stupid. And he almost always uses other drugs, anything he can lay hands on: alcohol, benzedrine, opiates, marijuana. Barbiturate users are looked down on in addict society: "Goof ball bums. They got no class to them." . . . It seems to me that barbiturates cause the worst possible form of addiction, unsightly, deteriorating, difficult to treat.
—William Burroughs, *Naked Lunch* (1959)

"Do you ever hear voices?" Ziporyn asked.

. . . After a long pause [Richard] Speck said, "Well, sometimes."
He paused again and added, "When I take drugs." . . .

"What kind of drugs?"

"Yellow-jackets and red-birds." [Slang names for habituating barbiturates (Nembutal and Seconal) capable of causing hallucinations
and bizarre actions.]

"And then sometimes I shoot myself with Inhalers. You know,
glue and stuff."

"And do you drink?"

"Boy, do I drink."

"What?"

"Anything I can lay my hands on—wine, beer, whiskey, gin, you
name it. I drink from the time I get up till I get drunk and fall back into
bed. Sometimes it makes me feel real good. But sometimes it puts me in
a real bad temper, and then I get into fights." . . .

"Look, I was drinking that day. I told you how I drink. I had six
red-birds. To tell you the truth, I don't know nothing about anything
from eight o'clock that night till I came to, about eleven o'clock the next
day. All I remember is I met three sailors in a tavern on the South Side
in the afternoon. We had some drinks, then we went off some place and
had a fix—a shot in the arm. I don't know what it was exactly, but it
wasn't heroin. It was something in a blue bottle, I think, I don't
remember a thing after that. I couldn't tell you or anybody else what
any of those nurses looked like." . . .

He talked of his rages. "I got mad at just about everything. When I
was a kid, just a teenager, in East Dallas, I was with some guys and we
got some red-birds. Whew, they made me wild. We were watching a
parade once, and we had some blockbusters [white barbiturate pills
with a yellow stripe (Nembutal)]. I just passed out, and they took me to
a juvenile home. I don't remember exactly what happened after that,
but I've been told that when my mother came to get me she says I was
talking nice and polite, then suddenly I went wild. Started swinging
and kicking at everybody. But I don't remember a thing about it
myself." . . .

"I pepped myself up on a few red-birds, six of them, and took a
walk by one of the little lakes out there, then went back to the bar for a
drink. I had some whiskey and a pint of wine and got talking to these
sailors, like I told you before. They took me to their room. It was dark.
They had this disposable syringe and took this stuff from a bottle and
started 'popping.' I tied a handkerchief around my left arm and stuck it
in. All the way. Before I had even got the needle out I could feel, you
know, feel—Zzzoommm—a buzzing all over me, and I was feeling real,
real good.

"The next thing I know I was back in my own room and it was morning. I had a gun, and I don't know where I got it. I just sat there wondering where the hell I got that gun."
—Jack Altman and Marvin Ziporyn, M.D., *Born to Raise Hell: The Untold Story of Richard Speck* (1967)

barbs. *1.* BARBITURATES. *2.* the jagged edges on an old hypodermic needle.

B-bomb. [since the 1940s] BENZEDRINE inhaler. Manufacturer (Smith Kline & French Laboratories) removed them from the market in 1949 after widespread abuse. The Benzedrine-impregnated wad inside the inhaler was removed and soaked in liquid to extract the Benzedrine. One inhaler contained the equivalent of twenty-five tablets.

B.C. birth control pills, as in "Half the girls in high school were on *B.C.*"

beast, the. [Harlem, since around 1965] LSD-25.

beat. *1.* [since around 1850, to rob—*EP*] to rob or cheat someone out of money, usually money owed to the cheated person, as in "to *beat* a whore out of her dough." *2.* counterfeit, as in "That was a *beat* bag of pot."

bee. *1.* [since around 1950] an addict's habit. *Obsolete. 2.* [from *box;* originally an amount of MARIJUANA sufficient to fill a penny matchbox, a measure for purposes of sale] box or BAG of marijuana.

behind acid. using LSD-25.

beinsa. [Burma] a plant, *Mitragyna speciosa*, chewed or drunk as an infusion, like tea, and thought to have narcotic effects, although little is known about it. Compare KRATOM.

belladonna. [from Italian *bella donna*, beautiful lady; the drug causes pupillary dilation, considered a mark of beauty among Romans] a plant, *Atropa belladonna*, belonging to the potato family *(Solanaceae)* and containing the alkaloids ATROPINE, SCOPOLAMINE, and HYOSCYAMINE. Also known as deadly nightshade, belladonna has been used as a poison and sedative since ancient times and, among certain cults, for the bizarre mental effects produced by toxic doses, e.g., witchcraft and devil-worship rites in the Middle Ages.

Tinctures of belladonna root and leaves and the pure atropine are most commonly used today, in combination with other ingredients, as a smooth-muscle relaxant which inhibits gastric secretions controlled by the vagus nerve in treating stomach disorders, peptic ulcers, vomiting, etc. Some closely related plants are mandrake, *Mandragora officinarum;* jimsonweed, or thorn apple, DATURA STRAMONIUM; henbane, *Hyocyamus niger;* and PITURI, *Duboisia hopwoodii.* Compare DATURA.

belly habit. [one WITHDRAWAL SYMPTOM characteristic of OPIUM is a gnawing pain or cramps in the stomach] *1.* opium ADDICTION subjectively centered in the area of the stomach. *Obsolete? 2.* a drug habit that is satisfied by taking drugs orally; usually refers to METHADONE.

belt. the HIGH or euphoria following the ingestion of a drug, as in "I shot up and felt the *belt.*"

belted. HIGH.

bennies. BENZEDRINE pills.

bent. [from the idea that the mind is warped, altered] HIGH or intoxicated from a HALLUCINOGEN or NARCOTIC.

benz. [since around 1944; perhaps the slang word dates from the widespread issuance of BENZEDRINE to combat troops in World War II] Benzedrine.

Benzedrine. [AMPHETAMINE sulfate, Smith Kline & French Laboratories] a central nervous system stimulant synthesized in 1927, first used in 1932 as an inhaler decongestant and in the treatment of narcolepsy (involuntary sleep). It was also issued in ships' survival kits and to German paratroopers in the Spanish Civil War. During World War II, it was issued to troops on both sides to counteract fatigue among frontline units or prior to missions requiring unusual exertion.

Manufacturer recommends dosages from 10 to 100 milligrams daily for (1) depressive states, (2) obesity (to depress appetite as an aid to dieting), (3) alcoholism, (4) narcolepsy, and (5) postencephalitic parkinsonism. Benzedrine is sold in flat pink, three-sided 5- and 10-milligram tablets with a groove down the middle; also in 15-milligram sustained-release capsules. Slang names: BENZ, BENNIES.

benzene. a toxic hydrocarbon, either chemically pure or (when derived from the distillation of crude naphtha) containing also xylene and toluene. Benzene is toxic in both forms. Prolonged inhalation or entry into the body by any other route results in acute poisoning, which can cause death by central nervous system depression and respiratory failure, or chronic poisoning, which results mainly from the action of benzene on the bone marrow over a period of months or even years, a serious (often fatal) blood disease being the ultimate result of the chemical's action. Because repeated inhalations of relatively small amounts over long periods of time may result in toxicity, most countries legally regulate the allowable exposure and concentration of the fumes in industrial use of benzene. For an abuse of benzene, see SCRUBWOMAN'S KICK. Compare BENZINE.

benzine. a product obtained by the distillation of petroleum and similar to kerosene and GASOLINE. Long used as a cleaning fluid, benzine has been also inhaled for its intoxicative effects.

> Benzinomaniac glove-cleaners have also been observed. The statement of a man who used *benzine* in his business apprises us of the sensations experienced after the inhalation of the vapour. He declared that he had previously consumed considerable amounts of liquor, but for six months not a drop had passed his lips. He had inhaled petrol vapour instead, this being abundantly at his disposal in his profession as bandage maker, and these inhalations completely substituted for alcohol. He said that he had experienced a wonderful feeling of peace, and agreeable delicious dreams. . . . But the agreeable effects of benzine diminished after some time. Hallucinations appeared, the patient heard the unpleasant music of barrel-organs and unharmonious singing by voices known to him; red ants crept about on his body, he saw several figures of animals and dwarfs, and once the whole room seemed to be full of colored silk threads which fluttered to and fro. In all probability these symptoms were due to the effects of benzine and cannot be explained by the cessation of the use of alcohol.
>
> —Louis Lewin, *Phantastica:*
> *Narcotic and Stimulating Drugs* (1964)

benzodiazepine. the chemical source whose derivatives are used as MINOR TRANQUILIZERS. Among these derivatives are chlordiazepoxide (LIBRIUM) and diazepam (VALIUM), which are used as nonhypnotic sedatives in minor anxiety states and as muscle relaxants.

In potency (as determined by performance-impairment tests) the benzodiazepines are intermediate between MEPROBAMATE (e.g., MILTOWN) and the MAJOR TRANQUILIZERS derived from phenothiazine, e.g., THORAZINE. Since they are classified as minor tranquilizers, they are not used in severe psychotic states. They are reported to produce less euphoria than the BARBITURATES, meprobamate, and NARCOTICS, and so the danger of PSYCHIC DEPENDENCE may be somewhat less, though it is a matter of degree, not kind. They are dangerous when used in conjunction with alcohol, barbiturates, phenothiazines, or MONOAMINE OXIDASE INHIBITORS, all of which POTENTIATE their effects.

PHYSICAL DEPENDENCE can occur after prolonged heavy use (300 to 600 milligrams daily), and identifiable WITHDRAWAL SYMPTOMS will result if use of the drug is abruptly ceased. They include convulsions, depression, abdominal and muscle cramps, vomiting, sweating, agitation, insomnia, loss of appetite, and aggravation of underlying neurotic states.

bernies. COCAINE.

bhang. *1.* leaves, stem, and sometimes fruit of the MARIJUANA plant, CANNABIS SATIVA *2.* a drink made from an infusion in soft drinks, milk, or water of the plant. It is drunk in India for its mild hallucinogenic effects, as a counteractant to fatigue, and in Hindu religious ceremonies. The leaves are pounded into a fine powder, a little black pepper added, and then it is brewed, filtered through a cloth, and drunk. When smoked, the leaves, etc., are also known as bhang. Bhang contains only about 2 percent of the resin containing TETRAHYDROCANNABINOL, the plant's ACTIVE PRINCIPLE. Compare CHARAS and GHANJA, which are more potent.

big bags. five- to ten-dollar BAGS of HEROIN.

big chief, the. MESCALINE.

big con. LONG CON.

Big D, the. LSD-25.

big man, the. high-level narcotics dealer; generally, the wholesaler who supplies the PUSHER. Compare SOURCE, PEOPLE, KILO, CONNECTION.

big supplier. BIG MAN.

bing. [a thinning of *bung*, purse or pocket—*EP*. Since around 1930] *1.* solitary confinement, as in "I did thirty days in the *bing*." *2.* jail. *3.* (variant of BANG?) an injection of narcotics.

Biphetamine. [*d*- and *dl*-AMPHETAMINE, Strasenburg Laboratories] a direct central nervous system stimulant. Sold in 7 1/2, 12 1/2, and

20-milligram capsules containing half *d*-amphetamine and half *dl*-amphetamine. The 12 1/2-milligram capsule has a black top and white bottom, the 20-milligram is an all-black capsule, and the 7 1/2 is all white; all are inscribed "RJS RJS." Manufacturer's recommended dose: one capsule daily. Slang name: black beauties.

bit. *1.* time served in jail, as in "I did a five-year *bit* on a pot bust." *2.* one's favorite drug, as in "His *bit* is pot."

biz. paraphernalia for injecting drugs. WORKS.

black beauties. [from the color] BIPHETAMINE capsules.

black gunion. [corruption of GUNGEON (?)] extra potent, thick, dark gummy MARIJUANA.

black pills. [from the color and shape of OPIUM that is prepared for smoking; since around 1910] pellets of opium heated over a flame, placed in a pipe, and smoked.

black russian. dark-colored, very potent HASHISH.

black stuff. [from the color] OPIUM.

blank. [perhaps from the expression "I drew a *blank*"] a container filled with a nonnarcotic powder, such as talcum powder, baking soda, or cleanser, and sold to the addict as heroin. Compare DUMMY, LEMON.

blast. [since around 1940?] to smoke MARIJUANA, as in "They were *blasting* pot." Compare BLOW.

blast party. a group gathered to smoke MARIJUANA.

blind munchies. the strong appetite for food or sweets that is part of the MARIJUANA HIGH.

block. *1.* a cube of MORPHINE sold by the can or ounce. *2.* crude OPIUM.

blockbusters. white, yellow-striped BARBITURATE pills (possibly 50-milligram NEMBUTAL, which are half yellow, half white).

blond hash. golden brown-colored HASHISH, said to be less potent than darker-colored varieties such as BLACK RUSSIAN.

blow. [to *blow* COCAINE or MORPHINE has meant to inhale it, since around 1920—*EP*] *1.* to smoke MARIJUANA, as in "*blow* pot." *2.* to miss the vein while injecting HEROIN and thereby "waste" some of the shot. *3.* to sniff heroin.

"There," Hank said finally, squeezing the eye dropper. "A good hit. Next time be more careful. You keep *blowing* shots like that and all you'll have for an arm is abscesses."
—James Mills, *The Panic in Needle Park* (1966)

blow a fill. smoke OPIUM.

blow a stick. [from *blow,* smoke, and *stick,* marijuana cigarette] to smoke MARIJUANA.

blow your mind. *1.* to drastically alter your consciousness, become HIGH on a HALLUCINOGENIC drug. *2.* to achieve a transcendent, ecstatic mental state or any abnormal state. *3.* to lose mental control or be extremely surprised, as in "It will *blow* your mind."

blow-your-mind roulette. a game played with depressant or stimulant pills.

A group of people turn out the lights and throw a large assortment of pills and capsules on the floor. They grope around and swallow the first pill they touch, then everyone waits to see if they got an uppie or downie, an innie or outie, or a carpet tack.
—Howard Smith, *Village Voice* (1966)

blue. condition resulting from an OVERDOSE; to become cyanotic from respiratory depression caused by a drug.

blues. *1.* NUMORPHAN. *2.* AMYTAL capsules.

blue acid. [from the pale blue color of the liquid drug in large amounts] LSD-25. Some users also report blue-tinged hallucinations.

bluebirds. [from the color] AMYTAL SODIUM capsules.

blue heavens. [from the color of the capsule] AMYTAL capsules.

blue morning glory seeds. hallucinogenic MORNING GLORY SEEDS of the HEAVENLY BLUE variety.

blue velvet. a combination of elixir terpin hydrate (a turpentine derivative in a high percentage of ALCOHOL), CODEINE, and tripelennamine, an ANTIHISTAMINE. The ingredients are combined and taken for the sedative and minor euphoric effects.

body drugs. [probably because they depress the consciousness and induce PHYSICAL DEPENDENCE; invidious term among users of HALLUCINOGENS: "I'll never get hooked on *body drugs* like a junkie"] drugs of the OPIATE and BARBITURATE type. The antonym is HEAD DRUGS. Compare HARD NARCOTICS, SICK.

bogart. to monopolize a MARIJUANA cigarette rather than passing it around, as is customary.

bogue. *1.* sickness from withdrawal of drugs. *2.* the first stages of WITHDRAWAL SYMPTOMS, as in "I've got the *bogue.*" Compare JONES, YENNING.

BOL-148. [*d*-2-bromolysergic acid tartrate] a hallucinogenic congener of LSD-25.

bolsa. [from Spanish *bolsa,* pouch, bag] a BAG (DECK) of HEROIN.

bomb. [from the connotation of explosive, perhaps a lethal one, if the dose is of a potency greater than that to which the addict has developed TOLERANCE; since around 1950] *1.* high-potency, relatively undiluted HEROIN. *2.* a fat, prerolled MARIJUANA cigarette resembling a king-size cigarette.

bombed out. HIGH or intoxicated on a drug.

bomber. *1.* [since around 1944] a BARBITURATE. *Obsolete? 2.* a (fat) MARIJUANA cigarette.

> Besides, I had bought some pot with the five left over and rolled some good-size *bombers* that immediately put me into business. . . . I was selling pot—smoking it, too—regularly. A bomber here, a bomber there; it kept me going inside and out.
> —Piri Thomas, *Down These Mean Streets* (1967)

bombita. [Spanish; little bomb] *1.* ampul of DESOXYN. *2.* by extension, perhaps any AMPHETAMINE in solution. Addicts often inject amphetamines in conjunction with their HEROIN injection to enhance the RUSH of the drug and to counteract its depressant effect. *3.* COCAINE in liquid form. Compare SPEEDBALL.

bonita. MILK SUGAR used in diluting pure HEROIN.

book, the. [the analogy is the Bible] Physician's Desk Reference, an annual compendium of commercial drug preparations manufactured in the United States, with descriptions by their manufacturers intended both as an aid to the physician in looking up drugs he intends to prescribe and as publicity for the manufacturers' products. Published by Medical Economics, Inc., it is given free to physicians, updated yearly, and sells for $10 a copy. Pill users refer to it frequently for identification and descriptions of the pills they are taking.

boost. [from *booster,* a shoplifter; to be a shoplifter, to steal goods from a store—*EP;* since the 1930s] to break, enter, and steal, as in "I *boosted* supermarkets for meat and sold it to buy drugs."

boot and shoot. a HEROIN addict who steals to pay for drugs.

booting. [from (?) *boot,* a strong pleasurable sensation; analogous to *kick—EP*] the technique of injecting HEROIN intravenously a little at a time, letting it back up in the eye dropper, injecting a little more, letting the blood–heroin mixture back up, and so on. The addict believes that this technique prolongs the initial pleasurable sensation of the heroin as it first takes effect—a feeling of warmth in the abdomen, euphoria, and sometimes a sensation similar to an orgasm. Compare DROPPER, GET OFF, GRAVY, and JERK OFF.

boss. [perhaps a deference to the authority and domination of a drug] *1.* high-potency, relatively unadulterated drugs, as in "That was really *boss* HEROIN." *2.* by extension, a dominant feeling of pleasure related to taking drugs, or anything that is the best, the strongest, etc., as in "*boss* clothes," "*boss* feeling," etc. Addicts say "horse (heroin) is *boss,*" meaning both that it runs (bosses) their lives and that it is the superior drug.

> "When you got that *boss* feeling, man, like you're your own boss, there isn't nobody can tell you what to do in this world."
> —addict, quoted in Jeremy Larner and Ralph Tefferteller, *The Addict in the Street* (1964)

B.O.T. balance of time. Sentence given to a parole violator; he must serve out his full original sentence, which his parole had, of course, curtailed.

bouncing powder. COCAINE. *Obsolete?*

boxed. HIGH or intoxicated on a drug.

boy. [since around 1920] HEROIN. Also HIM, BROTHER. Compare GIRL, HER.

brain ticklers. BARBITURATE or AMPHETAMINE pills. Compare CRASH (quotation).

brick. [from the shape] *1.* pressed block of gum OPIUM or MORPHINE for shipment. *2.* pressed block of MARIJUANA, weighing 1 pound or 1 kilogram (2.2 pounds), which is shipped by mail or freight in this form. *3.* intercepted marijuana (often used by narcotics police). Compare BAR.

brick, throw a big. *1.* to commit a crime. *2.* to do something violent.

"I know I had to go and *throw* just one *big brick*—kill myself, take an overdose; or something."
—Claude Brown, *Manchild in the Promised Land* (1965)

bring down. [to restore to sanity. "When a customer gets ready to 'cut out' (of the MARIJUANA den) Chappy *'brings* him *down'* with milk . . . to hasten clearing of the brain."—Meyer Berger, *The New Yorker* (1938), quoted in *EP*] *1.* to cause to lose the drug exhilaration; to depress. *2.* to cause or induce a mundane, "square," or depressed state, whether one was using a drug or not. *3.* the complex of social forces antithetical to an ecstatic state of mind, specifically, the narcotics laws which harass the drug user in his search for such ecstasy.

First Manifesto to End the Bringdown.
—Title of an *Atlantic Monthly* article,
by Allen Ginsberg, in favor of legalizing marijuana (1966)

British system, the. the rubric for the narcotics laws and treatment of addiction in Great Britain. It is not really a system, and when it was adopted, Great Britain had no addiction problem. Up to 1961, the addict population was small (around 300), most of whom were medical addicts. British doctors can legally prescribe HEROIN and COCAINE to addicts who are registered with the government, in order to prevent WITHDRAWAL SYMPTOMS, and also in decreasing amounts as an adjunct to voluntary withdrawal by an addict. The addict might also be maintained on drugs indefinitely if the doctor believed he would "lead a useful and fairly normal life" when so maintained. (A study found that 50 percent of maintained addicts were unemployed, so that this last criterion was at best a half fiction.)

The system became subject to abuse (overprescriptions, which enabled the addicts to sell their surplus to unregistered users), and the number of narcotics addicts increased from 300 in 1960 to 2,000 in 1966 (many of these, however, were immigrants from countries with stricter narcotics laws, such as the United States). This rate of increase held steadily upward, the number of new addicts roughly doubling every nineteen months. Addicts were also active in proselytizing among the young, who often bought their drugs illicitly rather than register as addicts (yet organized narcotics traffic, crime, and prostitution to obtain narcotics is otherwise nonexistent). As a result, the ready availability of drugs at low prices or under the National Health Service did not end the practice of PUSHING (selling drugs illicitly at an inflated price). Though the absolute number of addicts is still a tiny percentage of the population—less than in the

United States, for example—the increase in addiction led the government in 1967 to tighten the law.

No longer can general practitioners prescribe to addicts; prescriptions are issued only through designated hospitals (teaching hospitals with psychiatric centers). The drugs can be prescribed only through the National Health Service. Although this provision is not expected to end completely the practice of overprescription and illicit sales at inflated prices, it has prevented doctors from prescribing for money with the attendant risk of unscrupulous doctors' prescribing excessive amounts.

brody. pretending to be sick in order to obtain a prescription for drugs from a doctor.

brother. *1.* HEROIN. *2.* a male of the same race, usually black.

brown. HEROIN of a brown color. Mexican heroin is brown because it is diluted with brown milk sugar; heroin originating in the Middle East and Southeast Asia is white.

brown rock. granules of 50 percent HEROIN for smoking.

brownies. [from the color of the timed-release capsule, which has a brown cap] AMPHETAMINES; perhaps specifically, DEXEDRINE Spansules.

brown stuff. [from the color; as differentiated from WHITE STUFF, HEROIN; since around 1920] OPIUM.

bufotenine. [2-methylserotonin (5-hydroxydimethyltryptamine)] a substance first isolated from the skin of toads and used medically to raise blood pressure. It has also been isolated in two hallucinogenic plants, *Piptadenia peregrina* (see PIPTADENIA), a member of the mimosa family (*Leguminosae*), from whose seeds the hallucinogenic snuff COHOBA is extracted, and from the hallucinogenic mushroom FLY AGARIC, *Amanita muscaria*. While it is not absolutely certain that bufotenine is the active ingredient of these plants, when taken alone, it does have consciousness-altering effects. In an experiment, 16 milligrams of injected bufotenine caused color hallucinations in the form of reddish and red-purple spots and a yellowish haze, an impairment of time and space perception, and mental confusion and cloudiness. The effects disappeared after forty minutes. Bufotenine is close in structure to SEROTONIN, which in turn is similar, structurally, to a part of the molecular structure of LSD.

bum bend. [from *bent*, HIGH or intoxicated from a drug] a psychotic or panic reaction to LSD-25 or STP. Compare BAD TRIP, BUM TRIP.

> This (THORAZINE) is not the way for an STP user to mend a *bum bend*.
> —*Los Angeles Oracle* (1967)

bum kicks. [from *bum*, bad or malfunctional, and *kicks*, enjoyment, thrills] troubled, worried, depressed. Compare DOWN TRIP.

> I once gave marijuana to a guest who was mildly anxious about something ("*On bum kicks*" as he put it). After smoking half a cigarette he suddenly leapt to his feet screaming "I got the fear!" and rushed out of the house. —William Burroughs, *Naked Lunch* (1959)

bummer. BUM TRIP.

bum trip. [from *bum*, bad or malfunctional, and *trip*, a drug experience] an adverse reaction to a drug, usually a HALLUCINOGEN, characterized by panic, fear, etc. Compare BAD TRIP.

bundle. a package of twenty-five $5 bags of heroin, stacked and held together by a rubber band. The PUSHER buys them from the wholesaler in this form, then resells them individually to the addict in the street at a profit, retaining some bags for use if he is an addict. Compare PIECE.

bunk habit. [*bunk*, a couch for reclining while smoking OPIUM; since around 1930—*EP*] the practice of lying around in a place where others are smoking opium for the purpose of inhaling the fumes, although not smoking oneself. *Obsolete*. Compare CONTACT HIGH.

burese. COCAINE. *Obsolete*.

burn. [from *burn*, to cheat, or to be *burned*, to have someone run out on you with the money; since the 1920s; from *burner*, a card or dice cheat, about 1850—*EP*] *1*. to cheat or to be cheated through taking money for drugs, then absconding without delivering them or selling short weight or phony narcotics. *2*. to inform or be informed upon in connection with drug activity.

burn artist. *1*. anyone, especially a drug peddler, noted for employing the BURN technique in order to cheat others. *2*. a police informer, a stool pigeon.

burned. *1*. to be revealed as a drug peddler by a police informer. *2*. to be revealed to drug users as a police informer or undercover agent. *3*. to have been cheated in a drug sale.

burned out. *1.* collapsed, as in a *"burned out* vein." *2.* tired. *3.* a junkie who has kicked the habit.

burning. smoking MARIJUANA. Compare BLOW, BLAST.

> And *burning* marijuana, that's just like smoking a cigarette, the only thing you inhale it, you don't let it out, you just try to hold it in.
> —addict, quoted in Jeremy Larner and Ralph Tefferteller,
> *The Addict in the Street* (1964)

burn out. to overexploit a source of stolen goods. Compare BURNED OUT.

> If he [the addict] is a booster [thief] he will recognize the fact that he can *"burn out"* a certain department store. He will therefore respect the store detectives and move from place to place as the days pass.
> —Seymour Fiddle, *Portraits from a Shooting Gallery* (1967)

bush. MARIJUANA.

businessman's lunchtime high (drug). [so-called because its effects last only thirty minutes] DMT.

bust. [from Harlem slang for a police raid; a raid on drug addicts' parlors or clubs; since the 1930s—*EP*] *1.* to arrest or to be arrested, as in "The cop *busted* George"; "I was *busted* on a possession rap"; "The cops set me up for a *bust.*" Compare SET UP.

Butisol Sodium. [butabarbital sodium, McNeil Laboratories, Inc.] a short- to intermediate-acting BARBITURATE hypnotic and sedative. The maximum sedative dosage is 120 milligrams a day, taken three times a day. The hypnotic (sleep-producing) dose is 100 milligrams, at bedtime. Butisol Sodium comes in flat, round green, orange, pink or lavender tablets inscribed "McNeil." Subject to Schedule III of the CONTROLLED SUBSTANCES ACT.

button, the. [from peyote *buttons,* the surface growth of the peyote cactus] PEYOTE.

buy. a purchase of narcotics from a peddler, as in "I'm going out to make a *buy.*" Compare COP, SCORE.

buzz. [onomatopoetic equivalent of subjective feeling] *1.* feeling at the onset of a MARIJUANA high: buzzing in the ears, dizziness, blurring of perceptions, and cottony sounds. *2.* by extension, a moderate, pleasant HIGH from any drug, without hallucinations. *3.* a HEROIN high.

buzz, rolling. a moderate HIGH continuing after intake of drugs has ceased.

> Gnossos had stopped smoking anything but was still high enough for a *rolling buzz.*—Richard Fariña, *Been Down So Long It Looks Like Up to Me* (1966)

C c

C. COCAINE.

caapi. [Name used by Indians in northwestern Brazil and Colombia] *1.* a hallucinogenic tea made from the vine BANISTERIOPSIS CAAPI. *2.* the vine itself. Compare AYAHUASCA.

caballo. [Spanish, *horse;* translation of the American term for heroin] HEROIN.

ca-ca. [Puerto Rican slang for SHIT] shit, counterfeit HEROIN. Compare BLANK, CRAP, FLEA POWDER, GARBAGE, LEMON, DUMMY.

> Everybody was buying and nobody was selling except the gyps, and they were mixing milk-sugar with quinine and selling this *ca-ca* for the real thing.   —Piri Thomas, *Down These Mean Streets* (1967)

cactus. [from the peyote cactus plant] PEYOTE.

cahoba. see COHOBA.

came down. see COME DOWN.

can. *1.* a car. *2.* [one ounce of MORPHINE, so-called because it was sold in tins, around 1930; also convicts' word for a 1/2 pound of tobacco—*EP.*] MARIJUANA was sometimes measured for sale in Prince Albert pipe tobacco tins or coffee cans in the western United States, 1 ounce of marijuana costing $15 to $25. Compare LID, TIN.

Canadian black. [from the color] a variety of MARIJUANA grown in Canada.

C and H. COCAINE and HEROIN mixed. *Obsolete.* See SPEEDBALL.

C and M. COCAINE and MORPHINE mixed. *Obsolete.* See SPEEDBALL.

canceled stick. a cigarette filled with MARIJUANA.

candy. drugs.

candy man. [from (?) *nose candy,* COCAINE or HEROIN sniffed] a PUSHER or peddler of drugs.

cannabis. [from Greek *kannabis*] general international term for the flowering or fruiting tops of the hemp plant (CANNABIS SATIVA), the leaves, and sometimes the stems and seeds, of which are taken for their mild hallucinogenic effects by smoking, drinking in an infusion, or eating. American cannabis, i.e., MARIJUANA, differs in pharmacological potency and modes of preparation and ingestion from Indian or North African cannabis, though the species is the same. According to the WHO's definition, cannabis does not encompass the resin alone, which is the most potent product of the plant and is known as HASHISH. Compare BHANG, CANNABIS INDICA, CANNABIS SATIVA, CHARAS, GHANJA, KIF.

Cannabis indica. [correctly CANNABIS SATIVA] the Indian hemp plant. *Obsolete.* The pharmaceutical name for (1) the powder made from the dried, sifted flowering tops of the female *Cannabis sativa,* (2) the tincture made from that powder, or (3) the pure resin, used in the nineteenth century as a remedy for asthma, nasal catarrh, nervous coughs, colds, tuberculosis, facial neuralgia, and insomnia. Also called by its English name, Indian hemp.

It was apparently introduced into European medicine by doctors with Napoleon's forces in Egypt, who were impressed by its sedative and analgesic potentials. Now (except in India, where it is an ingredient in certain patent medicines) cannabis has little medical use, and it is no longer in the United States Pharmacopoeia. Despite its antibiotic properties, few people advocate its use for this purpose. The WHO advises against such use, asserting that it is not so effective as existing antibiotics.

Experiments with cannabis and its semisynthetic derivatives, e.g., PYRAHEXYL, were conducted with some success in the 1930s among mental patients suffering from depression; however, it has apparently been dropped in favor of TRANQUILIZERS, perhaps because the latter are more predictable in their effects and do not alter the consciousness. Another disadvantage of cannabis is that in powder form it tends to deteriorate so that its potency is unstable. The potency also varies with the geographic origin of the plant.

> The fact is undeniable that smoking cigarettes made of the leaves of this plant [cannabis] produces a rapid modification in the state of asthmatic patients. The difficulty of breathing, the stertorous respiration, the tightness of the chest, and the wheezing are promptly relieved; an abundant expectoration most frequently follows almost immediately, the breathing becomes easier, the cough gets moist and a refreshing sleep soon removes all the alarming symptoms. . . . To facilitate the use of Indian Cigarettes and enable the patient to benefit by them under all circumstances, whether travelling or walking, they are sold in elegant little cigar cases which can be carried in a breast-pocket with the least inconvenience. Each can contains a dozen cigarettes. . . . The

smoke must be gently inhaled and allowed to flow through the respiratory passages, so as to be brought in contact with the larynx and the lungs, and then be blown out through the nose. It is essential to do this slowly by short aspirations. . . . It has been observed that the cigarettes act most powerfully when smoked in a close room, the patient sitting quietly in a chair or reclining in a sofa.

—brochure for "Indian Cigarettes,"
Grimault & Co. Chemists (ca. 1860)

Cannabis sativa. a hemp plant which exudes a resin containing a HALLUCINOGEN, TETRAHYDROCANNABINOL. The use of the plant for its hallucinogenic effects probably originated in central Asia or China, where it was mentioned in a pharmacy book by Emperor Shun Nung in 3000 B.C., and spread through India and the Near East (in the fourth century B.C. the historian Herodotus described its use among the Scythians) and Africa, and thence to Europe and the Western Hemisphere.

The plant grows wild in most parts of the world, even in countries where attempts to eradicate it have been going on for centuries. *Cannabis sativa* is a tall annual plant which at maturity ranges in height from 3 to 16 feet and grows on the average to 6 to 8 feet. The leaves, usually seven to a stem, are dark green on top, hairy, with sawtooth edges. The stalks are fluted. The male and female plants are similar in appearance until maturity, when their flowers differ. The male plant produces prominent flowers which shed pollen freely. The female flowers grow amidst a profusion of small leaves and stems at the tip of the plant. The male plant yields fibers, or hemp, but is no longer cultivated for this purpose in the United States, imported Manila hemp or synthetics such as nylon being used instead. The female plant yields hard-hulled fruit containing seeds and, more copiously than the male, produces the resin containing tetrahydrocannabinol, the ACTIVE PRINCIPLE with hallucinogenic properties. The resin is most abundant at maturity.

These flowering tops, twigs, and leaves of the female plant are dried (either naturally in the sun, or artificially by low-temperature baking in a stove) and are smoked like tobacco for their hallucinogenic effects. This dried product is known in North America as MARIJUANA and in India as BHANG. Specially cultivated, unfertilized female hemp plants yield a higher resin content, which coats the fruiting tops of the plant, as a result of being unable to set seeds freely. The pure resin, with its much greater concentration of the active principle, is known as HASHISH, or CHARAS in India. It is related to the soporific yellow powder lupulin, found in the female hop plant, *Humulus lupulus,* used in making beer, which may account for its mild soporific effect. The Indians also use the unfertilized, resin-coated flowering tops, leaves, young twigs, and bark of specially cultivated female plants in making GHANJA, a byproduct that is more potent than bhang but less so than charas. Ghanja is smoked or eaten in cakes or candy.

Cannabis sativa varies in resin content, and hence potency, with the area in which it is grown (hence, the loose and obsolete application of such local names as *Cannabis americana* and *Cannabis indica*). Nevertheless, the Federal Bureau of Narcotics held that there is only one species and that seeds from one part of the world planted in another will, after several generations, assume the characteristics of the local variety of *Cannabis sativa*. (Some other experiments apparently contradict this.) See also CANNABIS.

canned sativa. HASHISH.

canned stuff. packaged smoking OPIUM. Compare CAN, TIN, LID.

carbona. a brand of CLEANING FLUID, the fumes of which are inhaled for their deliriant effect. Compare CARBON TETRACHLORIDE, GLUE SNIFFING. See DELIRIANTS.

carbon tetrachloride. [tetrachloromethane] a heavy, colorless, highly toxic liquid (which alcohol POTENTIATES) with a strong odor used in CLEANING FLUIDS and the source of the deliriant effect sought by drug abusers who sniff them. Toxic reactions to the fumes include headache, mental confusion, depression, fatigue, loss of appetite, vomiting, coma, and death. Some of these symptoms do not appear until after the passage of several hours. Both the vapor and the liquid irritate the skin and eyes. It can also cause damage to the liver, kidney, heart, and nervous system if inhaled in large quantities over a long period of time, or if swallowed. Compare GLUE SNIFFING, BENZINE. See DELIRIANTS.

carry. to have drugs on the person, as in the drug users' admonition "never *carry* when you can STASH." Compare ANYWHERE, HOLD.

carrying. possessing narcotics on the person, as in "are you *carrying?*"

cartwheels [from the scoring, in the form of a plus sign, on the round tablet, which gives it a resemblance to a wheel] AMPHETAMINE tablets. Compare CROSSROADS.

cat. *1.* any male. *2.* HEROIN. Compare BOY, CHICK, BROTHER.

catnip. the strong-smelling herb *Nepeta cataria,* sometimes sold as

MARIJUANA to an unsuspecting buyer and sometimes actually smoked for alleged hallucinogenic effects.

CB. [condensation of CIBA, a drug manufacturer's name] DORIDEN (GLUTETHIMIDE) pill.

cent. one dollar. (In drug parlance a nickel is $5 and a dime is $10.) Compare NICKEL BAG, DIME, QUARTER.

cephalotropic. modifying the physiological functioning of the brain; antonym of PSYCHOTROPIC.

chalk. [from the white color and chalky consistency] AMPHETAMINE tablets.

change. short jail or prison sentence.

changes. *1.* alterations, unexpected events which interrupt the addict's habitual life pattern, or routine, and which he characteristically finds unpleasant. *2.* interruptions in his drug-acquisition pattern, e.g., his PUSHER is not there at the appointed time, causing him to do without his needed drugs. *3.* periods during which no drugs are available. Compare HASSLE, PANIC. *4.* bizarre, surprising reactions to, and personality alteration from, a drug by another, as in "he's going through *changes.*" *5.* alterations in life style, values, perceptions of the world; becoming a different person.

channel. *1.* a vein for injecting HEROIN. Compare LINE, PIT. *2.* a source of narcotics.

charas. [Hindu word for the unadulterated resin] resin exuded by the flowering tops of the female hemp plant, CANNABIS SATIVA. Cultivation in India, Nepal, and Sinkiang, China, was brought to a fine art. Special techniques included preventing pollination of the female plants so that they produced more resin, trimming off the top leaves and dwarfing the plant, growing the plants in upland areas under hot sun (which seems to increase the pharmacological potency of the resin), and laboriously collecting the resin on cheesecloth by hand and scraping it off so that none is wasted.

Since only the resin is used (in contrast to GHANJA, another form of Indian cannabis, in which the resin-covered flowers, leaves, and twigs are ground up for smoking), charas represents the ACTIVE PRINCIPLE of cannabis in its most concentrated state. It is some eight times as potent as ordinary MARIJUANA from the United States (or what the Indians call BHANG) made from flowers, leaves, and seeds, whether resinous or not.

When freshly exuded, the resin is yellowish and smells like mint; it later hardens and turns brown or black. It is customarily smoked in a water pipe (HOOKAH) or eaten in confections. When smoked, the drug's intake can be better regulated than when it is swallowed. By the latter mode, charas can equal, in hallucinogenic effects, a small amount of LSD-25. Charas is commonly known as HASHISH in other parts of the world. Compare CANNABIS SATIVA.

charge. [a dose, especially by injection of a narcotic drug, around the 1930s; a MARIJUANA cigarette, perhaps a specialization of the first sense, circa 1943—*EP*; derived from (?) electric *charge*] *1.* the sudden, euphoric onset of the effects of an OPIATE drug following injection. *2.* an injection of drugs. *3.* a marijuana cigarette. *4.* (rare) COCAINE. Compare FLASH, RUSH.

charged. somnolent from an excess amount of a depressant drug. Compare OVERCHARGED.

charles. [since the 1920s] COCAINE. *Obsolete?*

charlie. a dollar; five *charlies* is $5, etc.

chasing the bag. [BAG, packet of heroin] *1.* hustling for HEROIN. *2.* addicted. *Compare* GLOBETROTTER.

chasing the dragon. [translation from the Chinese] a favored mode of taking HEROIN in Hong Kong among Chinese addicts. The heroin along with BARBITURATE powder is placed on a flat piece of tinfoil over the flame of a match or candle. The fumes that result are inhaled through a paper tube (usually a rolled matchbook cover) or directly. As it melts, the heroin resembles a small black snake and slides about on the tinfoil as if alive; hence the name: the user "chases" the heroin "dragon" in order to inhale the fumes (the dragon's smoke).

chemical. any illicitly used drug.

chicharra. [Puerto Rican slang] a marijuana–tobacco cigarette that is passed around communally.

chick shit habit. a small habit; not considered addicted. Compare CHIPPYING, WEEKEND HABIT.

chick. *1.* a female. *2.* HEROIN. Compare BOY, CAT, BROTHER.

chill. [from the idea of *freeze,* to ignore, to "cut" someone] *1.* to refuse to sell drugs to an addict who is suspected of being a police informer, as in "I *chilled* Charlie today." *2.* such a refusal, as in "the *chill's* on Charlie." *3.* to kill.

chillum. a clay pipe, with a short straight stem issuing from the bottom of the bowl, used in India for smoking GHANJA.

Chinese white. very potent white HEROIN.

Chinese cure. an addict's way of gradually withdrawing himself from HEROIN: opium in daily decreasing amounts is mixed with a tonic, until finally the addict is drinking only the tonic.

chip. [from CHIPPYING] to take drugs irregularly in such quantities as not to become addicted.

chipping. CHIPPYING.

chippying. [from *chippy,* a girl of easy virtue; *chippying,* dallying with such a girl; hence *chippy user,* one who uses narcotics infrequently, sporadically, rather than steadily, for kicks, rather than because of physical dependence—*EP*. Partridge adds, regarding the connection between the sexual and narcotic meanings, "to numerous men, women are but sexual narcotics"] *1.* infrequent, irregular use of narcotics for pleasure and without physical dependency. *2.* in states where opiate derivatives such as CODEINE or PAREGORIC can be bought without a prescription if the purchaser signs a register at the druggist, the practice of making the rounds of several druggists and buying the legal amount from each. Compare CHICK SHIT HABIT, WEEKEND HABIT.

chloral hydrate. [trichloroacetaldehyde] a nonbarbiturate hypnotic and sedative. Combined with alcohol, liquid chloral hydrate can induce acute intoxication, resembling an overdose of BARBITURATES, and coma. In this illicit use it is known as a MICKEY FINN or KNOCKOUT DROPS. Excessive, long-term use of chloral hydrate can result in both PSYCHIC DEPENDENCE and PHYSICAL DEPENDENCE, with a characteristic pattern of WITHDRAWAL SYMPTOMS when the drug is abruptly stopped. The toxic oral dose is approximately 10 grams, while the hypnotic (sleep-inducing) dose is 0.5 to 1 gram. A Schedule IV drug under the CONTROLLED SUBSTANCES ACT.

chlorpromazine. a MAJOR TRANQUILIZER chemically derived from phenothiazine, chlorpromazine is a dimethylaminopropyl compound. Its derivatives include trifluoperazine and perphenazine. Sold under the name THORAZINE and used in treating severe psychoses, it acts to reduce the patient's fear and hostility, thus preventing acts of violence. It also reduces hallucinations and delusions, or at least the patient's apprehension arising from them. Chlorpromazine is by the same action effective in reversing an LSD-induced panic psychosis by antagonizing the drug's effects, and enabling the subject to return to a normal state of consciousness.

In 1967 the self-administration of chlorpromazine, with which most LSD users are familiar, took an untoward turn. While experimenting with the powerful new hallucinogen STP, which induces a more profound and longer-lasting experience than LSD, several people took chlorpromazine, evidently in an attempt to reverse an unfavorable experience. But instead of reversing STP, it POTENTIATES its effect with possibly fatal results. This is because STP is believed to be similar to ATROPINE, to which chlorpromazine is also similar in chemical structure. Chlorpromazine has a central sedative effect but, unlike the BARBITURATES, large doses do not induce coma or anesthesia. PSYCHIC DEPENDENCE and PHYSICAL DEPENDENCE do not seem to occur.

chota. [Puerto Rican addicts' slang] RAT, an informer.

Christmas trees. DEXAMYL capsules.

chuck habit. [from *chuck*, food, as in chuck wagon] a ravenous appetite for food after one has been detoxified from HEROIN. Also chuck horrors, chuckers.

ciba. [from the manufacturer's name, CIBA Pharmaceutical Company, inscribed on the capsule] DORIDEN (GLUTETHIMIDE). Compare MERCK.

clean. [to rid oneself of stolen property; hence, free from suspicion, carrying no firearms; around the 1920s—*EP*] *1.* not carrying narcotics. *2.* not using narcotics. *3.* MARIJUANA with the twigs and seeds removed. These are considered undesirable by some users, because less potent, but others brew a tea from this "waste." "A very *clean* NICKEL (i.e., $5) BAG" means, in essence, more for your money, since the marijuana contains a minimum of waste. *4.* the act of removing this waste, often performed by a dealer—the cleaner his lot, the less bulk and the lower his profits.

cleaning fluids. inhaled for the deliriant effects. When sniffed (usually from a rag or a plastic bag), the fumes produce an intoxication, initially accompanied by exhilaration and excitement, uncoordinated actions, slurred speech, double vision, buzzing in the ears, and rarely, hallucinations. After thirty to thirty-five minutes, drowsiness, stupor, and unconsciousness ensue. The fumes are irritating to the mucous membranes, are extremely toxic, and can cause damage to the kidney, liver, brain, and bone marrow, but only after long, heavy exposure to the fumes. In their delirium users have been known to fall from heights with fatal results. Death can also result (especially among young people, the chief abusers) from the toxicity of the vapors themselves. Compare CARBONA, CARBON TETRACHLORIDE, GLUE SNIFFING, DELIRIANTS.

> A boy would pour the *cleaning fluid* into a rag and then hold it to his nose, and inhale deeply until he was intoxicated. Each boy would do this until they were all high, and then they would stagger around the lot playing schoolboy games until they became drowsy and lost interest.
> —eyewitness account of cleaning-fluid sniffing,
> *World Journal Tribune* (Nov. 6, 1966)

cleared up. to be detoxified or stop using drugs.

clitch. the decisive factor, the clincher.

> S.F.: I wondered whether you thought that drug addicts are under more pressure than people who are not drug addicts.
> M. [an addict]: Yes. Sure! There's more pressure, but there's a compen—there's a compensation here that . . . that's when you take off. This is the—that's the *clitch*—this is what keeps you in this.
> —Seymour Fiddle, *Portraits from a Shooting Gallery* (1967)

coast. to be in the somnolent, nodding state of the HEROIN addict, as in "he'd shot up and started to *coast.*"

coca. a bush, *Erythroxylon coca,* grown on mountain slopes or terraced ground in the uplands of Bolivia, Peru, and Java. Its leaves contain the alkaloid COCAINE in amounts ranging from 0.65 to 1.25 percent by weight. Because of its cocaine content, coca has been consumed for centuries by Indians of the Andean regions of South America, who seek its stimulant and appetite-depressant effects (which are more manifest in the high altitudes of the region) while performing heavy labor, making long treks or climbs, and the like. The Indians traditionally chew the leaves mixed with an alkali (lime) obtained from bricks of pressed ashes, usually from quinoa, a local pigweed, *Chinopodium quinoa,* with cornstarch added for adhesion or wrapped around bird droppings (guano). The alkali acts with saliva to release the cocaine from the leaves.

Such small amounts of cocaine are actually consumed that the coca habit is not considered a dangerous drug abuse, or addictive, but rather analogous to coffee drinking in this country. It has been estimated that coca is used by 90 percent of the Indians in the Andes. (The Indian user who chews 2 ounces of the leaf ingests about 0.7 grain of cocaine per day, while the cocaine addict may consume up to 6 to 8 grains per day.) The Peruvian government, nevertheless, is trying to discourage the use of coca so that the Indians will replant the land now used for coca bushes in more profitable, licit crops. Before the arrival of Spanish explorers, the Incas chewed coca leaves and considered them divine. In Paris, the leaves were infused into wine by Angelo Mariani, who called his mixture *vin coca mariana,* a popular nineteenth-century beverage in Europe. It was also an ingredient of the soft drink Coca-Cola until 1904, when federal authorities proscribed such use.

God is a substance   —Peruvian Indian saying about coca

cocaine. [from COCA and -*ine*] benzoylmethyl ecognine. The alkaloid or ACTIVE PRINCIPLE contained in the leaves of the coca bush, *Erythroxylon coca,* which has a pronounced stimulative effect on the central nervous system. In its pure form, cocaine is a white crystalline powder. The bush is grown in Bolivia, Peru, and Java, and most of the cocaine in illicit traffic originates in these countries. Cocaine was first isolated in 1884; in 1883 it was issued to Bavarian soldiers to increase endurance and wakefulness. It was used in medicine in various tonics as a stimulant and also as a local anesthetic. Sigmund Freud experimented with the drug extensively and for a time touted it for its beneficial effects in countering fatigue, increasing the ability to work, in combating depression, for stomach disorders, and as an aid to withdrawal from MORPHINE, to which a friend of his was addicted. When he learned of the drug's addictive nature, Freud gave it up.

The effect of the drug is a quick, intense euphoria, accompanied by a decrease in hunger, indifference to pain and fatigue, and illusions of great physical strength and mental capacity. Drug users take it for its violently stimulant and euphoric effects, the favored modes of ingestion being sniffing and injection (cocaine loses its potency when taken by mouth). Cocaine is either taken on its own or in combination with HEROIN or other depressant drugs. Those who inject cocaine either mix it with heroin or inject the latter subsequently in order to dampen the hyperexcitability the cocaine induces. The euphoria is relatively short-lived, and habitual users of the drug inject it as often as every ten minutes, and tend to escalate the dosages. When injected in small doses at frequent intervals, as much as 10 grams has been taken in a day. On the other hand, some authorities consider a single dose of around 1.2 grams (1,200 milli-grams) as lethal to most human beings. Lesser doses have been fatal, however; and when an injected toxic dose reaches the heart, death comes too rapidly for any effective therapy.

The body does not develop significant TOLERANCE to cocaine, though there is a tendency among users to increase the dose, i.e., the lethal dose remains constant, while the same injection will produce a similar effect even after long-term use. PHYSICAL DEPENDENCE on cocaine similar to that on HEROIN does not occur; however, a strong PSYCHIC DEPENDENCE can develop with a form of psychological "WITHDRAWAL SYMPTOMS" that occur even though the drug is still used. The user compulsively seeks the extreme mood elevation, elation, and grandiose feelings of heightened mental and physical prowess induced by the drug. When the drug's effects begin to wane, a corresponding deep depression is felt, which is in such marked contrast to the user's previous state that he is strongly motivated to repeat the dose and restore his euphoria, thus becoming psychically dependent upon the drug. If the habitual user tries to stop he will often be plunged into a severe depression, from which only cocaine will arouse him. Chronic use, however, will engender an increasingly unpleasant hyperstimulation (causing a resort to depressant drugs), accompanied by digestive disorders, nausea, loss of appetite, loss of weight, occasional convulsions; as with the AMPHETAMINES, long-term, heavy use will produce a paranoid psychosis with delusions of persecution. Another phenomenon, which amphetamine users also experience, is formication—the feeling that ants, insects, or snakes are crawling under or on one's skin. With the user in such a state, the possibility of violence cannot be discounted. Long-term injection also produces abscesses on the skin, and prolonged sniffing also results in deterioration of the lining of the nose (it shrinks the mucous membranes) and ultimately of the bone. Since prolonged use of cocaine depresses the appetite, the user may suffer from malnutrition and anemia. The drug also acts to raise the body temperature; this effect is preceded by a dramatic lowering of body temperature and a sensation of cold. In his weakened state, the user may be more susceptible to a lethal overdose of cocaine. Those who find it necessary to combine cocaine with depressant drugs also run the risk of becoming physically dependent upon the latter.

With the advent of new drug regulations limiting the amount of amphetamines manufactured, drug abusers seeking this kind of sensation have turned to cocaine, which, because it is imported, tends to be more expensive in illicit channels. Cocaine was errone-ously classified as narcotic by the old Federal Bureau of Narcotics, but of course it is a stimulant, very close to the amphetamines in its effects and not physically addicting, as are the OPIATES. Slang names: coke, snow, C, girl, stardust. A Schedule II drug under the CONTROLLED SUBSTANCES ACT. See *Addenda*.

> I smelled the sharp sickly-sweet odor of the cocaine. My palms were dripping sweat. He had the "spike" in his right hand. He grabbed my forearm with his left hand. I turned my head and closed my eyes. I bit down on my bottom lip waiting for the stabbing plunge of the needle.
> He said, "Damn! You got some beautiful lines [veins]." I shivered when it daggered in. I opened my eyes and looked. My blood had shot up into the dropper. He was pressing the bulb. I saw the blood-streaked liquid draining into me. It was like a ton of nitro exploded inside me. My ticker went berserk. I could feel it clawing up my throat. It was like I had a million "swipes" in every pore from head to toe. It was like they were all popping off together in a nerve-shredding climax.
> I was quivering like a joker in the hot seat at the first jolt. I tried to open my talc-dry mouth. I couldn't. I was paralyzed. I could feel a hot ball of puke racing up from my careening guts. I saw the green, stinking puke rope arch into the black mouth of the waste basket. . . .
> I felt like the top of my skull had been crushed in. It was like I had been blown apart and all that was left were my eyes. Then tiny prickly feet of ecstasy started dancing through me. I heard melodious bells tolling softly inside my skull.
> I looked down at my hands and thighs. A thrill shot through me. Surely they were the most beautiful in the Universe. I felt a superman's surge of power. —"Iceberg Slim," *Pimp. The Story of My Life* (1967)

codeine. [from Greek *kodeia,* poppyhead] also called methylmorphine. An alkaloid of OPIUM naturally occurring in the juices of the unripe pod of the white poppy, *Papaver somniferum.* It is usually extracted by methylization of MORPHINE, another natural alkaloid. In its general pharmacological action, codeine resembles morphine, but the effects are much milder. Since it has only about one-sixth to one-tenth the analgesic action of an equivalent amount of morphine, it is used only in minor pain. The usual recommended dose is 30 to 60 milligrams; 120 milligrams gives analgesia equal to that of 10 milligrams of morphine, the minimal analgesic dosage.

As an effective antitussive, codeine, like morphine, is a common ingredient in cough medicines. Other side effects of codeine are constipation and sometimes nausea. Large doses have a paradoxical stimulant effect. It is considered only mildly addictive, instances of codeine addiction being rare, though not unknown. When PHYSICAL DEPENDENCE on codeine develops, the WITHDRAWAL SYMPTOMS upon cessation of the drug are much milder than those connected with morphine or HEROIN dependence. PSYCHIC DEPENDENCE, however, is more common, as users seek out the drug's mild euphoric and sedative properties. As with any opiate drug, tolerance to the drug's action develops, necessitating increasing doses to repeat the initially pleasurable effects. Addicts seeking to withdraw themselves from heroin, or unable to obtain heroin, may use codeine to alleviate their withdrawal symptoms. In sufficient quantities this is effective, but when the codeine is stopped, the withdrawal symptoms have the same severity as those of heroin dependence. A Schedule II drug under the CONTROLLED SUBSTANCES ACT. Slang name: schoolboy.

> Codeinists have the same abnormal desires, sensations, and sufferings as morphinists. Their number is small in comparison with the latter, but nevertheless considerable. One such, an extremely neuropathic young man, on account of his mental erethism, was prescribed *codeine* pills, one of 0.03 gr. to be taken three times a day. He experienced one day a euphoric state after taking a large number of them at once. He continued to augment the dose, increasing it to 50 pills or nearly 2 gr. of codeine per day. Without these pills life seemed impossible to him. The attempt to escape from this necessity produced depression, restlessness and weariness of life. After a year five pills every hour or two did not suffice him. His restlessness increased. On leaving his bed he travelled purposelessly in street cars and by rail. At last he was consuming one hundred pills or nearly 3 gr. of codeine daily. He then procured opium pills and took that fraudulent preparation "Anti-morphine," which contains morphia as well as other narcotics. He lost weight considerably, became extremely pale, and talked slowly and hesitatingly. Withdrawal treatment produced, besides the craving for codeine, restlessness, irritability, depression, life-weariness, and physical disturbances. The wretched man sacrificed his fortune of 10,000 marks to this expensive passion.
> —Louis Lewin, *Phantastica: Narcotic and Stimulating Drugs* (1964)

cohoba. [Arawak Indian name] hallucinogenic snuff prepared from PIPTADENIA by the Indians of Trinidad. The hallucinogenic ACTIVE PRINCIPLE is thought to be BUFOTENINE. Compare YOPO.

coke. [since 1900] COCAINE.

coke head. [since around 1920; HEAD, one frequently under the influence of a drug whose mind (*head*) is therefore more or less permanently under its sway] habitual COCAINE user.

cold. *1.* COLD TURKEY. *2.* abruptly, as in "he quit *cold.*"

cold shot. [opposite of HOT SHOT?] a bad deal, a dirty trick.

cold turkey. [from the gooseflesh that is one of the WITHDRAWAL SYMPTOMS of HEROIN or MORPHINE] abrupt withdrawal from narcotics, when PHYSICAL DEPENDENCE is present, so that the addict goes through the withdrawal symptoms; as opposed to tapering off with gradually decreasing doses of the drug addicted to or a similar drug and other medication. The latter procedure will considerably lessen the withdrawal symptoms; however, it is agreed that cold turkey is not quite the agonizing process it used to be because the highly diluted heroin most addicts purchase gives them only a mild addiction; also, they often employ BARBITURATES or TRANQUILIZERS or METHADONE pills to allay their symptoms. Nevertheless some addicts undergo cold turkey at one time or another because they have no money for drugs, have lost their connection, or the source of supply has dried up. They do not fear the withdrawal symptoms and their alleged fear is not the prime reason for using drugs. Compare A LA CANONA, KICKING.

collapsed veins. venous thrombosis, swollen and blocked veins; a condition, common among long-term HEROIN addicts, resulting from frequent injections in a vein. When the arm vein has collapsed, the addict starts on a new one in the leg, hand, neck, or foot, sometimes continuing until he has none left. Some old addicts then revert to subcutaneous injection (SKIN POPPING).

collar. *1.* an arrest.

> "Who's given you every decent *collar* you've had in the past four weeks?" —addict-informer in James Mills, *The Panic in Needle Park* (1966)

2. to arrest *3.* a strip of paper or rubber band wrapped around an eyedropper tip to ensure a tight fit where it is joined to the needle. Compare DROPPER, WORKS.

Colombian. a kind of MARIJUANA from Colombia, considered a very potent grade.

come down. *1.* to lose the effects of the drug and be restored to a normal state. *2.* invidiously, a depressed, mundane, unpleasant state. *3.* in heroin addicts, to develop withdrawal symptoms. Compare BRING DOWN, HIGH.

> He had to go out on the street somewhat "sick" because during the nighttime his habit "*came down*," that is to say he developed symptoms. —Seymour Fiddle, *Portraits from a Shooting Gallery* (1967)

coming down. beginning to lose the effects of a drug. Compare BRING DOWN.

> In despair where the lids were swollen
> The heart that was pounding and writhing
> And ears where the sounds were screaming
> And the mind that was ashen and still.
> Cocaine, cocaine
> I'm a *comin' down*
> I'm a comin' down.   —Ed Sanders, "Coming Down" (1966)

Compazine. [prochlorperazine, Smith Kline & French Laboratories] a MAJOR TRANQUILIZER, chemically derived from phenothiazine. Manufacturer recommends it be used to control nausea, to alleviate anxiety, agitation, and confusion, in chronic alcoholism, and to control unruly behavior in disturbed children. The usual recommended daily dose is 40 milligrams, but in severe psychotic states up to 100 milligrams may be necessary. As a result of overdosage or individual sensitivity to Compazine, unpleasant side effects may occur, including lowered blood pressure (which can lead to fatal cardiac arrest), liver damage, allergic reactions, convulsions, and pseudo parkinsonism (drooling, tremors, shuffling gait). TOLERANCE and PHYSICAL DEPENDENCE do not develop.

The drug may act to POTENTIATE the effects of central nervous system depressants, i.e., alcohol, OPIATES, ANTIHISTAMINES, BARBITURATES, ANALGESICS, ATROPINE, and should not be used in conjunction with them lest respiratory depression and death result. Sold in 5-, 10-, and 25-milligram tablets, sustained-release capsules, suppositories, syrup, and solutions for injection. Compare CHLORPROMAZINE, THORAZINE.

Conar. [The S. E. Massengill Company] a cough syrup containing, among other ingredients, NOSCAPINE, a nonaddicting alkaloid of OPIUM. Each 5 cubic centimeters contains 10 milligrams of noscapine. Manufacturer recommends for coughs, congestion, and dry, nonproductive coughs. No prescription.

connect. *1.* to find a source of drugs. *2.* to buy drugs. Compare COP, SCORE.

connection. [convicts' word for a liaison with the "outside"—*EP;* narcotic connotation since around 1920] *1.* a person from whom one can buy narcotics. *2.* a PUSHER. *3.* a wholesaler, the pusher's source; a high-level dealer. *4.* one's source of supply of narcotics, one's CONTACT.

connection dough. money needed to pay a CONNECTION.

contact. *1.* a drug supplier, the PUSHER you know. *2.* on college campuses, the source of drugs. Compare SOURCE, MAN.

contact habit. vicariously experiencing some of the effects of drug addiction though not oneself addicted; said satirically by addicts of PUSHERS and narcotics agents.

> "Selling is more of a habit than using," Lupita [a pusher] says. Nonusing pushers have a *contact habit,* and that's one you can't kick. Agents get it too. Take Bradley the Buyer. . . . Well, the Buyer comes to look more and more like a junky. He can't drink. He can't get it up. His teeth fall out. . . . The Buyer takes on an ominous grey-green color. Fact is his body is making its own junk or equivalent.
> —William Burroughs, *Naked Lunch* (1959)

contact high. [compare BUNK HABIT] *1.* among jazz musicians, the player who is HIGH on MARIJUANA communicates his mental state through his music to other players who are not high, affecting their playing accordingly. *2.* the mild (if it exists at all) high obtained by inhaling smoke from another's marijuana cigarette. *3.* becoming high just from being around those who are using drugs, i.e., their mood communicates itself to the nonuser.

Controlled Substances Act. the omnibus federal act regulating drugs likely to be abused. Successor to the Narcotics Act and the Drug Abuse Control Amendments. The drugs are listed in five schedules according to medical usage and abuse potential. Drugs are placed on the list by the Drug Enforcement Agency and the Justice Department in conjunction with the Food and Drug Administration and the Secretary of Health, Education and Welfare. The schedules and drugs regulated are as follows:

> *Schedule I:* drugs deemed to have great abuse potential and no legitimate medical use; includes HEROIN and HALLUCINOGENS such as LSD, MESCALINE, PSILOCYBIN, and MARIJUANA; use is forbidden except for highly restricted research purposes.
> *Schedule II:* drugs with great abuse potential that have legitimate medical uses; includes OPIATES and SYNTHETIC OPIATES such as MORPHINE, METHADONE, and DEMEROL, certain BARBITURATES of the short-acting type, METHAQUALONE, and AMPHETAMINES. Under Schedule II, production quotas may be set, stringent import–export quotas are imposed, and telephone and refillable prescriptions are prohibited.

Schedule III: drugs with some abuse potential; includes DORIDEN and NOLUDAR 300, barbiturates, and PAREGORIC. Schedule III provides for no production quotas, looser regulations, and no prescription restrictions except prohibition of refills after six months.

Schedules IV and V: differ very little from Schedule III and from each other; they are defined to include drugs with less abuse potential than the next highest schedule. Schedule IV includes long-acting barbiturates such as phenobarbital, PLACIDYL, and CHLORAL HYDRATE, and minor tranquilizers such as MEPROBAMATE. (LIBRIUM and VALIUM were included but manufacturers contested.) Schedule V includes cough medicines with CODEINE; they may be sold without prescription under certain regulations (e.g., buyer must be over 18, drug must be sold by pharmacist, and purchaser's name must be recorded).

cook. to heat the mixture of HEROIN powder and water in the COOKER over a lighted match until the powder has dissolved for injection.

cooker. a small receptacle, e.g., a whiskey-bottle top, bottle cap, or spoon, in which the HEROIN addict heats up a mixture of heroin powder and water in order to dissolve the heroin, draw it up through a cotton filter, and inject it. Often a thin wire is wrapped around the whiskey-bottle cap so that it can be held without burning the fingers. The handle of the spoon may be bent for the same reason. Compare WORKS.

cook up. to COOK.

cool. trustworthy, safe, careful; having controlled emotions.

cop. [to buy; from to take, lay hold of. Since the 1800s—*EP*] to buy narcotics, as in "he went out to *cop*" or "I was *copping* on 125th Street at that time." Compare SCORE.

cope. to function more or less normally though intoxicated by a drug. But with HEROIN addicts, the ability to cope is a "normal" state, which only an injection of heroin can restore. See HOOKED (quotation).

copilot. one who sits with someone who has taken LSD and cares for him if necessary. Compare GUIDE.

copilots. DEXEDRINE tablets.

cop man. *1.* a PUSHER. *2.* the middleman in a drug sale.

cop sickness. the anxiety, discomfort, and incipient WITHDRAWAL

SYMPTOMS experienced by an addict needing his next FIX. See HEROIN, YENNING.

> And when you're hooked, it gets so that every time someone goes out to score [buy drugs] for you even though it's maybe three or four hours until you're due, you get sick. First you get severe cramps in your stomach. It's just like a tiny sick backache, then headache, then sweating, shaking, cigarettes start tasting bad, you can't sit still, you can't sleep, you can't rest, you can't do anything, you're just frantic, and you feel ill, quite ill.
>
> —Helen MacGill Hughes (ed.), *The Fantastic Lodge* (1961)

corrine. COCAINE. *Obsolete.*

corrine and the girl. COCAINE. Compare GIRL. *Obsolete.*

Coryz. [Marion Laboratories, Inc.] a cough syrup containing NOSCAPINE, a nonaddicting alkaloid of OPIUM. Each 5 cubic centimeters (1 teaspoonful) contains 30 milligrams of noscapine. No prescription.

Cosanyl [Parke, Davis & Company] a cough syrup containing CODEINE. One ounce contains 1 grain (60 milligrams) of codeine. No prescription necessary in most states. (Often misspelled as "Cocinol," etc.).

cotton. wisp of cotton through which the "cooked" HEROIN is drawn into the hypodermic to filter out impurities.

cotton habit. a mild habit; irregular use of narcotics.

cotton shooter. a hardup addict who shoots the residue from COTTONS.

count. the weight or volume of drugs in a sale. Compare WEIGHT.

courage pills. BARBITURATES or other sedative pills.

cracking shorts. [from *crack,* to break into, to burglarize, and SHORT, car, since around 1930—*EP*] breaking into cars, a common form of theft among addicts.

crank. AMPHETAMINES.

crank bugs. hallucinations, after heavy use of AMPHETAMINES or COCAINE, that bugs are crawling under one's skin (formication).

crap. [addicts' expression of contempt applied to the highly diluted HEROIN which started appearing on the illicit market in the 1920s:

"this is *crap*"—*EP*] *1.* low-quality, diluted heroin. *2.* heroin, however diluted. Compare CA-CA, SHIT.

crash. *1.* to fall asleep suddenly and profoundly after an extended JAG on a stimulant drug such as AMPHETAMINE. *2.* to return abruptly to normal from a state of drug intoxication, to COME DOWN, either due to a willed effort in order to appear STRAIGHT or because of a shock, such as the appearance of a policeman. *3.* simply to sleep, as in "looking for a place to *crash.*" Compare BRING DOWN, COME DOWN.

> Several times when I was looking for somebody I was told, "He's hiding to *crash.*" For a while I thought the term had something to do with an overdose of brain-ticklers—the maddened victim having slunk off in the woods like a sick animal, to ride out his delirium without disturbing the others. But crashing means nothing more sinister than going on the nod, either from booze or simple fatigue. When this happens—if the unfortunate has not found a safe hiding place—the others will immediately begin tormenting him. The most common penalty for crashing is the urine shower; those still on their feet gather quietly around the sleeper and soak him from head to foot.
> —Hunter S. Thompson, *Hell's Angels* (1966)

crater. a gaping hole in the flesh at a vein caused by repeated intravenous injections of a drug at the same spot. Compare PIT.

> I had cultivated a *crater* and always shot through the same hole. It sure looked awful, though.
> —Piri Thomas, *Down These Mean Streets* (1967)

creep. an addict who, because of fear, incompetence, or isolation, does not engage in risky, criminal activities to raise money for drugs but rather begs them, does errands, or lends out a hypodermic needle in exchange for a TASTE of someone else's drugs. On some days the creep may acquire a large amount of drugs in this manner and on others very little. Hence, if during his successful period he acquires a large habit, he is forced, during lean periods, to support it by (for him) desperate measures such as stealing. Since he is inexperienced and probably unskilled at this, he is more likely to be arrested than the more skilled hustlers. Compare FLUNKY, HUSTLER, HUSTLING.

crib. *1.* one's home or apartment. *2.* a place where drugs are injected. Compare SHOOTING GALLERY.

croaker. [from convict's term for the prison doctor, from *croak,* to die; the death rattles of a dying man; since 1850—*EP*] any doctor with whom the addict deals, e.g., in narcotics hospital, or *2.* a private practitioner who will illegally prescribe drugs for addicts in exchange for money. Compare MAKING A CROAKER FOR A READER, BRODY.

crossroads. [from the scoring on the pills] AMPHETAMINE tablets. Compare CARTWHEELS.

cross-tolerance. among certain pharmacologically related drugs, TOLERANCE built up to the effects of one will carry over to the others; thus, if one has acquired a tolerance to LSD and takes MESCALINE, one will experience no effects from the latter; similarly, one who has taken a large dose of METHADONE will perceive no effects from HEROIN. This is the basis of the METHADONE TREATMENT.

crumbs. small change.

crutch. rolled matchbook cover, hairpin, tweezers, etc., used for holding a MARIJUANA butt (ROACH) that has been smoked down too far to be held between the fingers. Compare ROACH HOLDER.

crystal. [the drug is supplied in white crystals] METHEDRINE or DESOXYN; any soluble AMPHETAMINE for injection.

crystal palace. a place where SPEED users congregate.

cube, the. [from the practice of ingesting tiny quantities of the liquid absorbed by a sugar cube] LSD-25.

cura. [from Spanish *cura,* cure] a shot of HEROIN.

cure. length of stay of volunteers in a United States Public Health Service narcotics hospital.

cut. [from bootlegger's term for diluting liquor with water or grain alcohol—*EP*] to adulterate HEROIN with MILK SUGAR, mannite, or quinine. Quinine is used because its appearance and bitter taste are identical with those of heroin, and because it is believed to enhance the RUSH. The purchaser cannot tell by taste or sight how much pure heroin he is getting, and the PUSHER can take a larger profit. Pure heroin diluted five times by half yields a mixture containing about 5 percent heroin, the usual proportion sold to the addict. Compare WHACKED.

cut ounces. further diluted.

cutting. the process of diluting heroin with MILK SUGAR, mannite, or quinine. Compare DECK UP, FIVE-DOLLAR BAG, SPOON, WHACKED, PIECE.

We would have a mirror, some sugar-milk or quinine, a teaspoon, a woman's stocking and a hanger. You take the quinine, measure out how many spoons you want for each spoon of heroin, then run 'em together through the woman's stocking out onto the mirror. You make a diamond-shape of the wire hanger and you stretch the stocking tight over that. You run a spoon through and it falls right back on the mirror. You rake it back and forth with the spoon, and when it falls on the mirror it's mixed. From there you have a measure: like for a $5.00 bag, an eighth of a spoon.

—pusher, quoted in Jeremy Larner and Ralph Tefferteller,
The Addict in the Street (1964)

"The different piles there," Santo [a heroin wholesaler] went on, pointing as he spoke, "are heroin, quinine, and milk sugar. We work a four-to-one *cut* here—about four parts of milk sugar or quinine to one part heroin. Actually, of course, the heroin has already been cut way down before we even get it. So the guy on the street gets maybe five percent. The quinine is just to cut the sweet taste of the sugar. Heroin itself has a bitter taste and if a junkie tastes some stuff before he uses it and it's real sweet he figures he's bought a blank and gets upset. So we put in the quinine to make it bitter. The rest is pretty much obvious. You can see how it works just by watching. Any questions just ask. That guy over there is gonna cut Bobby's [a pusher] stuff now."

Bobby had managed to get three pieces out of Santo and one of the men started cutting it. He took a wire coat hanger that had been spread open and covered with nylon from a stocking, and put it in front of him on the glass-topped table. Then he opened one of the ounce envelopes and carefully emptied the contents onto the nylon. He lifted the coat-hanger-and-nylon sieve and shook it gently, sifting the heroin through the nylon onto the table. He shook it slowly, almost tenderly, taking great care not to let the sifted heroin spread too much. When he was through, the heroin sat in a high fluffy mound, almost twice the volume he had started with. He took a razor blade and carefully scraped the heroin that had drifted away from the edge of the mound back toward the center. Next he took a whisky shot glass, filled it once with heroin, and emptied it onto the coat-hanger–nylon sifter. He added two shots each of milk sugar and quinine. He mixed the chemicals together on the nylon, then sifted the whole mess again.

Now everyone pitched in. The three men at the table and Santo and Bobby each took baby measuring spoons and dipped them into the mound of cut heroin. When each had a spoonful, he leveled it off with a razor blade and dumped it in a neat pile on the glass. After they had about ten piles, one of the men started shoveling each pile into one of the stamp-sized bags. Everyone else measured, and the one man bagged. When everything was in bags, Bobby and Santo started folding them over and sealing them shut with Scotch tape. The others went to work on Bobby's second and third ounces. Finally everything was cut and all the bags were rubber-banded together in bundles of twenty-five bags each. Hundreds of bundles were stacked up on the table. Each bundle would sell for $75—and sell as easily as water in hell.

—James Mills, *The Panic in Needle Park* (1966)

cyc. CYCLAZOCINE.

cyclazocine. a long-acting narcotic antagonist, which, administered either orally or by injection in given amounts, will reduce the psychological and physiological effects of a corresponding amount of any morphine-like drug. Cyclazocine, like other narcotic antagonists, will precipitate WITHDRAWAL SYMPTOMS when administered to someone physically dependent upon narcotics. Doses of 0.25 to 2 milligrams have the analgesic effects of 10 milligrams of MORPHINE.

Experiments conducted with cyclazocine in curing narcotics addiction, although limited, have been encouraging, although METHADONE remains the preferred drug. The addict is first withdrawn from HEROIN. Then he is given regular maintenance shots of cyclazocine, which acts to build up a large degree of tolerance to heroin in his system. As long as he continues taking the cyclazocine, a heroin injection will have little or no effect on him, except in large amounts. Thus, under medical supervision, on an outpatient basis, the patient can be effectively weaned from his dependence upon heroin, making it easier for him to break out of the addict's heroin-centered life pattern.

Most patients find the drug subjectively pleasant—more like MARIJUANA or BARBITURATES than heroin—and are motivated to continue the treatment. PHYSICAL DEPENDENCE on cyclazocine develops, but the withdrawal symptoms are much milder than those of heroin, and the patient has no craving for cyclazocine during or after the withdrawal.

D d

D. DORIDEN (GLUTETHIMIDE).

dabbling. [since the 1950s] using narcotics moderately, irregularly. Compare CHIPPYING, WEEKEND HABIT, CHICK SHIT habit.

dagga. [from the Hottentot *dachab,* to smoke gladly, to tread down gladly and frequently] CANNABIS in South Africa, where employers give it to laborers to stimulate their production and increase their endurance (a similar practice is followed in Jamaica). It is also used as medicine for headache and snakebite, as an anesthetic in childbirth, and to wean children.

dapped. HIGH on DAPRISAL.

Daprisal. [aspirin, phenacetin, amobarbital, dextroamphetamine, Smith Kline & French Laboratories] an AMPHETAMINE–BARBITURATE combination, with analgesics, recommended for relief of mild to moderate pain in headache, sinusitis, bursitis, and muscle pain. The amphetamine is supposed to enhance the activity of the painkillers—aspirin and phenacetin—while the amobarbital counteracts the excitation and wakefulness produced by the amphetamine. The Food and Drug Administration does not approve of amphetamine–barbiturate combinations (compare DEXAMYL). Abuse of Daprisal has been reported among professional football players. PSYCHIC DEPENDENCE occurs with prolonged use of such combinations and, if used heavily, exhaustion and depression might result from abrupt withdrawal of the amphetamine. In addition, PHYSICAL DEPENDENCE on the barbiturate could occur after long-term, heavy usage. Each tablet contains 162 milligrams of aspirin, 162 milligrams of phenacetin, 32 milligrams of amobarbital, and 5 milligrams of dextroamphetamine. Sold in yellow, oblong tablets with "SKF, D34" inscribed. A Schedule II drug under the CONTROLLED SUBSTANCES ACT.

Darvon. [propoxyphene hydrochloride, Eli Lilly & Company] a synthetic narcotic analgesic (pain-reliever). Darvon is recommended by the manufacturer for mild to moderate pain and was once touted as a nonaddictive analgesic. Subsequent experience with the drug has proved this not to be the case and Darvon has found its way into the drug subculture.

Darvon is chemically related to METHADONE and in potency and addiction-potential is closest to CODEINE. The usual dose is 65 milligrams, orally, three or four times daily. The drug is also sold in combinations with aspirin, phenacetin, and caffeine; propoxyphene napsylate is a variation which is more soluble and slightly less potent, so that 100 milligrams is the equivalent dosage. Darvon can cause drowsiness and impair driving; some users experience euphoria. Overdosages result in convulsions, coma, respiratory depression, and circulatory collapse. Narcotics antagonists such as NALLINE, rather than stimulants such as AMPHETAMINE or caffeine, are the recommended treatment for overdoses.

TOLERANCE develops to the drug, as well as PHYSICAL DE-PENDENCE, after long-term use, accompanied by WITHDRAWAL SYMPTOMS if the drug is abruptly stopped. If Darvon is administered to someone dependent upon an OPIATE drug such as HEROIN, it may trigger withdrawal symptoms. Darvon is sold in light pink, football-shaped pills, capsules with red body and light-gray cap, and red body and light pink cap. Despite its abuse potential, Darvon is not subject to the CONTROLLED SUBSTANCES ACT. Compare TALWIN.

datura. [from Hindi for jimsonweed, DATURA STRAMONIUM] in India, thieves surreptitiously mixed datura with HASHISH and offered it to their victims. The interaction of the two drugs causes mental derangement followed by coma. In addition to *Datura stramonium,* several other species are found in the southwestern United States and Mexico, the main ones being *D. meteloides,* known as *tolgucha* in Mexico and used as a narcotic since ancient times, and *D. inoxia.* The species found in the Andes include *D. candida, D. sanguinea, D. aurea, D. dolichocarpa,* and *D. vulcanicola.*

The Indians of these regions often pulverize the seeds and mix them with locally brewed beers. The intoxication produced begins with the characteristic excitation, sometimes so extreme that the drinker becomes violent and has to be forcibly restrained. This is followed by a deep sleep, marred by dreams and hallucinations, which the witch doctor often interprets as an aid to diagnosing diseases, discovering culprits, or predicting the future.

Datura stramonium. a plant of the potato family *(Solanaceae)* containing poisonous alkaloids with narcotic and hallucinogenic properties. In the United States it is known variously as jimsonweed, stinkweed, thorn apple, and devil's-apple. It contains the alkaloids STRAMONIUM, HYOSCYAMINE, and ATROPINE.

This [jimsonweed] being an early Plant, was gather'd very young for a boil'd salad, by some of the Soldiers sent thither, to pacifie the troubles of Bacon; and some of them ate plentifully of it, the effect of which was a very pleasant Comedy; for they turned natural Fools upon it for several Days. One would blow a Feather in the Air; another would dart straws at it with much Fury; and another stark naked was sitting up in a Corner, like a Monkey grinning and making Mows at them; a Fourth would fondly kiss and paw his Companions, and snear in their Faces, with a Countenance more antik than any in a Dutch Droll. In this frantik Condition they were confined, lest they in their Folly should destroy themselves; though it was observed that all their Actions were full of Innocence and Good Nature. Indeed, they were not very cleanly; for they would have wallow'd in their own Excrements, if they had not been prevented. A Thousand such simple Tricks they play'd and after Eleven Days, return'd themselves again, not remembering anything that had pass'd.

—Robert Beverley, *History and Present State of Virginia* (1705)

Magic ointments or witches' philtres procured for some reason and applied with or without intention produced effects which the subjects themselves believed in, even stating that they had intercourse with evil spirits, had been on the Brocken and danced at the Sabbat with their lovers, or caused damage to others by witchcraft. The mental disorder caused by substances of this kind, for instance *Datura,* has even instigated some persons to accuse themselves before a tribunal. The peculiar hallucinations evoked by the drug had been so powerfully transmitted from the unconscious mind to the consciousness that mentally uncultivated persons nourished in the absurd superstitions of the Church, believed them to be reality. . . .

Besides other disagreeable symptoms these *solanaceae* and their active elements, especially atropine and scopolamine, give rise to hallucinations of sight, hearing and taste, which differ, however, from those produced by the other Phantastica. They are not of an agreeable but on the contrary of a terrifying and distrustful kind.

—Louis Lewin, *Phantastica: Narcotic and Stimulating Drugs* (1964)

dawamesk. a small, green aromatic cake composed of CANNABIS plant tops, sugar, orange juice, cinnamon, cloves, cardamom, NUTMEG, musk, pistachios, and pine kernels. Eaten in North Africa for the hallucinogenic effects of the cannabis. Cannabis was introduced to Europe from North Africa in this form through Le club des HASCHISCHINS, a group of Paris intellectuals, in the 1840s. Compare MAJOON.

day-glo paint. paint with an iridescent sheen suggesting the intensification of colors during an LSD experience. LSD users sometimes paint their bodies with it and also wear clothing in such colors, which sometimes can trigger, in the frequent user, a brief state of altered consciousness, as if he had taken LSD.

> The next day [after taking LSD] we felt cold and remote, but got through a lot of work. Driving the children to school, I nearly crashed when a coloured girl came out of a grey house wearing *day-glo* orange trousers: they went off on my retina like a bomb in a free-church assembly. —Peter Laurie, *Drugs* (1967)

deadly nightshade. BELLADONNA.

deal. [from DEALER, a trafficker in narcotics; since around 1925—*EP*] to peddle narcotics.

dealer. trafficker in narcotics, PUSHER.

dealer's band. a rubber band securing packets of HEROIN to the wrist in such a manner that if flipped it will send the packets flying. Used by peddlers so that they can rid their person of narcotics quickly the moment they spot a police officer.

dealing. peddling narcotics.

deck. [from its resemblance to a deck of cards; a small packet, a thin paper fold of some drug; since 1890. Since the 1940s it generally has implied HEROIN—*EP*] a folded paper or glassine envelope containing heroin. Compare BAG, PAPER, BUNDLE.

deck up. to fill the DECK with diluted HEROIN. Compare CUTTING.

> We just take it [heroin] and put it in the bag. It's a special bag that they use mostly for stamp collecting. We could *deck up* 2-300 in an evening's time. It all depends on how much you got and how fast you deck up.
> —pusher, quoted in Jeremy Larner and Ralph Tefferteller, *The Addict in the Street* (1964)

deeda. [from D, diminution of LSD; Harlem since around 1964] LSD-25.

deliriants. volatile substances, the fumes of which are inhaled for intoxicating effects. There are two general types of these substances: vaporous anesthetics including NITROUS OXIDE, chloroform, and ether, and organic solvents derived from petroleum. The effects of the anesthetics include giddiness, hilarity (hence "laughing gas"), euphoria, and sleep—sometimes death from respiratory failure, if too much is inhaled. The effects usually last about five minutes;

ether, which is a distillate of alcohol and sulfuric acid, also produces these effects if drunk.

Abuse of the organic solvents, which are found in a wide variety of household products, increased in the early sixties after much adverse publicity was given to an epidemic of GLUE SNIFFING that had broken out in Denver, Colorado, and other cities. The publicity, it seemed, while warning of dire effects from such practices, actually alerted potential drug abusers and contributed to the spread of the phenomenon. Also contributing was the accessibility of a large number of products capable of producing the desired effects, in addition to glue (which contains toluene). The users tended to be teen-aged or sub-teens, perhaps because more conventional drugs were unavailable to them.

At any rate, products sniffed for their effects include gasoline, CARBON TETRACHLORIDE, BENZINE, paint thinners, lacquers, enamels, varnishes, varnish removers, glues, cigarette lighter fluid, charcoal lighter fluids, finger nail polishes and polish removers, spot removers, freezing preparations (Freon) and all kinds of aerosol sprays. The usual effects of inhalation of these substances include incoordination, restlessness, excitement, confusion, disorientation, ataxia, delirium, and finally coma. The effects resemble alcohol intoxication, while if enough is sniffed hallucinations will result. Deaths have been reported but some of the evidence is conflicting. For example, a series of deaths from glue sniffing were actually attributable to the practice of inhaling the glue while the head was encased in a plastic, dry-cleaning bag; suffocation from the bag, not the glue, caused the death. Similarly, there were repeated warnings of brain, liver, and kidney damage from the practice, but it turned out that these had been based upon industrial data and involved men who had inhaled the vapors eight hours a day over months or years. Consequently, the hazards have perhaps been exaggerated, although such studies as have been made of casual sniffing are so inconclusive and inadequate in their data that neither can it be said that the practice is totally harmless. Deaths by accidents caused by loss of coordination are said to have also occurred, e.g., the user falls off a roof. Deaths attributable to inhaling freezing preparations have been definitely established.

Demerol. [MEPERIDINE hydrochloride, Winthrop Laboratories] a SYNTHETIC OPIATE used as an analgesic and sedative, Demerol is one of the most widely used of the synthetic opiates, especially as an analgesic in childbirth. It is also, perhaps because of this accessibility in hospitals and the mistaken view that it is not addictive, the most frequent choice of medical personnel who became addicts and who prefer it to MORPHINE. Demerol does cause PHYSICAL DEPENDENCE.

The usual clinical dosage is 50 to 100 milligrams repeated at three- to four-hour intervals. Demerol does not produce so much sedation as morphine, nor is it so effective in severe pain, but it causes less nausea, constipation, or vomiting. Danger of respiratory depression is relatively small except when administered intravenously. A Schedule II drug under the CONTROLLED SUBSTANCES ACT.

dependence, drug. the World Health Organization's Expert Committee on Addiction-producing Drugs recommended in its Thirteenth Report (1964) that the terms *drug addiction* or *drug habituation* be dropped because they were too general and imprecise. WHO recommended that the term *drug dependence* be substituted, defining it as follows:

> *Drug dependence* is a state of psychic or physical dependence, or both, on a drug, arising in a person following administration of that drug on a periodic or continuing basis. The characteristics of such state will vary with the agent involved, and these characteristics must always be made clear by designating the particular type of drug dependence in each specific case; for example, drug dependence of morphine type, of amphetamine type, etc.

See PHYSICAL DEPENDENCE and PSYCHIC DEPENDENCE.

deprivation roll. using any drug at hand (such as NUTMEG, MACE, ANTIHISTAMINE) to achieve a HIGH. Compare GARBAGE HEAD.

Desbutal. [methamphetamine hydrochloride and pentobarbital sodium, Abbott Laboratories] an AMPHETAMINE and BARBITURATE in combination, developed as a mood elevator and an aid in dieting. The amphetamine stimulates the central nervous system and acts to depress the appetite; the barbiturate provides sedation and enhances the mood elevation of the amphetamine while minimizing some of its undesirable effects, e.g., hyperexcitement, insomnia, and nervousness. TOLERANCE may develop both to the amphetamine and the barbiturate, so that increasing dosages are a temptation. PSYCHIC DEPENDENCE accompanied by frequent and prolonged usage may also develop. If taken in large amounts over prolonged periods, PHYSICAL DEPENDENCE will occur, accompanied by chronic barbiturate and amphetamine intoxication and resulting in severe WITHDRAWAL SYMPTOMS if the drug is suddenly stopped. The F.D.A. does not consider amphetamine–barbiturate combinations desirable.

Desbutal is sold as green capsules containing 5 milligrams of methamphetamine hydrochloride (DESOXYN) and 30 milligrams of pentobarbital sodium (NEMBUTAL) and in Desbutal Gradumet delayed-release 10- and 15-milligram tablets. Desbutal 10 Gradumet (orange top half, pale blue bottom half) contains 10 milligrams of methamphetamine hydrochloride and 60 milligrams of pentobarbital sodium; the Desbutal 15 Gradumet (yellow top half, pale blue bottom) contains 15 milligrams of methamphetamine hydrochloride and 90 milligrams of pentobarbital sodium. Manufacturer's recommended dosages are one capsule, two to three times daily, or one Desbutal 10 or 15 Gradumet once daily, in the morning. A Schedule II drug under the CONTROLLED SUBSTANCES ACT. Compare DEXAMYL.

Desoxyn. [methamphetamine hydrochloride, Abbott Laboratories] a direct central nervous system stimulant of the AMPHETAMINE type. Recommended by the manufacturer in short-term dieting. Dose is 2.5 to 5 milligrams, up to three times daily. (Manufacturer warns against exceeding 15 milligrams in a single dose.) Sold in ampuls and tablets, upon which is inscribed the Abbott symbol *a*. A Schedule II drug under the CONTROLLED SUBSTANCES ACT. Compare METHEDRINE.

> Tolerance to the drug may develop during prolonged administration. In such cases careful supervision is essential to avoid excessive dosage or abuse which can lead to chronic intoxication and addiction. If this should occur, psychotic manifestations of chronic amphetamine intoxication may require temporary sedation. The drug should be withdrawn without delay. Lethargy, which may persist for some weeks, has been seen following withdrawal. Methamphetamine should not be used to combat fatigue or to replace rest in normal persons. The occurrence of paradoxically increased depression or agitation in mentally depressed patients is an indication for withdrawing the drug.
> —Abbott Laboratories (1967)

DET. [N,N-diethyltryptamine] a synthetic HALLUCINOGEN chemically related to DMT, which in turn is similar in structure to psilocin, the hallucinogenic substance to which PSILOCYBIN, the active ingredient in the hallucinogenic mushrooms, is converted in the body. The effects of a dose of 50 to 60 milligrams of DET produce hallucinogenic effects which last longer than DMT—about two or three hours. The effects include visual distortions, distortions in time and space, dizziness, and other effects such as are produced by LSD. The state of Oregon Mental Health Division reports that panic reactions to the drug have resulted in illusions of invulnerability, acts of violence, suicide, and acute and chronic psychosis. A Schedule I drug under the CONTROLLED SUBSTANCES ACT.

Dexamyl. [*d*-amphetamine sulfate and amobarbital, Smith Kline & French Laboratories] a central nervous system stimulant of the AMPHETAMINE type combined with a central nervous system depressant. The BARBITURATE ingredient acts to dampen down any overstimulation produced by the amphetamine ingredient without counteracting its appetite-depressant and euphoric properties. Manufacturer recommends as an aid in short-term dieting. Recommended maximum daily dose 15 milligrams of *d*-amphetamine sulfate and 97 milligrams of amobarbital. It is sold as elixir, sustained-release capsules (Spansules), or tablets, with contents as follows:

form	*d-amphetamine* sulfate, mg	*amobarbital,* mg
Spansule:		
No. 1	10	65
No. 2	15	97
tablet	5	32
elixir, 1 tsp	5	32

The Spansules have a green cap and a clear body showing green and white pellets. The tablets are flat, three-sided, green, and scored down the middle. Long-term use may result in PSYCHIC DEPENDENCE and PHYSICAL DEPENDENCE (on the amobarbital) and increasing TOLERANCE to both ingredients. Psychic dependence on the amphetamine ingredient may also occur. Overdose may result in excessive stimulation or excessive depression, which may reach the point of shock in severe cases. In Great Britain this combination is sold as Drinamyl ("purple hearts" or "French blues"), a purple tablet. The Food and Drug Administration has banned Dexamyl as ineffective, but manufacturer has appealed. Slang names: dex, dexies, Christmas trees. A Schedule II drug under the CONTROLLED SUBSTANCES ACT.

Dexedrine. [*d*-amphetamine sulfate, Smith Kline & French Laboratories] a central nervous system stimulant of the AMPHETAMINE type considered twice as potent as other amphetamines. Manufacturer recommends as an appetite depressant in dieting, as a mood elevator in minor depression, and for alcoholism and narcolepsy (involuntary sleep). Recommended dosages range from

30 to 50 milligrams total a day. As with all amphetamines, TOL-
ERANCE and PSYCHIC DEPENDENCE may develop.

Sold as elixir, timed-release capsules, or tablets. The timed-
release capsules (Spansules) come in three sizes: 5, 10, and 15 milligrams. They have a brown lid and a clear bottom showing orange
and white pellets and are inscribed "SKF." Two dots by the "SKF"
means 15 milligrams; one dot, 10 milligrams; and no dots, 5 milligrams. The tablets contain 5 milligrams of *d*-amphetamine sulfate.
They are pale orange in color, three-sided, flat, and scored down the
middle. A Schedule II drug under the CONTROLLED SUBSTANCES
ACT.

dexies. DEXEDRINE tablets; DEXAMYL.

dextromoramide. a SYNTHETIC OPIATE analgesic, dextromoramide
has a somewhat higher pain-relieving potency than MORPHINE: 5 to
7.5 milligrams injected equal the analgesic effects of 10 milligrams of
morphine, with the effects lasting four to five hours. PHYSICAL
DEPENDENCE occurs after prolonged use, but WITHDRAWAL SYMP-
TOMS are similar to those of METHADONE dependency and less severe
than those of morphine or HEROIN. Dextromoramide is sold under
the trade name PALFIUM. A Schedule II drug under the CONTROLLED
SUBSTANCES ACT.

dihydrocodeine. a semisynthetic derivative of MORPHINE, about
twice as potent as CODEINE. A dosage of 60 milligrams produces the
analgesia of 10 milligrams of morphine, lasting four to five hours.
Dihydrocodeine is generally prescribed for minor pain and as an
ingredient in cough medicines. Prolonged use will result in PHYSICAL
DEPENDENCE, with WITHDRAWAL SYMPTOMS somewhere between
those of codeine and morphine in severity. A Schedule III drug
under the CONTROLLED SUBSTANCES ACT. Compare DROCOGESIC
No. 3, SYNALGOS-DC, TUSSANIL-DH.

dihydrocodeinone. HYDROCODONE.

dihydromorphinone. HYDROMORPHONE.

Dilaudid. [HYDROMORPHONE (dihydromorphinone), Knoll Pharmaceutical Company] a semisynthetic derivative of MORPHINE. Although derived from morphine, Dilaudid is a much more potent
pain reliever. Injections of 2 milligrams provide the analgesia of 10
to 15 milligrams of morphine or 100 milligrams of MEPERIDINE, with
effects lasting four to five hours. There is less nausea, vomiting, and
sedation than with morphine. PHYSICAL DEPENDENCE develops after

prolonged use, and the WITHDRAWAL SYMPTOMS are similar to those of morphine in severity.

Dilaudid is sold in small, white, saccharinelike tablets (1, 2, 3, or 4 milligrams), as rectal suppositories (yellow, shaped like the upper half of a bowling ball), and ampuls for injection. Dilaudid Cough Syrup contains 1 milligram of Dilaudid hydrochloride and 100 milligrams of glyceryl guaiacolate per teaspoonful, in a reddish-orange peach-flavored syrup. Recommended adult dosage is 1 teaspoonful repeated in three to four hours. Both Dilaudid and Dilaudid Cough Syrup are Schedule II drugs under the CONTROLLED SUBSTANCES ACT.

> And any doctor who wasn't suspicious would write out a script for twenty or thirty Dilaudids. Possibly one, definitely two would get me straight. But that's no good either. I mean a Dialudid habit is no good. First of all, your habit on Dilaudid you get it much faster than you do on stuff [heroin]. Your body tolerances build up fast and before you know it you're taking fifteen or twenty Dilaudids at once, where maybe three days before, one or two would help. It goes up fantastically high. Second, there isn't a doctor in New York that isn't hip to junkies. But I'll tell you that if a doctor can be conned by anyone, I can do it. I can con anyone.   —addict in James Mills, *The Panic in Needle Park* (1966)

dill. dill weed, dried and smoked, is alleged to produce a mild HIGH.

dillies. DILAUDID.

Dilocol. [(HYDROMORPHONE) hydrochloride and other ingredients, Table Rock Laboratories, Inc.] cough syrup containing a semisynthetic derivative of MORPHINE. Each 30 cubic centimeters (6 teaspoonsful) contains 6 milligrams of dihydromorphinone hydrochloride, upon which PHYSICAL DEPENDENCE can develop after prolonged use. Recommended for coughs, reducing mucous irritation, and liquefying phlegm. Recommended dose is 1 teaspoonful every three or four hours. A Schedule II drug under the CONTROLLED SUBSTANCES ACT.

dime. [codeword formerly used in discussing prices during narcotics transactions] ten dollars, as in "sell me a *dime* bag." Compare CENT, NICKEL, QUARTER, DOLLAR.

Dionin. [Merck Sharp & Dohme] ethylmorphine hydrochloride.

Diosan. [commercial name in Spain] ethylmorphine hydrochloride.

dip and dab. experiment with HEROIN, use it occasionally. Compare CHIPPYING.

dipipanone. a SYNTHETIC OPIATE analgesic somewhat less potent than MORPHINE. A 20-milligram injection gives the analgesic effects of 10 milligrams of morphine, lasting four to five hours. PHYSICAL DEPEN-DENCE develops after prolonged use, with WITHDRAWAL SYMPTOMS similar to those of METHADONE dependence and considerably less severe than those of morphine or HEROIN. A Schedule II drug under the CONTROLLED SUBSTANCES ACT.

dirty. [antonym of CLEAN] *1.* carrying narcotics on the person. *2.* applied to MARIJUANA from which the stems, twigs, and seeds have not been removed.

discon. disorderly conduct charge or conviction.

> "What happened to you?" I asked.
> "Discon. Helen said she told you. The judge threw it out. He said the cop never should have busted me while I was in the phone booth. Like how could I be disorderly if I was just standing in the booth talking to someone on the phone? Which is right. The cop was a real jerk."
> —addict in James Mills, *The Panic in Needle Park* (1966)

Ditran. [piperidyl benzilate, Lakeside Laboratories, Inc.] a HALLUCINOGEN and PSYCHOTOMIMETIC drug. Experiments with Di-tran induced clear psychotic symptoms, toxic organic symptoms, hallucinations (mainly auditory), delusions, and a catatonic state.

The drug produced the following sequence of reaction in one experiment: (1) upon injection: odd sensations, heaviness of limbs; (2) after fifteen to twenty minutes: slurred speech, inertia, sensory cloudiness; and (3) one hour after injection: unresponsiveness both to questions by the examiner and to environmental occurrences. Subjects would have brief lucid intervals of ten to thirty seconds approximately every three minutes, when they responded to questions with fair coherence; then they would sink back into a withdrawn state. Other mental disorganization occurred, especially disorientation as to time and place. Changes in perception altered the form, distance, movement, and color of objects. Subjects sank into a state of immobility, occasionally making slow, aimless movements of the hands and mouth. The drug's effects are markedly different from those of LSD; there are no visual hallucinations, and the loss of contact with the surrounding environment is more nearly total.

djamba. [Brazil] CANNABIS. See DJOMA.

djoma. [central Africa; the similarity of this word to the Brazilian word for cannabis lends credence to the theory that the use of cannabis was introduced to the Western Hemisphere by African slaves] CANNABIS. Also called diamba, liamba, lianda, and maconha.

DMT. [N,N-dimethyltryptamine] a semisynthetic, fast-acting hallucinogenic chemical very similar in structure to psilocin, the hallucinogenic substance to which PSILOCYBIN, the active ingredient in the hallucinogenic mushrooms, is converted in the body. DMT is also thought to be the active ingredient of the hallucinogenic plants PIPTADENIA and BANISTERIOPSIS CAAPI. It is easily synthesized with rudimentary equipment and common ingredients, and there is evidence that illicit use is on the increase. Several close chemical variants, including DPT and DET, are also hallucinogenic. The onset of the drug occurs within two minutes, and its effects last upward of thirty minutes. The usual mode of ingestion is to soak parsley in the drug, let it dry, then smoke it in a pipe or cigarette. PHYSICAL DEPENDENCE does not develop, but TOLERANCE probably does, as is the case with psilocybin.

> My desperate attempts to climb toward sunlight and release from horror occupied the remainder of the experience—barely thirty minutes by clock time, but an infinite eternity subjectively during which I experienced total evolution, from the primary amoeboid stage, crawling and grasping for something to hold onto even though I was on the floor, slowly and then ever more rapidly growing and hurtling through both time and space.
> —anonymous DMT user, quoted in Dr. Donald Louria,
> *Nightmare Drugs* (1966)

do. use (a drug), as in "he was *doing* pot."

D.O.E. [origin obscure] taking drugs.

dogie. HEROIN. Also doojee, duji.

> Yet there is something about *dogie*—heroin—it's a superduper tranquilizer. All your troubles become a bunch of bleary blurred memories when you're in a nod of your own special dimension.
> —Piri Thomas, *Down These Mean Streets* (1967)

dollar. one hundred dollars. Compare CENT, DIME, NICKEL, QUARTER.

dollies. DOLOPHINE (METHADONE) pills. Often secured by addicts to alleviate WITHDRAWAL SYMPTOMS when there is a shortage of HEROIN, when they wish to withdraw from heroin, or when they are about to be imprisoned.

dolls. [coined by Jacqueline Susann, author of *Valley of the Dolls;* not true slang] BARBITURATE or AMPHETAMINE pills.

Dolophine. [METHADONE hydrochloride, Eli Lilly and Company] a SYNTHETIC OPIATE analgesic slightly more potent than MORPHINE. An injection of 10 milligrams gives analgesic action equivalent to that of 15 milligrams of morphine. Dolophine produces considerably less euphoria than morphine. It may also cause dizziness, dryness of the mouth, and vomiting. Even when the first doses are well tolerated, nausea may appear after several doses. Overdosage can cause drowsiness, sweating, mental depression, delirium, hallucinations, circulatory collapse, and coma. PHYSICAL DEPENDENCE occurs after prolonged use, but WITHDRAWAL SYMPTOMS are considerably less severe than those of morphine dependency. Sold in ampuls, in syrup containing 33.33 milligrams of Dolophine per 100 cubic centimeters, and tablets of 5, 7.5, or 10 milligrams. A Schedule II drug under the CONTROLLED SUBSTANCES ACT.

DOM. see STP.

doojee. HEROIN. Also dogie, duji.

dope. any narcotic. The word is also applied to MARIJUANA, HALLUCINOGENS, AMPHETAMINES, and BARBITURATES.

dope fiend. a term applied with defiant irony by addicts or other drug users to themselves (less frequently, by society to addicts).

Doriden. [GLUTETHIMIDE, CIBA Pharmaceutical Company] a non-barbiturate hypnotic and sedative, comparable to short-acting BARBITURATES in onset and duration of sedative action. Manufacturer recommends for simple insomnia, calming ambulatory patients suffering from insomnia, in preoperative sedation, and as a daytime sedative (TRANQUILIZER).

Recommended doses range from 125 milligrams (for sedation) up to 500 milligrams for sleep. Doses of thirty times the hypnotic dose (15,000 milligrams) have been taken in suicide attempts, resulting in prolonged coma, absence of reflexes, high fever, and death. Taken in combination with alcohol or other sedatives (which POTENTIATE its action), Doriden has caused fatal respiratory and circulatory failure.

TOLERANCE to the drug's effects develops; PHYSICAL DEPENDENCE also develops relatively rapidly; 2,000 to 2,500 milligrams taken daily can produce dependence. WITHDRAWAL SYMPTOMS are comparable to those of barbiturate dependence in severity, if the drug is abruptly ceased and, if untreated, fatal in 20–25 percent of the cases. Symptoms range from anxiety to grand mal (major epilepticlike) seizures. Chronic Doriden intoxication, which can appear when amounts of 1,500 milligrams and more are taken daily for several months, resembles chronic barbiturate intoxication and manifests itself in unsteadiness, tremors, slurred speech, loss of memory, irritability, delirium, etc. Doriden is supplied in tablets of 0.125, 0.25, and 0.5 gram (white, round, flat with "CIBA" inscribed) and in capsules of 0.5 gram (white bottom, blue cap bearing inscription "CIBA"). Slang names: CB, Ciba. A Schedule III drug under the CONTROLLED SUBSTANCES ACT.

do rights. first-time patients at LEXINGTON who are considered good prospects for a cure.

double trouble. BARBITURATES or barbiturate–AMPHETAMINE combination.

do up. [analogous to *fix;* from *tie up,* to tie a cord around an arm to distend the vein, thus making injection easier] to inject HEROIN.

down. DOWNIE.

downer. DOWNIE.

downie. [from *down,* antonym of HIGH] a BARBITURATE or TRANQUILIZER pill, often taken by AMPHETAMINE users to reverse the stimulant action of the drug when it becomes uncomfortable. Compare COMING DOWN, UP, UPPER.

down trip. [from *down,* antonym of HIGH, and TRIP, hallucinogenic drug experience] boring; depressing. Compare BRING DOWN, BUM KICKS.

drag. a BAD TRIP, a BUM TRIP.

dragged. frightened, hysterical after smoking MARIJUANA.

dreamer. *1.* MORPHINE. *2.* any depressant drug.

dried out. detoxified, withdrawn from a drug, usually in a hospital, as in "I went into Beth Israel and got *dried out.*" A process of at least ten days.

Drinamyl. [British drug] see DEXAMYL.

dripper. DROPPER.

Drocogesic No. 3 [DIHYDROCODEINE bitartrate with other ingredients, Carrtone Laboratories, Inc.] an analgesic preparation containing dihydrocodeine, an addictive MORPHINE derivative. A dose of 60 milligrams of dihydrocodeine gives analgesia equivalent to 10 milligrams of morphine; PHYSICAL DEPENDENCE can occur after prolonged use, with WITHDRAWAL SYMPTOMS less severe than those of morphine.

Each Drocogesic tablet contains 30 milligrams of dihydrocodeine. Manufacturer recommends it for headaches, neuralgia, and pain connected with upper respiratory infection. Recommended dosage is one to two tablets every three to four hours. A Schedule III drug under the CONTROLLED SUBSTANCES ACT. Compare CODEINE.

drop. to swallow (a pill), as in "they were sitting around *dropping* acid."

drop it. to conceal a drug.

dropper. medicine dropper used as a hypodermic syringe for injection of HEROIN. The needle is fastened to the tip of the dropper, with the glass part acting as the barrel of a hypodermic and the rubber bulb as the plunger. Most addicts find an eyedropper less clumsy than a regular hypodermic. Held upright, the bulb between thumb and forefinger, the dropper is easily manipulated, and the addict can inject the drugs in graduated amounts—injecting a little, withdrawing a little mixed with blood, and so on—thus prolonging and graduating the pleasure of the heroin's initial onset. Compare BOOTING, COLLAR, FIX.

drug automatism. ingestion of drugs without conscious awareness of the amount being taken or previously taken. This state occurs with heavy BARBITURATE users. Taken in large amounts, the drug clouds the mind and paralyzes the judgment. When sleep fails to come, because of TOLERANCE to the drug's effects, the users take more of the pills. This practice may result in a fatal overdose.

druggies. college students who experiment widely and frequently with a variety of drugs. Compare HEADS.

> On campus they cluster into three distinct groups. The *"druggies"* try anything, mix pills, and are high much of the time. They are steady LSD users. The casual potheads dabble in pills and "hash" and try acid once or twice. The fringe majority, friends, roommates of "heads," puff pot a couple of times and use amphetamines before exams.
> —*Look* (Aug. 8, 1967)

dry up. stop using drugs temporarily.

duby. MARIJUANA.

duji. HEROIN. Also spelled dogie, doojie, dugee.

dummies. DUMMY.

dummy. [from *dummy,* a phony, not the real thing] counterfeit HEROIN; white powder such as kitchen cleanser, talcum, or quinine placed in a BAG and sold to the addict as heroin. The addict rarely can tell whether he has bought heroin until he injects the purchase. Compare BLANK, GARBAGE, LEMON.

> "I saw a guy get caught dealing *dummies* [fake heroin] in a vestibule. This other cat took a taste from the bag, and he began yelling. 'You sold me a dummy!' He took out a gun, the rest of us hit the wall like postage stamps, and he blew the dealer away."
> —addict, quoted in Tom Alexander,
> *The Drug Takers* (1965)

duster. a cigarette with HEROIN mixed with the tobacco.

dusting. [from *dust,* tobacco; and *dust,* narcotics, as in *happy dust,* COCAINE—*EP*] mixing HEROIN in a MARIJUANA cigarette (OPIUM or DMT are also used). Compare A-BOMB.

dynamite. *1.* COCAINE and HEROIN taken in combination (see SPEEDBALL, BOMBITA). *2.* relatively undiluted high-potency heroin. *3.* any potent drug, especially MARIJUANA. Compare DYNO.

dyno. relatively undiluted, high-potency HEROIN, often stronger than the addict is tolerant to. Insufficient TOLERANCE can result in a fatal overdose.

E e

eater. an addict who ingests his drugs orally. Compare BELLY HABIT.

ecognine. the principal part of the COCAINE molecule. Obtained by hydrolysis of cocaine and other COCA alkaloids. Cocaine can also be synthesized from ecognine.

eighth, an. *1.* one-eighth ounce (approximately) of diluted HEROIN. *2.* a rough measure for the purpose of sale. Compare PIECE, CUTTING, SIXTEENTH, SPOON.

electric. influenced by or containing a PSYCHEDELIC drug, as in ELECTRIC KOOL-ADE.

electric Kool-Ade. a punch containing LSD-25, frequently served at ACID TESTS.

elemicin. [3,4,5-trimethoxyallylbenzene] a compound present in oil of NUTMEG and thought to be the ACTIVE PRINCIPLE causing its hallucinogenic effects. It is very similar in structure to TMA, another HALLUCINOGEN. See MDA, MMDA.

elephant. PHENCYCLIDINE, an animal tranquilizer.

embalao. [Puerto Rican addicts' slang] strongly addicted, with accompanying physical debilitation; STRUNG OUT.

embroidery. scars on the veins from frequent injections of drugs. Compare TRACKS.

enchaioui. [Arabic] a man who has centered his life around KIF (CANNABIS).

epeña. a hallucinogenic snuff used by the Waika Indians of northern Brazil and made from the bark of the *epeña* and *amasita* trees, which is ground up to produce a fine powder. One end of a long hollow tube containing the snuff is held to the nose, and another person blows through the other end, driving the snuff up the nasal passages. At onset, the effects are nausea and vomiting. Then the user straightens up and struts about, emitting an occasional laugh or yell. He experiences hallucinations in which everything is seen in giant size and he becomes a giant towering into the clouds, where he converses with the Indian deities.

Equanil. [MEPROBAMATE, Wyeth Laboratories] a nonhypnotic muscle relaxant and MINOR TRANQUILIZER. Manufacturer recommends in conditions involving muscle spasm, neuromuscular disorders, anxiety, and tension, as adjunctive therapy in rehabilitation of alcoholics, in minor epilepsy (petit mal), and as an aid to sleep. Recommended dosages are 400 milligrams, three or four times a day. Sold as white scored 200- and 400-milligram tablets, yellow-coated 400-milligram tablets, in a liquid base (200 milligrams per teaspoonful), and continuous-release 200-milligram capsules.

   A danger of Equanil, as with many minor tranquilizers, is that PSYCHIC DEPENDENCE will occur, the drug being a "crutch" for the user seeking to alleviate deep-set anxieties. PHYSICAL DEPENDENCE also develops after prolonged, excessive use. After excessive use, if the user's crutch is abruptly withdrawn, his underlying symptoms (anxiety, insomnia, poor appetite) will characteristically return with greatly increased severity. Large amounts will produce a state very similar to BARBITURATE intoxication. In some cases of excessive use, WITHDRAWAL SYMPTOMS have included vomiting, loss of bodily equilibrium, muscle twitching, and epilepticlike seizures. Equanil has been used in a number of suicide attempts, with amounts up to 20 to 40 grams (20,000 to 40,000 milligrams) being taken (the manufacturer's maximum recommended total daily dose is 2,400 milligrams). Fatalities in such attempts have been rare, but such dosages produce coma, shock, and respiratory collapse. Alcohol POTENTIATES the drug's effects. A Schedule IV drug under the CONTROLLED SUBSTANCES ACT. See also MILTOWN.

esrar. [Turkish, meaning secret preparation, evidently from the practice of mixing cannabis with tobacco to avoid detection; cannabis smoking was outlawed in Turkey in the nineteenth century] CANNABIS.

ethanol. ethyl ALCOHOL.

ethchlorvynol. a nonbarbiturate hypnotic and sedative compounded of a carboamic acid ester of alicylic alcohol. Its onset and effects are similar to those of secobarbital, a short-acting BARBITURATE. Like the other nonbarbiturate sedatives, ethchlorvynol has not proved to be the "safe alternative" to barbiturates. Prolonged excessive use can result in PSYCHIC DEPENDENCE, accompanied by increasing doses, PHYSICAL DEPENDENCE, and WITHDRAWAL SYMPTOMS when the drug is abruptly stopped. The latter may include convulsions and epilepticlike seizures similar to those accompanying barbiturate dependence. However, ethchlorvynol is useful as a sedative for patients who are allergic to the barbiturates.

Since it is a less potent central nervous system depressant than the barbiturates, larger amounts (500 milligrams) are needed to produce sleep, and only extremely large doses produce fatal respiratory failure. Dosages ranging from twenty to fifty times the hypnotic (sleep-inducing) dose of 500 milligrams have produced comas lasting a week, and sometimes death. Alcohol taken in conjunction with ethchlorvynol POTENTIATES its effects and hence its dangers. A Schedule IV drug under the CONTROLLED SUBSTANCES ACT. See also ETHINAMATE, PLACIDYL, TRANQUILIZERS.

ethinamate. a nonbarbiturate hypnotic and sedative, compounded of a carboamic acid ester of alicylic alcohol. Its onset and effects are similar to those of secobarbital, a short-acting BARBITURATE, though of shorter duration. Prolonged, excessive use can result in PSYCHIC DEPENDENCE requiring increased dosages, PHYSICAL DEPENDENCE, and WITHDRAWAL SYMPTOMS similar to those of barbiturate dependency when the drug is abruptly halted.

Overdosage can be fatal, but the lethal dose of ethinamate is unknown, a dose of 15 grams proving fatal while a dose of 28 grams was not. The usual sedative dose is 0.5 to 1 gram (500 to 1,000 milligrams), and one experiment showed that 0.5 gram was equal in sedative effect to 100 milligrams of secobarbital with some persons, while with others it performed scarcely better than a placebo used as a control. A Schedule IV drug under the CONTROLLED SUBSTANCES ACT.

ethyl alcohol. See ALCOHOL.

Eucodal. [OXYCODONE hydrochloride] a semisynthetic derivative of MORPHINE. A Schedule II drug under the CONTROLLED SUBSTANCES ACT.

eye opener. the first narcotics shot of the day. Without it, the addict cannot engage in the necessary HUSTLING. Compare MORNING SHOT, WAKE-UP.

F f

factory. a clandestine location where illicit drugs are processed in preparation for sale, e.g., pure HEROIN is diluted with quinine and milk sugar and packaged; MARIJUANA is cleaned and packaged. The word is used mainly by police and newspaper reporters.

fake a blast. to simulate drugged behavior. Compare BRODY.

falling out. dozing off while under the influence of a drug; going into a half sleep. Compare OVERCHARGED.

fatty. a thickly rolled MARIJUANA cigarette. Compare BOMBER.

feds. [traditionally applied by criminals to members of any federal law-enforcement agency] federal narcotics authorities. Compare UNCLES.

feeling the habit (monkey) coming on. preliminary signs of WITHDRAWAL SYMPTOMS. See COP SICKNESS (quotation).

fiend. an addict who uses drugs excessively, messily, who is not COOL.

finger. a condom filled with a drug and hidden in the rectum or even swallowed, and later excreted, for purposes of smuggling. Compare BALLOON.

fingers. HASHISH of Mediterranean origin that comes in finger-shaped sticks.

firing the ack-ack gun. [translation of the Chinese] a mode of taking HEROIN prevalent in Hong Kong. Heroin is applied to the tip of a cigarette, which is then smoked. Compare DUSTING.

fish. a patient newly admitted to a narcotics hospital.

fit. [shortening of *outfit*] equipment for injecting drugs. See WORKS.

five-cent paper. [from the folded PAPER in which HEROIN is sometimes packaged] a quantity of heroin in a folded piece of paper sold for $5. Compare FIVE-DOLLAR BAG.

five-dollar bag. a glassine envelope of HEROIN sold for $5 and containing perhaps 5 grains (0.011 ounce) of heroin diluted with MILK SUGAR or quinine; about 1/8 teaspoon. The proportion of heroin varies from 0 to 80 percent; however, it is usually around 1 to 5 percent, or 3 to 15 milligrams. This is equal in potency to 9 to 45 milligrams of MORPHINE, the amount given medically for moderate to very severe pain. Also: NICKEL BAG.

fives. tablets containing 5 milligrams of the active ingredient; usually refers to BENZEDRINE or other AMPHETAMINE tablets.

fix. [from *fix-up*, a shot of narcotics; since the 1920s. A ration of drugs since the 1930s. Just enough to *fix up* or satisfy the addict—*EP*] *1.* to inject oneself with narcotics, as in "I *fixed.*" *2.* an injection, a dose of narcotics, as in "I gave myself a *fix*" or "I need a *fix.*" *3.* the amount of drugs in the BAG or packet which make up the fix, as in "I couldn't find anybody to sell me a *fix.*"

> After an intravenous injection of morphine, former narcotics addicts report that they feel "*fixed.*" This term seems to denote a state of

gratification in which hunger, pain and sexual urges are greatly reduced or abolished. In addition, intravenous injection of morphine
results in a highly pleasurable "thrill" which is described as similar to
orgasm except that the sensation seems to be centered in the abdomen.
—Abraham Wikler, *Opiate Addiction. Psychological and
Neurophysical Aspects in Relation to Clinical Practice* (1953)

It's not only a question of kicks. The ritual itself, the powder in the
spoon, the little ball of cotton, the matches applied, the bubbling liquid
drawn up through the cotton filter into the eye-dropper, the tie round
the arm to make a vein stand out, the *fix* often slow because a man will
stand there with the needle in the vein and allow the level of the
eye-dropper to waver up and down, until there is more blood than
heroin in the dropper—all this is not for nothing; it is born of a respect
for the whole chemistry of alienation. When a man fixes he is turned on
almost instantaneously . . . you can speak of a flash, a tinily murmured
orgasm in the bloodstream, in the central nervous system. At once, and
regardless of preconditions, a man enters "Castle Keep." In "Castle
Keep" and even in the face of the enemy, a man can accept.
—Alexander Trocchi, *Cain's Book* (1960)

flake. COCAINE.

flaky. [addicted to COCAINE, since around 1925; from the flaky
appearance of the cocaine crystals—*EP*] general slang for being a bit
crazy, just as cocaine makes the user a bit crazy.

flash. [from the sense of the sudden light, combined with the idea of
a deliberately quick showing of something, e.g., the pea in the shell
game] *1.* the sudden onrush of pleasurable effects, euphoria following an injection of heroin. *2.* the pleasurable effects of any drug at
the moment they are first perceived. Compare FIX (quotation), RUSH,
FLUSH. *3.* to vomit after an injection of HEROIN. See GOOD SICK.

flashing. [from (?) FLASH] GLUE SNIFFING.

flea powder. inferior, highly diluted HEROIN. Compare DUMMY,
GARBAGE, LEMON, BLANK, etc.

flip out. *1.* a temporary or chronic psychotic reaction to a drug,
characterized by panic and loss of control over one's actions. *2.*
divine madness or ecstasy, a mystical experience, in which one tran-
scends one's normal state through the use of drugs, meditation, or
religious techniques such as yoga.

floating. HIGH or intoxicated on a drug.

flow. to relax and let the effects of a drug take over.

flowers. the buds that appear at the top of the MARIJUANA plant, containing a high amount of the psychoactive resin.

fluff. to filter HEROIN or COCAINE through a stocking to make it appear bulkier. See CUTTING.

flunky. also called fool. An addict who takes large risks in acquiring money for drugs, often in ways that will bring him only small amounts, either because he is a novice and lacks criminal know-how or because he is a convicted burglar known to the police. The only way he can obtain drugs is to carry drugs for PUSHERS, buy drugs for other addicts, or otherwise expose himself to risks that addicts and pushers prefer to avoid when they can afford to.

flush. [from FLASH, sudden drug euphoria; or perhaps *flush*, blushing, hot skin, etc., analogous to sudden physiological changes induced when the drug takes effect] *1.* the sudden onrush of euphoria. *2.* relief from withdrawal sickness after HEROIN is injected.

fly agaric. [the poison in the mushroom was used on flypaper] a hallucinogenic, poisonous mushroom, *Amanita muscaria,* which grows in North America, Siberia, and Europe. The North American variety has a whitish, yellowish, or orange-red cap from 3 to 8 inches wide, mottled with whitish, yellowish, or reddish warts; in Europe the cap is bright red or purple. The mushroom contains an alkaloid, MUSCARINE, which in sufficient quantities will stop the heart. Death usually follows the ingestion of one to three of the mushrooms unless the antidote ATROPINE is administered in time.

Death follows delirium, convulsions, and deep coma, and the action of the poison is rapid. In smaller toxic amounts the fly agaric induces vomiting, diarrhea, and rapid breathing. It also causes hallucinations, intoxication, gaiety, a form of perception distortion in which small objects such as pebbles seem large and the victim ludicrously tries to step over them, and sometimes paranoia and aggressive behavior. The intoxication always ends with a deep sleep. (Such doses, survivable by adults, are usually fatal to children.)

The action of the kidneys, as the drug passes through, seems not to affect it and even to enhance its potency. Consequently, the urine of persons who have eaten the mushroom contains powerful amounts of the ACTIVE PRINCIPLE. The Indians of northern Siberia, who call the mushroom *muchamor,* collect the urine and drink it for continued intoxication. It is believed that the mushroom's active principle is BUFOTENINE, which is chemically similar to the HAL-

LUCINOGENS PSILOCYBIN and DMT. A close relative of fly agaric is the death cup, *Amanita phalloides,* which is much deadlier, 60 to 100 percent fatal upon ingestion. It, too, has hallucinogenic properties and is found in North America.

> The poorer sort, who love mushroom broth to distraction as well as the rich, but cannot afford it at first hand, post themselves on these occasions around the huts of the rich and watch the opportunity of the ladies and gentlemen as they come down to pass their liquor, and holding a wooden bowl catch the delicious fluid, very little altered by filtration, being still strongly tinctured with the intoxicating quality. Of this they drink with the utmost satisfaction and thus they get as drunk and as jovial as their betters.   —Oliver Goldsmith (1762)

flying. in a state of drug intoxication, as in *"flying* on LSD." Compare COMING DOWN, HIGH, WINGS.

Flying Saucers. [trade name] a variety of morning glory, the seeds of which have hallucinogenic properties. See MORNING GLORY SEEDS.

fold up. to cease selling or taking drugs.

fool. FLUNKY.

footballs. *1.* [from the shape] Diphetamine pills. *2.* pill containing DILAUDID, a synthetic opiate.

forwards. AMPHETAMINE pills.

fours. [from the figure on the white, scored tablet] Tylenol with CODEINE tablets. The tablets, numbered 1, 2, 3, and 4, according to strength, have varying amounts of codeine in them; the 4s contain 60 milligrams plus acetaminophen, an aspirin-type pain killer.

freak. [from the sense of grotesque, bizarre, distorted in appearance; not necessarily ugly, except to the "squares" who come to gape, and certainly not to the freaks themselves] *1.* to hallucinate, implying a grotesque, grandiose, perhaps bizarrely beautiful or abnormally horrifying distortion of consciousness. *2.* a bad reaction to a hallucinogenic drug, as in "it's not so much the LSD trip that *freaks* me, it's getting back." See FREAK OUT. *3.* one who prefers a certain kind of drug, as in ACID FREAK or METH FREAK. *4.* by extension, one who is obsessed with a certain way of thinking, as in "political *freak"* or "flying-saucer *freak."* When the drug user refers to himself as a freak, he is either saying "Well, if that is what society calls me, that is what I'll be; if *we're* freaks, then freaks are better than ordinary people" *or* expressing criticism of grotesque, compulsive drug use.

When he refers to nonusers of drugs as freaks, he means that their mental set, prejudices, and view of life are altered under the influence of his drug, and the term becomes one of opprobrium. *5.* less pejoratively, someone who is unusual, out of the ordinary; not a "square."

freaking freely. spontaneous, random, LSD-induced behavior.

freak out. *1.* a panic reaction to LSD-25, causing the user to lose control of himself and his mind. *2.* [perhaps because the object of the LSD experience is to "lose one's mind," i.e., escape one's normal mental state] to take LSD, as in "to *freak out* on LSD." *3.* an LSD (or other hallucinogenic drug) experience, as in "I tried the LSD *freak out.*" Compare FLIP OUT.

> It is kicks man. It is The Kick. You *freak out* and there is nothing but greatness and madness. . . . It's Zen and Jesus Christ and all the mad magicians rolled into one big freak.
> —anonymous college student, quoted in W. R. Young and J. R. Hixon (eds.), *LSD on Campus* (1966)

freak up. *1.* deliberately to act in a bizarre, grotesque way, as in "the rock and roll group was *freaking* it *up* on stage." *2.* a kind of hoax, as in "the performance was a *freak-up* from first to last."

freaky. *1.* freakish. *2.* bizarre, abnormal behavior.

freeze. to refuse to sell drugs to an addict. Compare CHILL.

Frisco speedball. mixture of HEROIN, COCAINE, and LSD-25.

front. *1.* [from the sense of "putting up a *front*," i.e., a false display of respectability] a conventional set of clothing, as opposed to HIPPIE attire.

> Have three sets of clothes, including one *"front"* with which you can go back into the square world for a job—or an appearance in court if need be.
> —Doc Stanley, "How to Survive on the Streets," *Los Angeles Free Press* (1967)

2. [from the idea of "put the money *in front,* and the delivery will follow"] also front money. Payment in advance for drugs.

fruit salad. among teen-agers, a game in which each participant takes one pill from every bottle found in the family medicine cabinet.

full moon. *1.* a large PEYOTE chunk about 4 inches in diameter. *2.* the entire top of the peyote cactus (as opposed to the BUTTONS or slices).

fumo d'Angola. [Brazilian Portuguese, Angolan smoke] CANNABIS.

This reference to the Portuguese colony of Angola in Africa lends further credence to the theory that cannabis smoking was introduced to the Western Hemisphere by African slaves. Compare DJOMA.

fun. [Chinese unit of measure] a unit of measure of OPIUM.

fuzz. *1.* policeman or detective. *2.* [shortening of NARCO FUZZ] narcotics officer.

G g

gage. GAUGE.

gammon. one microgram (one-millionth of a gram), as in "500 *gammons* of LSD."

ganga. GUNGEON.

gangster. MARIJUANA.

gangster pills. BARBITURATES or other sedative pills.

gaping. [from the excessive yawning that is an early WITHDRAWAL SYMPTOM] experiencing OPIATE (HEROIN) withdrawal symptoms.

garbage. weak, heavily diluted HEROIN. Compare BLANK, FLEA POWDER, LEMON.

garbage head. one who will take anything to get high. Compare DEPRIVATION ROLL.

gasoline. the fumes, when inhaled, have a deliriant effect similar to GLUE SNIFFING or CLEANING FLUID and are highly toxic. Compare BENZINE. See DELIRIANTS.

gauge. [from *gauge butt,* a marijuana cigarette; since the 1930s. Tenuous definition is "marijuana sends people insane; *gauge* or measure of insanity"—*EP*; perhaps a corruption of GHANJA or GUNGEON] MARIJUANA.

gay. [a person who takes drugs for the exhilarating effect they produce is either "gay" or "high" or "sent"—*EP; since around 1945*] in a state of drug intoxication. *Obsolete*. The homosexual meaning seems dominant nowadays. But also note that prostitutes in nineteenth-century England were called "gay girls." "She is *gay*" meant she is a prostitute. So gay "homosexual" may have originated from the gay "prostitute" sense (prostitutes "cruise around" looking for clients, and homosexuals "cruise around" looking for someone of kindred sexual predilection).

G.B. [from GOOFBALL] a BARBITURATE pill.

gee head. [from thinning of P.G.?] a PAREGORIC addict.

geeze. to inject a drug.

geronimo. [from WILD GERONIMO] an alcoholic beverage, often wine, mixed with BARBITURATES.

get down. inject HEROIN.

get in the groove. [to become familiar with drug traffic or proficient in drug taking—*EP*; from the jazz sense of playing *in the groove,* with the right swinging beat] *Obsolete,* but see GROOVING.

get off. [related to *go off* in the sense a gun goes off, and perhaps from *get off,* have an orgasm, the sexual thrill HEROIN users feel when they inject into the vein] *1.* to inject heroin, as in "he *got off* right there in the hallway." Compare FIX, JERK OFF. *2.* to feel the effects of any drug.

get on. to take drugs for the first time, as in "he *got on* SPEED."

get one's yen off. [from *yen,* a craving for drugs] to satisfy one's desire for a drug, indulge.

get the habit off. to take a drug at a time when WITHDRAWAL SYMPTOMS are beginning to manifest themselves, or at one's regular time.

getting on. smoking MARIJUANA. Compare TURN ON.

ghanja. [Compare the Jamaican words GUNGEON, ganga] the flowering tops, twigs, leaves, and stems of the female hemp plant, CANNABIS SATIVA, covered with a sticky resinous exudate that contains TETRAHYDROCANNIBINOL, the hallucinogenic ACTIVE PRINCIPLE of the plant in highly concentrated form. Special techniques of cultivation are used in India to increase this resinous exudate. In India ghanja is usually smoked or mixed into cakes and sweetmeats. This form of CANNABIS is more potent than BHANG (the Indian form of MARIJUANA, consisting of the leaves, stems, and twigs) and somewhat less potent than CHARAS (HASHISH). Compare CANNABIS INDICA, FLOWERS.

ghost, the. LSD-25.

giggle weed. MARIJUANA.

gimmicks. [from a secret knack; any trick aiding the operations of a device or a game or a sales trick; pitchmen and criminals' slang—*EP*] equipment for injecting drugs. *Obsolete?* Compare WORKS, BIZ, KIT.

girl. [antonym of BOY, HEROIN, both in the slang usage and as a rough metaphor for their effects, since cocaine is a stimulant and heroin a depressant; probably rose out of the practice of taking the two drugs together, and perhaps from the quasi-sexual thrills obtained] COCAINE. Compare GET OFF, HIM, HER, SPEEDBALL.

globetrotter. an addict who circulates around a drug-selling area, making inquiries of PUSHERS, in order to select the best HEROIN.

glow. *1.* HIGH. *2.* drugged euphoria.

> You had to be a lot harder to be a pusher; you couldn't have a soft heart, like "no dough, no *glow*."
> —Piri Thomas, *Down These Mean Streets* (1967)

glue sniffing. sometimes called FLASHING. Inhaling the fumes of model-airplane glue (containing toluol) or any DELIRIANT for their intoxicating effect. Generally the user squeezes some of the glue into a paper bag, holds the bag tight over his nose, and inhales the fumes. These induce, in the first stage, a feeling of hazy euphoria something like that from alcohol. Soon there follows a disordering of perception: double vision, ringing in the ears, and even hallucinations. The user's speech becomes slurred, and he staggers around with poor coordination, as if he were drunk. After thirty-five to forty minutes he falls into a state of drowsiness or stupor lasting an hour, during which he is unable to recall what he was doing.

Occasionally sniffers erupt into violence or have delusions of grandeur, during which they think they can fly, or lie on railroad tracks; such impairment of judgment has resulted in serious or fatal accidents.

PHYSICAL DEPENDENCE does not develop in glue sniffing (though a case has been reported of a glue sniffer who experienced cramps and abdominal pains when withdrawn from the practice). A form of PSYCHIC DEPENDENCE can develop, and some users increase the amount sniffed each time in order to intensify their experience. Eventually, however, the user gives up the practice. Glue sniffing is regarded as "kid stuff" by many older adolescents (although cases have been reported of addicts unable to obtain their HEROIN supply who resorted to glue sniffing). Since most cases are in the twelve to fourteen age group, it appears that either the glue sniffer will outgrow his habit or will go on to more "adult" drugs, such as AMPHETAMINES, BARBITURATES, and even heroin.

Glue sniffing was first reported in the United States in 1955; the 1960s brought a sharp upsurge. In New York City there were 2,003 cases reported, compared to 779 in 1962. Although manufacturers no longer sell tubes of airplane glue separately from model kits, it is doubtful that this measure has reduced the practice in the slightest. Compare CARBONA, CARBON TETRACHLORIDE, CLEANING FLUID.

glutethimide. a nonbarbiturate hypnotic and sedative used to induce sleep and as a preoperative and daytime sedative (TRANQUILIZER). Glutethimide closely resembles phenobarbital in molecular structure; its effects resemble those of secobarbital, a short-acting BARBITURATE. Although glutethimide was once touted as being safer than barbiturates, the Council on Drugs of the American Medical Association says, "Glutethimide is now regarded as a typical general depressant having no special advantage over barbiturates, but constituting a satisfactory alternative to the latter if one is needed."

If taken in excessive amounts (above 2 grams, or 2,000 milligrams, per day) for 21 days, the drug produces PHYSICAL DEPENDENCE; glutethimide is more rapidly addicting than barbiturates. Abrupt withdrawal of the drug from one who has become physically dependent will cause serious WITHDRAWAL SYMPTOMS, ranging from anxiety to epileptic (grand mal) seizures, accompanied by abdominal cramping, chills, numbness of extremities, and difficulty in swallowing. These are delayed up to four days after the drug is stopped; the death rate for untreated withdrawal is 20 to 25 percent. Newborn infants of mothers dependent upon glutethimide may also suffer withdrawal symptoms. The drug often produces euphoria, as well as generalized sedation, which makes it similar to the barbiturates in its liability to induce PSYCHIC DEPENDENCE in the patient, especially habitual users of other drugs and alcohol, accompanied by a tendency to increase the frequency and amount of the dose.

The drug has been used in suicide attempts, in amounts averaging 15 grams, or thirty capsules, and is particularly difficult to cleanse from the system. Acute intoxication will result from doses of 3 grams (six times the usual therapeutic dose) or above; doses of 10 grams or more will include respiratory depression, coma, fever, sometimes cyanosis (blue skin), impairment of reflexes, and dilation of the pupils—followed by death in some cases. Fatalities are more apt to occur if glutethimide is used in combination with alcohol, barbiturates, or other depressant drugs. Chronic, heavy use of glutethimide, in addition to producing physical dependence, will result in behavior similar to that of the alcoholic or barbiturate addict—i.e., impairment of memory and ability to concentrate, impaired gait, ataxia, tremors, and slurring of speech. Since withdrawal symptoms can be fatal, a person physically dependent upon glutethimide must be gradually withdrawn from the drug by decreasing doses of glutethimide or pentobarbital. Compare DORIDEN.

go. to use drugs, as in "*going* on pot."

goblet of jam. [translation of Arabic m'jun-i akbar] MAJOON, a confection containing CANNABIS, eaten in North Africa for the hallucinogenic effects. See also DAWAMESK.

God's medicine. MORPHINE.

going down. *1.* going well. *2.* happening.

going high. a pleasurable, continuing state of drug intoxication, not necessitating ingestion of any further drugs for the time being.

> *How can I make out of this?* I was thinking. "Nay, dad, I've been blasting *yerba*; I have a *going high,* and I don't want to mess it up."
> —Piri Thomas, *Down These Mean Streets* (1967)

gold. ACAPULCO GOLD.

gold dust. [since the 1930s] COCAINE. *Obsolete.*

gold duster. [since the 1930s] COCAINE user. *Obsolete.*

golden leaf. ACAPULCO GOLD.

goods. *1.* narcotics. *2.* any drugs.

good sick. the nausea and vomiting that HEROIN sometimes induces soon after injection. Addicts do not consider it unpleasant, associated as it is with the drug's euphoria. Compare FLASH.

> "Just a minute," I said. I climbed off the bed, walked round him and across the kitchen to the bucket he used for a w.c. I vomited. It wasn't

painful. It's not like getting sick on alcohol. The little food I had eaten during the day was soon regurgitated. Geo was standing beside me with a saucepan full of water.

"Here."

I drank and regurgitated, drank and regurgitated, the spasms lessening as whatever nervousness caused the nausea was neutralized first by the thought of my transcendent immunity, and then by the extreme but indefinable ecstasy at my senses. There was a wet, prickly sweat at my belly and thighs and temples.

—Alexander Trocchi, *Cain's Book* (1960)

good stuff. [from STUFF, HEROIN] heroin of superior quality.

goofball. [from *goofy, goof,* a stupid, silly, or crazy person; hence a pill that makes one behave in this manner; since around 1940] *1.* BARBITURATE pill. *2.* [rare and erroneous] an AMPHETAMINE pill.

goofers. BARBITURATES; any sedatives.

goofing. *1.* under the influence of BARBITURATES and hence acting in a random, uncoordinated, drunken manner. *2.* conversely, sitting and staring dreamily into space. Compare NOD, NODDING.

gorilla pills. BARBITURATES or other sedative pills.

grass brownies. brownies containing MARIJUANA.

gravy. mixture of blood from the addict's vein and HEROIN which is reheated in the COOKER because it has coagulated and cannot be injected. Compare SHOOTING GRAVY.

greasy junky. a passive, indolent addict whose drug-hustling activities are at a minimum and who will make no great effort to get money to buy narcotics, relying on begging and personal services instead.

green. [from the color; generalized term for any MARIJUANA of that color, whatever the origin] a "grade" of marijuana of relatively low potency because it is low in resin content. Usually called MEXICAN GREEN, because of its origin. This is the cheapest grade.

grefa. [from the Spanish] MARIJUANA.

greta. [probably a variation of *grefa*] MARIJUANA.

grifa. [Mexican] MARIJUANA.

griffo. MARIJUANA.

groovers. teen-agers (thirteen- to seventeen-year-olds) who use drugs largely for thrills, especially sexual thrills and bizarre mental effects.

grooving. [from *in the groove,* musician's term for playing well, with a good beat, etc.] becoming intoxicated on a drug, as in "he was *grooving* ⌊on⌋ pot."

groovy. the euphoric, HIGH experience under a drug or like that under a drug, as in "feeling *groovy.*"

ground control. a person who attends an LSD user undergoing the drug's effects in case he has a panic reaction. Compare COPILOT.

ground man. GROUND CONTROL.

guide. an experienced LSD user who supervises a novice's first experience with the drug; literally, one who teaches another how to use LSD, controls and directs the TRIP, and administers tranquilizers when necessary. Compare GURU.

gum. gum OPIUM, the raw opium refined for smoking.

gun. [from *shoot,* to inject] a hypodermic needle used to inject narcotics. Compare BANG, POP.

gunga. [England; from "Gunga Din," meaning Indian hemp, i.e., marijuana—*EP*; since around 1945; but perhaps from the Indian *ghanga,* or the Jamaican word *ganga.* As in the United States, the practice of marijuana smoking began in England among colored minority groups] MARIJUANA.

gungeon. [An American spelling; it may be a variant of the Jamaican word *ganga;* Jamaica was a source for American MARIJUANA in the 1940s] *1.* especially potent marijuana from Jamaica or Africa. *2.* a cigarette containing gungeon.

gunja. [American, probably a variation of *ganga* or *gungeon*] MARIJUANA.

guru. [Hindi, a religious teacher, a spiritual master] an experienced LSD user who guides, directs, and sits with a novice during his first LSD experience. Compare GUIDE.

gutter. veins inside the elbow, where HEROIN is injected. Compare CHANNEL, MAINLINE.

H h

H. HEROIN.

habit. [a fierce craving for drugs; since around 1910—*EP*] the state of being physically dependent upon a drug, as in "he had a $50-a-day *habit*" or "he knew he had a *habit* when he started getting cramps and chills." (Since the addict cannot know the strength of the diluted heroin he buys, he cannot speak of a "2-grain-a-day" habit but must measure it by the amount he spends; this amount varies with the potency of the drug he purchases, i.e., how much it is diluted, which in turn determines how much is needed to forestall WITHDRAWAL SYMPTOMS.)

habit-forming. used by drug manufacturers, the familiar "Warning—May Be Habit-Forming" means that prolonged use will result in PHYSICAL DEPENDENCE and specifically that the medicine contains an OPIATE, opiate derivative, SYNTHETIC OPIATE, BARBITURATE, or other drug which can cause physical dependence. See also ADDICTION, HABITUATION.

habituation (habit), drug. a term formerly used by the WHO Expert Committee on Addiction-producing Drugs to describe compulsive drug abuse of a lesser degree than ADDICTION. The committee later decided that the distinction was unclear and the definition unscientific and has adopted the phrase "drug dependence of the [name of drug] type." The discarded definition read:

> Drug habituation (habit) is a condition resulting from the repeated consumption of a drug. Its characteristics include (1) a desire (but not a compulsion) to continue taking the drug for the sense of improved well-being which it engenders; (2) little or no tendency to increase the dose; (3) some degree of psychic dependence on the effect of the drug, but absence of physical dependence and hence, of an abstinence syndrome; (4) detrimental effects, if any, primarily on the individual [as distinguished from harmful effects upon society].

See DEPENDENCE.

hacks. [from prisoners' term for prison guards; since the 1920s—*EP*] attendants at the U.S. Public Health Service (Narcotics) Hospital, Lexington, Kentucky.

Haight, the. HAIGHT-ASHBURY.

Haight-Ashbury, the. [from intersecting streets in the center of the area] a decaying residential section in San Francisco to which bohemians (generally young) gravitated in 1966 and set up communal quarters in the area's large old houses. Buoyed on a wave of love and peace, they came singing "When You Come to San Francisco, Wear Flowers in Your Hair." Tied in with the new lifestyle was the use of drugs, at first the HALLUCINOGENS, which were accorded a mystic potential for enhancing a religious awakening.

The area thus became a mecca for those of this inclination, who were labeled HIPPIES. Because of the bizarre dress and lifestyle of the inhabitants, the area enjoyed a tourist boom, as out-of-towners rode around in sightseeing buses staring at the local freakiana, which stared back. Head shops—stores selling clothing, posters, MARI-JUANA pipes, bells, and other accouterments of the PSYCHEDELIC life—sprang up. Various loosely organized communal efforts, such as the Diggers' Free Store, sprang up among the hippies themselves as they attempted to deal with the area's growing health and crowding problems. There were employment centers, community kitchens dispensing free food, centers giving information about free lodgings, and even free medical care to deal with health problems peculiar to the area, including venereal disease, serum hepatitis (from using unsterile needles to inject drugs, mostly LSD or AMPHETAMINES), and panic psychoses resulting from bad LSD trips. Many of the runaway middle-class youths, often in their teens, could not cope with the new scene, and there were casualties—emotional and physical. Then, too, as the authorities clamped down on LSD and marijuana use, the drug of choice became amphetamines, which were much more destructive physically. The love and peace fled, to be replaced by the paranoia and the tendency to rip off one's fellows that characterize the SPEED FREAK. Haight-Ashbury became at last a psychedelic slum, and the original dream that had drawn the young to it like lemmings in that one brief "summer of love" was no more.

half. HALF LOAD.

half load. fifteen packages, or BAGS, of HEROIN wrapped together with a rubber band and purchased by the PUSHER from the wholesaler for resale to addicts. Compare BUNDLE, LOAD.

hallucinogen. [from Latin, *hallucinari*, to wander mentally, and *-gen* (from Greek *-genes*, be born), one that generates] a hallucination-producing drug, a category of drugs producing this effect. The hallucinations are dislocations of consciousness similar in some aspects to those suffered by psychotic patients; however, the user of a hallucinogenic drug is almost invariably aware that what he is seeing are hallucinations, or else they are recognized distortions of known objects in the physical environment, while the psychotic cannot distinguish the "real" from the "unreal," and his delusional world tends to be persistent, obsessive, and integral to the structure of his psychosis.

With the more powerful hallucinogenic drugs, such as LSD-25, the hallucinations can become startlingly real to the subject, and he may indeed be caught up fully in them for temporary periods. However, in the majority of users these powerful hallucinations pass and are recalled as such in the return to a normal state. In a small number of cases, the hallucinations persist or recur, to a troubling degree, for weeks or months after the drug has been taken; in this case, the users may enter a true psychotic state. As a descriptive term for the drugs or the experience they produce, hallucinogen is rejected by partisans of the drugs, who prefer PSYCHEDELIC (mind-manifesting). The term PSYCHOTOMIMETIC (psychosis-miming) is also employed, mainly by the psychiatric profession, but has fallen into disfavor; PSYCHOTOGENIC is more frequent. Hallucinogen has been adopted by journalists (with psychedelic a close second), doctors, and federal authorities. It acquired the government's imprimatur in the Drug Abuse Control Amendment of 1965, which outlawed possession of hallucinogenic drugs. The Food and Drug Administration's Drug Abuse Control Bureau named the following as hallucinogenic drugs under the terms of the statute:

DMT
LSD-25
mescaline and its salts
peyote
psilocybin
psilocin

Unlike the other categories of drugs, i.e., BARBITURATES and AMPHETAMINES, which were found by the FDA to be habit-forming, hallucinogens were brought under federal regulation because they have a "potential for abuse." They are continued under Schedule I of the CONTROLLED SUBSTANCES ACT.

hand to hand, go. to transfer narcotics at the point of sale, as opposed to "drop," where the buyer picks them up after paying his money.

hang tough. ["to tell him to hang on would be too square." —Seymour Fiddle] phrase used (e.g., at SYNANON) to encourage addict undergoing WITHDRAWAL SYMPTOMS COLD TURKEY to stick it out, hang on.

hara, la. [Puerto Rican addicts' slang] a policeman; the cop.

hard drugs. HARD NARCOTICS.

hard narcotics. [*hard*, in the sense of potentially painful, onerous; the term is becoming invidious] addictive drugs, the OPIUM and MORPHINE derivatives and their synthetics; COCAINE; usually opposed to soft drugs. Usually the narcotics falling under federal narcotics laws, although in common parlance MARIJUANA is considered a soft drug even though it is a narcotic by Federal Bureau of Narcotics definition. Compare BODY DRUGS, HEAD DRUGS.

hard stuff. HARD NARCOTICS.

harmaline. an alkaloid found in the seeds of *Peganum harmala,* which grows wild along the Mediterranean coast of Africa, Europe, and the Near East. It is also found in plants of the genus BANISTERIOPSIS, from which the HALLUCINOGENIC substances variously called yage, AYAHUASCA, and CAAPI are derived by South American Indians. Given in doses of 70 to 100 milligrams, the drug produces visions that are surprisingly similar among diverse persons. Among the recurring images are tigers and animals, birds or flying, dark-skinned men, death and circular patterns. To a psychiatrist these images would appear to be similar to the universal archetypes central to Jung's thought. Dr. Claudio Naranjo concluded that out of thirty subjects who took harmaline, fifteen showed some therapeutic benefit and ten showed a marked improvement. The symbols in the visions are functions of a sense of energy, of power, and of freedom that the subject feels, leading to a deeper sense of self. Untoward experiences with the drug include physical discomfort, fatigue, and half sleep; this may be a toxic reaction to the drug. Compare IBOGAINE.

I see a white bird. A cross. A lamp with violet teardrops—glass. I feel a ringing in the ears. I see two crystal balls, like glittering lamps. I see sand on a beach being tossed with shovels. I see a red rag. I see the image of an old and ugly man making globes with his mouth. Many lights are reflected, and then light and dark follow. Lights go on moving by in turquoise shades, green in the middle and turquoise all around. A black teardrop of a turning lamp. I see a radiant sun. I see the face of the beast in *Beauty and the Beast.* A large black blot. A map. I first see America and then Europe—Italy. I see some stained glass windows. I see only lights. I see glittering lights, many lanterns in red-green-yellow colors. A Persian carpet with a red background and shapes.   —visions of a harmaline subject in Claudio Naranjo, *The Healing Journey* (1974)

harmine. also called banisterine, telepathine, yageine, and yagenine. An alkaloid found in the South American vine BANISTERIOPSIS CAAPI and thought to be hallucinogenic. Harmine is an indole derivative originally identified in the seeds and roots of harmal, *Peganum harmala.* Recent investigations have uncovered two other active alkaloids in *Banisteriopsis caapi,* HARMALINE and d-tetrahydroharmine, which are thought to be more hallucinogenically active than harmine.

Harris-Dodd Act. Drug Abuse Control Amendment of 1965. (Superseded by the CONTROLLED SUBSTANCES ACT.)

Harrison Narcotics Act. the nation's first law regulating narcotics. When passed in 1914, it was basically a revenue measure designed to make narcotics transferals a matter of record. A nominal tax of 1 cent per ounce was imposed on the narcotics; forms were required to be kept recording all transfers of the drug between manufacturer, wholesaler, retailer, and doctor. Persons authorized to handle or manufacture drugs were required to register, pay a fee, and keep records of narcotics in their possession.

Under several Supreme Court decisions interpreting the basic law, however, it was expanded to prohibit possession of smuggled drugs by an addict, i.e., anyone, rather than, as some interpreted the law, merely establishing a presumption that any unregistered person who possessed drugs was guilty of illegal possession only if he was among those persons specifically required to register under the law. Further decisions of the court made it illegal for a doctor to prescribe narcotics to an addict to relieve WITHDRAWAL SYMPTOMS and keep him comfortable over a period of time (maintenance doses). These decisions were embodied in Treasury Department regulations even though the Supreme Court later modified its stand (1925) and implied that the physician should be the judge of what drugs, in what quantities, and in how many dosages be prescribed for the patient, if he does so in good faith, and he may do so to relieve an addict's withdrawal symptoms. The Federal Bureau of Narcotics ignored this decision, and physicians were prosecuted for giving addicts drugs, even though in good faith. In sum, the act said that only persons who have paid the tax on narcotics may possess, transfer, prescribe, or manufacture them, and only persons who are authorized to possess, transfer, prescribe, or manufacture them may pay the tax. The addict caught with such untaxed drugs in his possession was automatically a criminal and could receive medical treatment only as an adjunct to his incarceration. Two subsequent pieces of narcotics legislation, the Boggs Amendment of 1951 and the Narcotic Drug Control Act of 1956, supplemented the Harrison Act by making convictions under it easier and stiffening penalties. Penalties were as follows, according to Alfred Lindesmith in *The Addict and the Law:*

first possession offense	2-10 years; probation and parole permitted
second possession or first selling offense	mandatory 5-20 years with no probation or parole permitted
third possession or second selling and subsequent offenses	mandatory 10-40 years; no probation or parole permitted
sale of heroin to person under 18 by one over 18	10 years to life; no probation or parole; or death if jury recommends

Such mandatory sentences and prohibition of parole or probation limited the judge's flexibility in sentencing and gave the prosecution (the U.S. Department of Justice) all the discretion because it could manipulate charges and recommend sentences to the court. Superseded by the CONTROLLED SUBSTANCES ACT of 1970.

harry. HEROIN.

haschischins, Le club des. a group of French literary men who met periodically to eat HASHISH. The club was founded in 1844 by the novelist Théophile Gautier, author of the scandalous *Mademoiselle de Maupin,* a hedonist who extolled pleasure as the supreme good. Gautier had been introduced to the drug by Dr. Jacques Joseph Moreau, a specialist in mental illness, who noted similarities between mental disorientation produced by hashish and that produced by mental illness and sought to test the drug's effects on Gautier and his friends. These "experiments" were conducted in settings of exotic splendor, and the subjects' motives were, apparently, mainly sybaritic. The club's membership included Victor Hugo, Honoré de Balzac, Gerard de Nerval, Charles Baudelaire, and a number of other Paris intellectuals.

The meal drew to an end; already some of the more fervent members felt the effects of the green jam [MAJOON]: for my part, I had experienced a complete transformation in taste. The water I drank seemed the most exquisite wine, the meat, once in my mouth, became strawberries, the strawberries, meat. I could not have distinguished a fish from a cutlet. My neighbors began to appear somewhat strange. Their pupils became big as a screech owl's; their noses stretched into elongated proboscises; their mouths expanded like bell bottoms. Faces were shaded in supernatural light. One among them, a pale countenance in a black beard, laughed aloud at an invisible spectacle; another made incredible efforts to raise his glass to his lips and the resulting contortions aroused deafening hoots from his companions; a man, shaken with nervous convulsions, turned his thumbs with remarkable agility; another, fallen against the back of his chair, his eyes unseeing and his arms inert, let himself drift voluptuously in the bottomless sea of nothingness.

My elbows on the table, I considered all this with clarity and a vestige of reason which came and went by intervals, like the light of a lantern about to flicker and die. A deadening warmth pervaded my limbs, and dementia, like a wave which breaks foaming onto a rock, then withdraws to break again, invaded and left my brain, finally enveloping it altogether. That strange visitor, hallucination, had come to dwell within me.

"To the salon, to the salon!" cried one of the guests; "can't you hear those heavenly choirs? The musicians have been gathered for a long time." —Théophile Gautier, *Revue des Deux Mondes* (1846) (Translation by Polly Kraft, *The Drug Experience,* 1961)

hash. HASHISH.

Hashbury, the. [contraction of Haight and Ashbury, with the *hash* predominating, perhaps because of the connotation of HASH] the HAIGHT-ASHBURY section of San Francisco.

hashish. [Hasan-ibn-al-Sabbah, the first "Old Man of the Mountain," Persian founder of the Assassins in the eleventh century; both the word HASHISH and the term for his thugs, assassins, come from his name] the pure resinous exudate of the female hemp plant, CANNABIS SATIVA. In medical use hashish was sifted and powdered, sometimes prepared in a tincture with alcohol, and known as CANNABIS INDICA, or Indian hemp. Among drug users, it is usually seen as a hard, brown lump, the resin having hardened after being harvested from the plant at maturity. The darkness determines the strength: light ocher brown is least and deep cocoa brown or black most potent. It has a sweetish, minty smell and taste. Since the resin contains the ACTIVE PRINCIPLE, TETRAHYDROCANNABINOL, in highest concentration, hashish is the most powerful form of CANNABIS consumed. (The MARIJUANA used in the United States, for example, is considered about one-eighth as potent.)

In India hashish is known as CHARAS and is generally consumed by smoking, while in North Africa, it is smoked or eaten in a confection called MAJOON or DAWAMESK. When smoked, a water pipe (HOOKAH) is frequently used, for filtering through water regulates the intake and cools the smoke. Hashish intoxication has much in common with that produced by MESCALINE and, in sufficient quantities taken orally, that of LSD. These effects include distorted perceptions of various parts of the body, depersonalization or "double consciousness," the feeling of being here and there simultaneously, spatial and time distortions, intensification of scents, tastes, colors, and sounds, visual hallucinations, seeing faces as grotesque, synesthesia, i.e., the merging of the senses so that sounds are seen as colors, heightened suggestibility, grandiose delusions of being god-like, and anxiety, dread, and paranoia.

The effects of hashish are more violent when it is swallowed, for the smoker can regulate the degree of intoxication by spacing out his intake and, in effect, making it more gradual. The final stage of hashish intoxication is deep sleep. As with other hallucinogenic drugs, hashish can trigger acute or chronic psychosis in a small percentage of users.

The question of whether there is a "cannabis psychosis," i.e., that excessive use of hashish causes a psychosis characteristic of the drug, has been debated. Studies in Morocco and India, where hashish is used more widely than it is in the United States, have resulted in the identification of such a psychosis occurring among approximately five out of every thousand users. One Moroccan investigator has broken the psychosis down into three types: acute or subacute (the majority), resulting from a toxic overdose, sometimes erupting in violence, usually lasting for a few days; residual, resulting in schizophrenia, mental confusion, and mild recurring hallucinations, usually disappearing after a few months; and psychical deterioration resulting from prolonged, excessive use and producing premature senility, vagabondage, and other behavior reminiscent of the skid-row alcoholic in this country. Most American investigators doubt that marijuana produces psychoses of itself, believing instead that the psychosis was already latent, waiting to be born, and the drug acted the part of midwife. Conversely, the heavy user of cannabis (hashish or marijuana) may actually be masking a psychosis through the drug and preventing it from asserting its hold upon his mind.

TOLERANCE to hashish develops only to a slight degree, which may be partially a result of the user's learning to control its effects subjectively as he becomes more familiar with them. As a general rule, however, the same dose of cannabis, no matter how frequently taken, will have the same effects. PHYSICAL DEPENDENCE upon hashish does not develop; there are no characteristic WITHDRAWAL SYMPTOMS, although long-term, heavy hashish users do suffer some discomfort if they abruptly stop using the drug. These symptoms are of much less severity than those associated with physical dependence upon the OPIATE and BARBITURATE drugs.

Aside from the occasional transient or even chronic psychoses triggered by its use, the chief hazard of the drug is the debilitation of the will and mental deterioration resulting from PSYCHIC DEPENDENCE with prolonged, heavy usage. This deterioration from long-term involvement with the drug, often seen in North Africa and India and described above, appears to be almost nonexistent in the United States because heavy users of cannabis predominantly choose marijuana, a much milder form. Also, in the United States hashish is more expensive than marijuana ($40 to $100 an ounce, roughly the same as the cost of a pound of marijuana; 1 ounce of hashish, it is said, lasts the heavy smoker about as long as 1 pound of marijuana, though this could vary widely, depending on the habits of the smoker). Finally, although there was no tradition of hashish smoking in the United States to the extent there is in India and North Africa, hashish is increasingly appearing on the illicit market, most of it smuggled in by tourists from North Africa, Nepal, Afghanistan, and Lebanon.

> The earliest encroachments of the drug, like symptoms of a storm that hovers before it strikes, appear and multiply in the very bosom of . . . incredulity. The first of them is a sort of irrelevant and irresistible hilarity. Attacks of causeless mirth, of which you are almost ashamed, repeat themselves at frequent intervals, cutting across periods of stupor during which you try in vain to pull yourself together. . . . This mirth, with its alternating spells of languor and convulsion, this distress in the midst of delight, generally lasts only for a fairly short time. Soon

the coherence of your ideas becomes so vague, the conducting filament between your fancies becomes so thin, that only your accomplice can understand you. . . . One of the most noticeable sensations resulting from the use of hashish is that of benevolence; a flaccid, idle, dumb benevolence resulting from a softening of the nerves. . . . At this [next] phase of intoxication . . . a new subtlety or acuity manifests itself in all the senses. . . . The eyes behold the Infinite. The ear registers almost imperceptible sounds, even in the midst of the greatest din. This is when hallucinations set in. External objects acquire gradually, and one after another, strange new appearances; they become distorted or transformed. Next occur mistakes in the identities of objects, and transposals of ideas. Sounds clothe themselves in colors, and colors contain music. . . . It sometimes happens that your personality disappears, and you develop objectivity—that preserve of the pantheistic poets—to such an abnormal degree that the contemplation of outward objects makes you forget your own existence, and you soon melt into them. . . . A new stream of ideas carries you away; it will hurl you along in its living vortex for a further minute; and this minute, too, will be an eternity, for the normal relation between time and the individual has been completely upset by the multitude and intensity of sensations and ideas. You seem to live several men's lives in the space of an hour. You resemble, do you not?, a fantastic novel that is being lived instead of being written. There is no longer any fixed connection between your organs and their powers; and this fact above all, is what makes this dangerous exercise, in which you lose your freedom, so very blameworthy.   —Charles Baudelaire, *Les Paradis Artificiels* (1860)

hassle. *1.* annoyances, bother, exertion in obtaining drugs. *2.* to obtain drugs in a difficult, etc., manner, as in "*hassle* marijuana." *3.* to bargain over price.

Customers are funny. Some *hassle* for an hour before they buy and some don't even open the envelope.
—"Ric," "Confessions of a Campus Pot Dealer,"
Esquire (September, 1967)

"You get hung up with all the *hassle*," said one [marijuana dealer], "and it becomes a full-time profession. . . ."
Yet the typical dealer, although cautious, is nonchalant, and well aware that the first arrest is not likely to lead to prison. "It reaches the point where it's [avoiding arrest] not worth the *hassle* [elaborate precautions]," said a 19-year-old marijuana merchant. "If I get busted, I get busted."   —Don McNeill, *Village Voice* (Dec. 1, 1966)

hassling. *1.* buying drugs; used especially of a small-time dealer who must locate a wholesaler, meet him clandestinely to avoid being followed, argue the price with him, test the quality of what is offered him, and arrange the transferal. *2.* the process of doing this, as in "I got tired of the *hassling* all the time, so I'd buy MARIJUANA in large amounts so there'd be less of a hassle."

hawk, the. [the hawk, among Chicagoans, is the powerful wind that blows off Lake Michigan; hence, implying the drug's powerful, stormy effect on the mind] LSD-25.

hay. [from the appearance of marijuana prepared for sale] MARIJUANA. Compare BALE, TEA.

H-caps. HEROIN in gelatine capsules, each of which contains, roughly, 1 grain of CUT (diluted) heroin. From $^1/_4$ ounce of pure heroin the wholesaler could fill up to 100 capsules for resale to the addict. In the 1940s and 1950s this was the favored container for selling heroin, but it is less common today. See BAG.

head. [a drug addict; since the 1900s; especially HOPHEAD (OPIUM addict); also Veronal head (BARBITURATE addict); perhaps suggested by *deadhead,* a useless person—*EP.* The latter origin seems unlikely. Perhaps from the idea that the drug fills or alters one's consciousness, i.e., brain or head, and dominates it] *1.* a frequent, fairly heavy user of drugs, though not an addict; often qualified by the specific kind of drugs the head prefers, as in ACID HEAD, AMPHETAMINE head, POT head, etc. The word has the slight connotation that the head prefers his mental state while under the drug to his normal one. *2.* state of being HIGH, as in "he's really enjoying his *head.*"

head drugs. [used, often invidiously, in opposition to BODY DRUGS] *1.* drugs which produce higher, finer states of consciousness in the mind of the user and do not produce PHYSICAL DEPENDENCE. *2.* drugs that stimulate the brain. *3.* nondepressant drugs. In practice, HALLUCINOGENS and possibly AMPHETAMINES, but not OPIATES, ALCOHOL, or BARBITURATES.

hearts. AMPHETAMINES.

heat, the. [to *have a heat* is to be taking drugs; *with a heat on,* exhilarated by drugs, since the 1930s, and in trouble with or being sought by the police, since the 1920s—*EP*] the police or narcotics detectives.

heaven dust. COCAINE.

Heavenly Blue. [trade name] a variety of morning glory, the seeds of which produce hallucinogenic effects. See MORNING GLORY SEEDS.

heavy drugs. HARD NARCOTICS, i.e., addictive OPIATES and COCAINE, which come under the federal narcotics laws.

heavy stuff. [from *heavy*, onerous, weighty; the effects of these drugs, compared to LIGHT STUFF] HEROIN, COCAINE, other OPIATE drugs. Compare BODY DRUGS, HARD NARCOTICS, LOAD.

heeled. [from *heeled*, armed, weaponed; since the 1900s; the origin of that sense is the practice of arming a fighting cock with spurs on its feet—*EP*] possessing drugs. Compare CLEAN, DIRTY.

hemp. [from Middle English *hemp*, CANNABIS SATIVA, the Indian hemp plant] MARIJUANA.

henry. HEROIN. Compare HARRY.

her. COCAINE. Compare GIRL, HIM, BOY, BROTHER.

herb. MARIJUANA. Compare YERBA.

heroin. [from German, *heroisch*, heroic, powerful] (diacetyl-morphine) a semisynthetic derivative of MORPHINE obtained by the action of acetic anhydride or acetylchloride on morphine. The operation—which can be performed with chemical equipment costing less than $700—results in a white, odorless, crystalline powder with a bitter taste, which is soluble in water. (Some types of heroin from Mexico and Southeast Asia are brown because of the substances with which they are diluted.) Heroin was developed in 1898 by the Bayer Co., in Germany, as an analgesic more potent than morphine and a highly effective cough suppressant. When it was discovered that heroin relieved morphine WITHDRAWAL SYMPTOMS (then a perplexing medical problem because morphine and OPIUM were widely prescribed for a number of diseases and many people had become physically dependent), it was touted as a cure for morphine addiction. Heroin itself was considered to be nonaddictive. Twelve years passed before medical authorities discovered that, on the contrary, heroin was as addictive as morphine. By this time opium addicts (centered mainly among the criminal elite and Chinese immigrants) and novices alike, who had been turned away from opium by stringent controls, had discovered heroin's efficacy; the word "junk" had entered the underworld lexicon by the early 1900s.

The HARRISON NARCOTICS ACT of 1914 placed heroin under federal taxing powers and doctors were discouraged from prescribing it; by 1924, in a wave of reaction against heroin clinics that had been set up to treat addicts, Congress had prohibited the manufacture of heroin in the United States and turned the problem over to law-enforcement authorities; by 1956 all existing stocks on hand at pharmacies and manufacturers were surrendered. The League of Nations took action to discourage the export of heroin, and by 1963 it was used medically in only five countries and manufactured in three. Heroin is still used (and dispensed to addicts, see BRITISH SYSTEM) in Great Britain, and considered to be a more useful drug in combating pain than morphine. At the same time, heroin was steadily replacing opium and morphine as the drug of choice in the underworld of addicts. To understand this fact, it helps very little to understand the pharmacological action of the drug. Heroin is two to three times as potent, analgesically, as morphine (a widely accepted ratio is 4 milligrams of heroin equals 10 milligrams of morphine). In equipotent doses, however, the effects are very similar: analgesia, drowsiness, euphoria, constipation, vomiting, sedation, and respiratory depression in large doses and relief of anxiety and tension.

Experiments in which addicts were given "blind" intramuscular injections of morphine and heroin in equipotent doses revealed that the addicts were not able to tell the difference between the two and showed no preference for one drug over the other. (Tests employing METHADONE and heroin had similar results.) However, when the drugs were injected intravenously, most former addicts could identify the heroin. And once PHYSICAL DEPENDENCE had set in, five-eighths of the former addicts said they preferred heroin for continuing administration. Furthermore, though the withdrawal symptoms of heroin dependence are somewhat briefer in duration than those of morphine, they are qualitatively so similar in severity that there seems to be no real difference between them., Goodman and Gilman's standard text on pharmacology says that heroin produces more euphoria and stimulation and physical dependence develops more quickly than with morphine. Perhaps a key factor is the aura surrounding heroin: addicts *think* that it produces the greatest euphoria, while they could probably actually achieve their purposes just as well with intravenously injected morphine or any of the many SYNTHETIC OPIATES. At any rate, it is doubtful that the alleged euphoria is the main factor in continued administration of the drug; rather, the addict seeks release from the pain of oncoming withdrawal symptoms, this relief being a paradoxical pleasure.

Addicts' preference aside, the most significant factor in heroin's dominance lies in the logistics of the illicit traffic. Raw opium is ten times the weight of morphine; morphine, as a natural alkaloid of opium, before being refined into a soluble salt so that it can be injected, is also in the form of a solid block; and both are too bulky for long-distance smuggling to the United States, where the most lucrative black market is. Reduction to heroin provides the most potency with the least bulk (half the bulk of morphine even when the latter is in soluble powder form) and the greatest profits. Because it was more profitable, heroin usurped the market, at least in the United States, where injection is the leading mode of consumption, and addicts acquired a "taste" for it, even though its effects were roughly the same as those of morphine. Heroin has thus become the classic drug of addiction in the United States. (During World War II, when heroin shipments to the United States were cut off, addicts returned to morphine.)

This addiction consists of craving for the drug, which is used in quantities and settings considered abnormal by the culture, TOLERANCE to the effects of the drug, and the taking of increasing amounts, a compulsion to continue acquiring the drug even to the extent of adopting a criminal lifestyle, a preoccupation to the point where obtaining a supply dominates the user's entire life, and a high tendency to relapse after the drug is withdrawn and seek it again. Addiction is invariably accompanied by physical dependence which sustains and intensifies it, for the avoidance of withdrawal symptoms and related anxiety is a powerful motive—perhaps the most powerful—to continue taking the drug. Indeed, physical dependence is not the sole factor in addiction; the medical addict, i.e., one who has received prolonged treatment with morphine to relieve pain, becomes physically dependent after his pain has gone but has no other psychic motivation than the avoidance of withdrawal symptoms. In true addiction there must also be a craving for the drug's psychic effects, specifically, the sum of the conditioned interaction between the addict's personality and the pharmacology of the drug. In addition there is the high liability of relapse after the addict is withdrawn. This may be due less to the addict's lack of "willpower" and moral character than to the pharmacological effects of the drug. Taking the drug over a long period of time causes the cells to adapt to its presence; when it is removed, the cells still crave it. In any case, there is the phenomenon of the post-abstinence syndrome, in which the former addict feels depression, anxiety, and a continued craving for the drug, expressed even in dreams; to relieve the pain of this state the addict returns to the tranquilizing effects of the heroin.

To understand addiction better it might help to consider heroin (or rather morphine, since the latter is used medically and the effects are approximately the same) in a purely medical setting. Primarily, morphine is given for its analgesic actions; the side effects, ranging from drowsiness to constipation, are incidental. Morphine accomplishes three things: (1) it raises the threshold of pain, i.e., the patient is unable to perceive the pain he has; (2) it decreases the patient's anxiety about pain so that although he knows the pain is there, he feels detached from it; and (3) it appears to quiet the self-preservation drive, which takes up arms against the interloping pain regarded as an ego threat. Pain being regarded with drowsy equanimity, the ego is lulled into a sense of security that would be false, except that the disease which is the cause of the pain, the real threat it signals, is being treated, or, when terminal, is beyond treatment anyway. In the normal pain-free individual a therapeutic dose of morphine (or heroin) usually produces a predominately unpleasant reaction. Further, pain acts as an antidote to the drug, so that the greater the pain, the more tolerance there is to the action of the drug and the larger the necessary dose.

How then can we explain the action of a drug which the addict finds so necessary that he must repeat it again and again? In alleviating pain morphine often produces a state of euphoria, a subjective state of well-being produced by the patient's dramatic release from pain and the anxieties and tensions accompanying it. Since he has this state of well-being, even though his body is threatened by disease, in a sense his euphoria goes counter to the true situation: his body is frantically signalling that something is wrong, but the patient, lying in a narcotized half sleep, is at peace with the world.

An analogous cause-and-effect series must be at work in the addicts; they, too, seek that state of euphoria, of "escape" from the world and from themselves; or rather they seek to change their anxiety-ridden persons so that they can cope on normal terms with the world. The reasons for this need are probably as numerous as the individuals who use heroin. One might be a prosperous doctor who takes regular shots of morphine in order to cope with the strain and stress of a busy practice. Another might be a fifteen-year-old boy from the slums whose anxieties stem from both the conditions of his existence and an underlying neurosis. And the recent spread of heroin addiction to white middle-class youths suggests that poverty is not a controlling factor. All these addicts have in common is that they chose heroin rather than some other drug; further, many others of the same background and with similar personalities did not choose heroin. There was, in short, a factor of availability or peer-group pressure: the doctor with ready access to narcotics and practically no chance of being caught at it, the slum kid who lives in Harlem where pushers flourish and where his peers are also using drugs, or the suburban youth who may have listened to lecturers on drugs telling him that addiction can be cured and who runs with a drug-taking group and decides to try what is reputed to be the ultimate drug, thinking that if he becomes addicted he can become cured. So there must be both the pull of availability and the push of social-psychological "set," making heroin seem desirable, conjoining with some inner need which heroin satisfies and a tendency, partially determined by availability, to seek out escape in drugs.

Heroin addicts differ from other abusers in the lifestyle dictated by the drug they have chosen—or rather that has chosen them. ALCOHOL or BARBITURATES act to release inhibitions. They encourage aggressive drives that users cannot express in a sober state because of their inhibitions and because they are so conflicting and contradictory. Heroin acts to depress sex, aggression, even hunger; in their torpor, heroin users are free from conflicting motives, relaxed and detached. And the heroin addict suffering from some psychic pain due to inner anxiety arising from unrelievable subconscious drives and feelings of inadequacy or weak identity, palliates this pain by suppressing these drives at their source. Immediately the source of pain is deadened, a feeling of well-being returns, and addicts are detached from normal human hungers: they do not even desire to defecate. Yet the significant number of ex-heroin addicts and those undergoing the methadone treatment who use alcohol or barbiturates suggests that there is not necessarily a specific heroin hunger in addicts, though heroin may be the drug that works best for them, but rather a wider, pan-drug craving that can be assuaged as well by one depressant drug as another.

With many users, heroin injection has more positive aspects, a kind of sexual pleasure which they compare to an orgasm and which centers around a warm feeling in the stomach. In others the initial shock, when the drug is taken intravenously, is so powerful that it is akin to death, followed moments later by an immense relief at being alive. (Injection of a foreign substance—water alone would have a kindred effect—into the bloodstream destroys some blood cells, lowers the blood pressure suddenly, and induces a near state of shock.) In any case, users are "fixed," HIGH—high above it all, above all cares and hurts, above hungers that are doomed not to be satisfied subconsciously because they are felt to be wrong and tainted, above the fears that are nameless; in short, they are in a state of what to them is normality—"fixed," in a relationship of psychic equilibrium with the stresses of their environment (and it should be added that addicts, placed by society outside the law, have created for themselves an even more stressful environment; add to this the psychic pain caused by the ever-recurring incipient withdrawal symptoms; it is as though they have written themselves a scenario of pain, in order that pleasure—the release from pain—is continually assured).

The method of taking heroin is determined largely by economics: getting the most out of the least amount. Heroin is the only opiate that can, like COCAINE, be experienced through inhaling (SNIFFING), but this is somewhat wasteful (in Vietnam, where heroin was around 80 percent pure, users could afford to smoke it in cigarettes or even swallow it). Subcutaneous injection (SKIN POPPING) is usually the next step, but one also receives less of the effects (and less liability to addiction) by this method. Sniffing produces a euphoria all right, but the heroin has a bitter flavor, and many find it unpleasant. Skin popping will also do the job and is relatively more efficient. Some users—how many is uncertain—may remain at this level of using—CHIPPYING or JOY POPPING on weekends. But the majority go on to MAINLINING or intravenous injections. Heroin is most potent injected intravenously and, with the highly adulterated heroin available on the black market (an average of 5 milligrams of heroin in a FIVE-DOLLAR BAG), this is the most thrifty method, providing the most bang for the buck. It is after all a short step from injecting into the skin to injecting into the vein—especially when one has, or can borrow, the WORKS (the needle and so on), with all the necessity for secrecy and association with other addicts this entails. This necessity further alienates the user from normal society; indeed by some wickedly self-fulfilling prophecy this alienation is exactly what the addict is seeking—it feeds upon itself: getting high on a drug necessitates a way of life that necessitates getting high on a drug, to oversimplify. Mainlining is, as the name implies, the quickest, the most direct route to this state, for by prosaic medical fact, intravenous injection is thriftier: it takes about two-thirds as much of the drug to produce the effect of subcutaneous injection, and the initial thrill (RUSH) is more immediate. And since regular users are developing tolerance to the heroin and are well on their way to being HOOKED, they need heroin in its most potent form.

In a hospital, a patient can develop a mild physical dependence after about three weeks of daily injections of morphine, and the narcotic antagonist nalorphine (see NALLINE) will precipitate withdrawal symptoms after only *three days* of regular injections. In the STREET users shooting 30 milligrams a day (roughly six $5 bags) will acquire fairly substantial habits within two or three weeks. All this time, they have been undergoing a learning and conditioning process. First, they had to learn how to inject the drug. They were probably taught this by the friends who "turned them on." (Most addicts are introduced to the drug by friends, who may have a habit themselves and support it by low-level pushing.) As the learning experience continues, neophyte addicts learn to experience the effects of the drug—experience them as the answer to their underlying needs, the inner psychopathology that enhances the intense pleasure they experience with heroin from the beginning—and this satisfaction must continue, reinforcing their motivation to repeat. Thus, each time the drug relieves their anxieties, fears, and depression, their desire to use it again is strengthened. Also bound up in this motivation is a profound self-hatred and self-destructive drive. The addict is consciously committing suicide slowly! As one addict put it, heroin "has all the advantages of death without its permanence." Addiction, then, is a kind of suicide-in-life. Addicts learn that nothing else can quite do for them what heroin does. So, in addition to the need for the drug to relieve the anxieties associated with incipient withdrawal symptoms, a powerful conditioning has set in that will remain even after drug-taking is stopped. Former addicts visiting a place where they suffered withdrawal symptoms years before start yawning, their noses run, and so on, even though they have not taken drugs in the interim, and such a visit to their old haunts can set off an intense craving for the drug. A single shot after years of abstinence will set off withdrawal symptoms.

Some addicts are said to become so conditioned to the smell of the match they habitually use to COOK their heroin that just the smell of a burning match will set off preliminary withdrawal symptoms. Addicts have been conditioned to associate the smell of the match with both the symptoms that accompany their need and with the fiercely demanded relief their bodies know will automatically come when the cooking is finished and the drug injected. The bodily craving has become a demanding, autonomous entity, operating irrespective of the addict's conscious will or reason.

While this cycle is continuing, addicts' bodies are making a thousand minute cellular adjustments to the drug that is being regularly introduced into them. Now, they find they must take more to relieve their pain (pain is an antidote). They find, too, that they cannot reexperience quite the same intensity of that first intravenous shot and that, as one addict said bitterly, "horse [heroin] is a cheat": its effects are not quite what they first were. Perhaps then, in order to intensify the drug's initial rush, addicts will take to injecting SPEEDBALLS (heroin and cocaine) or BOMBITAS (heroin and AMPHETAMINES). Nevertheless they are hooked now: *they must continue to take the drug*, both physically and mentally. Frequently, a craving for the drug, akin to an intense hunger for food, but many times stronger, will accompany this compulsion. But physical dependence throws up new anxieties. Each time the effect of the drug starts to wear off, the addict can feel cramps and the other vague miseries (see COP SICKNESS, YENNING). Now, the anxieties of the psyche are overborne by the anxieties of anticipatory withdrawal. The habit is feeding upon itself. Euphoria, pleasure, whatever, are secondary, as avoidance of withdrawal becomes an end in itself. In this state, *addicts continue to take the drug*, for they have become conditioned to the drug, in the classic Pavlovian manner, as an alleviator of withdrawal anxiety. Their pleasure is lessened, but their desperation is increased. Now, they do not shoot for pleasure but to avoid pain, or, at best, to achieve what many addicts call a "normal state" or a satisfactory NOD.

If they are younger addicts from the slums, without solid careers, they are probably involved in HUSTLING for drugs, that is, devoting full time to stealing or perhaps small-time pushing in order to obtain money for drugs. In New York City an addict needs $10,000 a year to support a habit, meaning stealing and reselling, at one-fifth their value, $50,000 worth of goods. Drug users account for about one-fourth of the crimes against property, 1.2 percent of crimes against person, and a majority of the female prostitution in New York City. The relationship of addiction to crime has been overstated, however; some addicts do not engage in crime; most addicts do not engage in violent crime (barbiturate users have the highest rate of violent crime); and the majority of addicts engaged in criminal behavior before they got on drugs. The words of the thirties movies are half true: society has made addicts criminals, for crime is the only way they can obtain their drugs.

For all its stress and anxiety, the life of the street addict who has no easy access to drugs has compensations. There are the satisfactions from making daily rounds, hustling drugs, stealing—all that behavior addicts call "TAKING CARE OF BUSINESS"—the pride in one's ability to provide for oneself. But the police are not the only threat. There is the danger of INFECTION from unsterile needles, resulting in serum hepatitis, endocardic infection, abscesses, or tetanus. In the forties there was an epidemic of malaria from unsterile needles, so heroin began to be adulterated with quinine, a practice that has continued to the present day because quinine has a bitter taste—the taste of good heroin—which overcomes the sweetish taste of other usual adulterants such as MILK SUGAR (for bulk) and MANNITE (a mild laxative to overcome the drug's constipating effects). Some addicts think that quinine also enhances the rush. Gradually addicts' veins become scarred or thromboid (COLLAPSED VEINS) and they may resort to using those on their wrists, feet, and neck; older addicts who have run out of veins even revert to skin popping, and their bodies become covered with sores.

Then there is the constant fluctuation in supplies. Narcotics agents might intercept a large shipment of heroin, the heat may be on one's pusher. A drug PANIC is the result; addicts find their sources of supply suddenly dried up, and they must frantically search out another or else suffer withdrawal. This is perhaps overstated, though; however spectacular the police hauls, they seem to have little effect on the availability of heroin in the long run. There is always another source. Indeed, if federal narcotics authorities by some miracle managed to intercept all the heroin smuggled into the country, the sellers would then resort to synthetic opiates, which could be easily synthesized in clandestine laboratories. But there is at present no need for that; smuggled heroin continues to be sufficiently cheap to warrant bringing it in (the heroin in a $5 bag is worth about one-quarter of a cent).

The greatest danger is death from what is usually called in the newspapers OVERDOSE. It is conceivable (but unlikely) that addicts might get bags of heroin of such potency that it overcomes the tolerance they have built up to the drug and causes death by respiratory depression. Most cases of overdose, however, do not involve sufficiently large doses and the coroners prefer to call them "acute reactions." They may be associated with the quinine or other adulterants in the heroin or with the use of alcohol and barbiturates in conjunction with it. In any case, the risks of overdose are high and their unpredictability makes them that much worse. In New York City heroin overdose is the leading cause of death among youths aged fifteen to thirty-five, although the rate has dropped slightly, and methadone-induced deaths are on the rise.

The prognosis for addicts, in any case, is not good. Their death rate is over twice that for the normal population. At the age of forty they may begin gradually to slip out of the addicts' life (the phenomenon of "maturing out"); only about 10 percent of the addicts in the United States are over forty. Many addicts, however, continue their addiction until the day they die, and there is the story of the former addict who, bedridden, was forcibly kept off drugs for many years, yet who in his last words asked for a shot of heroin.

Numerous studies of addicts have demonstrated that heroin is not physiologically harmful; nor does it lower I.Q. or cause deterioration of the brain in any way. Functioning as a kind of tranquilizer (although its pharmacological actions are different from the drugs commonly known as tranquilizers), heroin might theoretically make certain persons more functional than they might be without it, though it is at best a crutch.

What is harmful about the drug is the addicts' lifestyle; if an overdose or unsterile needle does not get them, their characteristic neglect of their health will. Malnutrition is a common debilitation among addicts, though not by any means inevitable, a byproduct of the drug's suppression of hunger. Chronic bronchitis may also ensue because it deadens the cough reflex. Accidents and violent deaths also take their toll, and the addict and his pusher live on the fringes of the criminal underworld which controls the sale of heroin.

The prognosis for cure at the present time is not good. The three types of therapy now offered are incarceration (after which the addict usually heads straight for a fix), encounter therapy (including a kind of incarceration) in such voluntary groups as SYNANON and Phoenix House (in which the most effective cures come when ex-addicts exchange their addiction for addiction to the movement; Synanon has admitted a 90 percent relapse rate; most of Phoenix House's "cures" are engaged in working within the movement with other addicts), and chemotherapy, the use of narcotics-blocking drugs such as methadone or CYCLAZOCINE. The most promising of these is the methadone treatment, which manages to stabilize former addicts on the substituted drugs. Studies in New York City have shown as many as 85 percent of the participants remaining with the program and leading crime-free lives. If it is true that addiction is followed by a post-abstinence syndrome which impels the ex-addict to return to drugs (and the statistics bear this out), then it would seem that the best hope at present is to substitute another chemical which has demonstrated that it can quench this syndrome and at the same time wean the addict away from the heroin lifestyle.

Society's efforts to stamp out the illicit heroin trade have aimed a two-pronged legal effort at the traffickers and the addict in the streets—with little success. In 1914, before the passage of the Harrison Narcotics Act, there were an estimated 215,000 drug addicts in the country; at present there are 250,000 to 315,000, and some estimates put the number as high as 600,000. Harsh repressive laws against addicts have done little to decrease usage or rehabilitate addicts, for addicts are notoriously recidivistic and drugs are often freely available in prison.

As for controlling the traffic, it is doubtful that more than 10 percent of the heroin smuggled into this country is intercepted. Of an estimated 6,600 pounds of heroin smuggled into the United States in 1970, 311 pounds was seized by Customs; it is simply impossible to search each of the millions of persons entering the country each day. The occasional apprehension of low- and middle-level dealers has little effect because there is always someone eager to take over the lucrative traffic ($5,000 worth of heroin in Europe will sell for $1 million in the United States; these profits, of course, are siphoned off by several hands in the chain of smuggling). Indeed, making heroin illegal has only served to create a lucrative black market for it in the United States, which in turn makes it a desirable field for criminals to enter. More successful have been diplomatic pressures (e.g., persuading Turkey to ban the cultivation of the opium poppy) and police action against smugglers abroad (especially the Corsican gangs in Marseille).

The place of origin of 80 percent of United States heroin is Turkey; under pressure from the United States, along with subsidies to farmers, the Turkish government made the growing of the opium poppy (*Papaver somniferum*) illegal, but in 1974 the ban was lifted. Heroin also comes from Mexico, while the "Golden Triangle" area of Burma, Laos, and Thailand in Southeast Asia, where opium is cultivated by hill tribes living outside the pale of government, is another important source—producing half the world's opium. Heroin from the Middle East has traditionally been a Mafia operation; the crime syndicate, it is estimated, controls 80 percent of the heroin traffic, although blacks, Hispanics, and Chinese are entering the market in a major way.

No doubt law-enforcement agencies must continue an all-out war against the major importers and dealers before any dent can be made in the heroin traffic. But responsible groups have come to realize that the real target should be the consumers—the addicts in the street—and, further, that the only realistic hope of turning them off heroin is to substitute another drug such as methadone or even heroin itself, dispensed legally to them. Otherwise, the United States, the world's richest country and hence its most lucrative heroin market, will continue to pay a "tax" in the form of crime and theft to addicts forced to seek out their drug illegally. Slang names: H, harry, boy, brother, scag, schmeck, smack, horse, junk, poison, shit, crap, stuff, tecata, ca-ca, caballo.

The mind under *heroin* evades perception as it does ordinarily; one is aware only of contents. But that whole way of posing the question, of dividing the mind from what it's aware of, is fruitless. Nor is it that the objects of perception are intrusive in an electric way as they are under mescalin or lysergic acid, nor that things strike one with more intensity or in a more enchanted or detailed way as I have sometimes experienced under marijuana; it is that the perceiving turns inward, the eyelids droop, the blood is aware of itself, a slow phosphorescence in all fabric of flesh and nerve and bone; it is that the organism has a sense of being intact and unbrittle, and, above all, *inviolable.* For the attitude born in this sense of inviolability some Americans have used the word "cool."

At certain moments I find myself looking on my whole life as leading up to the present moment, the present being all I have to affirm. It's somehow undignified to speak of the past or to think about the future. I don't seriously occupy myself with the question in the "here-and-now," lying on my bunk, and, under the influence of heroin, inviolable. That is one of the virtues of the drug, that it empties such questions of all anguish, transports them to another region, a painless theoretical region, a play region, surprising, fertile, and unmoral. One is no longer grotesquely involved in the becoming. One simply is. —Alexander Trocchi, *Cain's Book* (1960)

high. [drug-exhilarated (from *high* spirits); since around 1920; from the sense of being at the top of one's form—*EP*. With LSD users, a literal sensation of being on an aerial voyage; also, perhaps, a sense of being "above it all"] in a state of drug euphoria. Compare TAKE OFF, COME DOWN, FLYING, UP.

him. HEROIN. Compare BOY, HER, GIRL.

hippie. [from *hep,* wise, informed, which is in turn from hep! hep!, encouragement of a team of horses, who "get hep"—*EP*. Also, *hepcat,* a connoisseur of swing music and jazz; *hip,* related to *hep,* but in a wider sense of *hip* to life, as well as to music, sophisticated; *hipster,* one who is *hip,* "cool," alienated, who lives in the present, a pure hedonist, who acts out psychopathically his drives of sex and aggression. *Hippie* is sort of the diminutive of hipster, i.e., the hipster's little brother, and descendant. But compare Laurie: *hip,* "addicts' jargon meaning to be an initiate, to have sores on the hips from lying on boards to smoke opium"; hence, a drug addict] a self-styled dropout from (usually middle-class) society; one whose life centers around hallucinogenic drugs, poverty, and hedonism, who rejects society's accepted means and ends, and who seeks to live a withdrawn life on as little money as possible, devoting himself to drug experiences, introspection, private ecstasy, religious quest, and love, sexual and fraternal.

The hippie subculture centered around the HAIGHT-ASHBURY section in San Francisco (where there were about 11,000 in 1967, at the movement's peak), the lower East Side in New York City (5,000), and various smaller pockets, rural and urban, scattered about the country. Most, but not all, hippies were young, dressed shabbily, had long hair, and wore beads (and other artifacts associated with Eastern religions) and colors inspired by the hallucinogenic experience.

Many supported themselves by DEALING in drugs. Hippies were oriented toward Eastern mysticism, a religion of quietism and withdrawal; they avoided aggression and power seeking and stressed meditation and pansexualism, in which the body is an instrument for union with others. Drugs were not considered the only means of achieving mystical enlightenment, the Zen Buddhist's *satori*, but they were considered valid shortcuts to the meditation and spiritual discipline of the mystics, and in practice the hippie's life centered around drug taking.

How many hippies achieved a profound and lasting religious experience is, of course, another question; jejune hedonism, escape, and KICKS may have been a dominant motive for many, who came from well-to-do middle-class homes and saw drugs as a way of rebelling against their parents, to whom HALLUCINOGENS and MARI-JUANA were unfamiliar and repugnant. The publicity surrounding the hippies was wide; their romantic image attractive abroad. Some observers saw the movement as a children's crusade for mass schizophrenia; certainly the mass movement of hippies into urban ghettos, where the rents are cheap, created new tensions and health problems.

hit. [*hit oneself,* take drugs; Australian addicts since 1944. *Hit, make, make the man,* purchase drugs, since around 1910; *hit it,* use a drug—*EP.* More probably from the sense of *hitting* a target] *1.* a successful injection of HEROIN into the vein. *2.* a shot, puff, sniff, dose, ingestion of a drug.

> You put the spike in slow, and the only way you know you got a *hit* is by watching the blood come up; then you take off the strap and squeeze it in.   —addict, quoted in Jeremy Larner and Ralph Tefferteller, *The Addict in the Street* (1964)

At the third attempt she found a vein and the blood rose up through the needle into the eye-dropper, and appeared as a dark red tongue in the colourless solution. *"Hit,"* she said softly, with a slow smile.
—Alexander Trocchi, *Cain's Book* (1960)

hog. PHENCYCLIDINE, an animal tranquilizer.

hold. [to have drugs for sale; since around 1910; compare *holding heavy,* having plenty of money—*EP*] *1.* to have drugs in one's possession (and thus be more liable to arrest) or in one's dwelling place for one's own use. *2.* to have drugs for sale. See STASH.

Never *hold* when you can stash. —drug user's saying (1966)

holding. possessing drugs, as in "are you holding?" Compare ANYWHERE.

homatropine. a semisynthetic derivative of ATROPINE considered to have fewer undesirable side effects and to be about one-fiftieth as toxic.

hookah. also hubbly bubbly. A pipe for smoking CANNABIS which bubbles the smoke through water, thus cooling it and softening the characteristic harshness of cannabis smoke. Compare NARGHILE.

hooked. [gripped by the drug habit; since 1925—*EP*] physically dependent upon a drug, usually an OPIATE drug. Compare ADDICTION, PHYSICAL DEPENDENCE.

When you're *hooked* it's different. The cool feeling you had when you're not hooked gradually diminishes, the amount that you have to take always getting larger, and with it less and less effect as you go on. . . . Then, as you go along that's when you begin to find out that horse [heroin] is a cheat, a real cheap cheat. Before this, you can have a whole evening or a whole day of wonderful I'm-great-and-the-world-is-all-cool feeling. But after you get hooked you have to take 8 or 10 caps to get that feeling and even after you take your 10 caps it is just sort of a recreation of that old relief. It isn't really there because for one thing just after you've taken off, you're already back in the position within an hour, maybe, you're going to look at things in the cold gray light of dawn already. And so, desperately hoping to hang on to this much nicer, much finer world, and in order to keep re-creating this capable-of-coping-with-things feeling you must keep opening a cap every few hours. . . . And then, finally, the third stage is when all you're trying to do is keep from getting ill, really.
—Helen MacGill Hughes (ed.), *The Fantastic Lodge* (1961)

hooking. [from a resident of "the Hook," Caesar's Hook section, in New York, where there were a number of brothels, hence the sailors called the prostitutes from that area *hookers—EP*] working as a prostitute to earn money for narcotics.

hop. [opium, narcotics; since around 1900; probably a corruption of some Chinese ideograph, but perhaps because it exhilarates—makes the addict *hop* (?)—*EP*] OPIUM.

hop dog. [also, *hop hog—EP*. "Anyone who uses more junk than you do. To use over five grains (300 milligrams) per day puts a user in the hog class."—William Burroughs, *Junkie* (1953)] an OPIUM addict.

hophead. [drug addict; since around 1900; compare HEAD—*EP*] HEROIN or OPIUM addict.

horn. to sniff a drug.

horror drug. any drug containing BELLADONNA alkaloids (mainly ATROPINE) or SCOPOLAMINE, a related alkaloid.

horrors. an unfavorable reaction to a drug, a BAD TRIP.

horse. [heroin; since around 1940; one "rides high"—*EP*. But also perhaps from the initial *h* sound, like HIM, HARRY, and the idea of a powerful steed carrying the rider where it will] HEROIN. Compare CABALLO.

> *Horse* is boss.   —addicts' saying

hot shot. a lethal injection which the addict thinks contains heroin but actually contains a poison—often strychnine, which looks and tastes like heroin.

> "Ever see a *hot shot* hit, kid? I saw the Gimp catch one in Philly. We rigged his room with a one-way whorehouse mirror and charged a sawski to watch it. He never got the needle out of his arm. They don't if the shot is right. That's the way they find them, dropper full of clotted blood hanging out of a blue arm. The look in his eyes when it hit—kid, it was tasty."   —William Burroughs, *Naked Lunch* (1959)

House of D. Women's House of Detention, New York City (closed).

> "But she's been booked now, she's in the *House of D* right now, so what can he do? It's got to go to court now."
> —addict in James Mills, *The Panic in Needle Park* (1966)

hubbly bubbly. HOOKAH.

huffer. user of DELIRIANTS (e.g., glue, cleaning fluid, etc).

hump. see OVER THE HUMP.

hungry croaker. [from *hungry,* i.e., in need of money, or eager to take money, and CROAKER, convicts' term for prison doctor] a doctor who will prescribe narcotics for addicts in exchange for money.

hustler, good, ace boss, five-star. general term of admiration, variously employing all the listed adjectives, for an addict who aggressively and successively engages in a variety of activities, mostly criminal, to obtain money for drugs. According to the mores of the addict subculture, good, etc., hustlers are go-getters, sharp entrepreneurs, admired for their success at supporting their habits and their skill in outwitting the law and the square world. Compare HUSTLING, GREASY JUNKY.

hustling. *1.* obtaining money for drugs by theft, prostitution, pimping, small-time narcotics peddling, con games, etc. *2.* prostitution. *3.* the addict's characteristic behavior pattern revolving around illicitly obtaining money and drugs, a way of life inextricable from the narcotics habit for many. Compare STREET, ON THE; TAKING CARE OF BUSINESS.

Hycodan. [dihydrocodeinone bitartrate, Endo Laboratories Inc.] a cough syrup containing HYDROCODONE, a semisynthetic derivative of OPIUM, in amounts of 5 milligrams per teaspoonful or tablet, and 1.5 milligrams of HOMATROPINE methylbromide. Prolonged use will result in PHYSICAL DEPENDENCE. Manufacturer's recommended dosage is 1 teaspoonful, four times a day. A Schedule III drug under the CONTROLLED SUBSTANCES ACT.

Hycomine. [dihydrocodeinone, bitartrate, and other ingredients, Endo Laboratories Inc.] a cough syrup containing HYDROCODONE. Compare HYCODAN.

hydrocodone. also called dihydrocodeinone; a semisynthetic derivative of MORPHINE. Taken orally, 5 to 10 milligrams of hydrocodone gives analgesia equal to that produced by 10 milligrams of morphine, lasting from four to six hours. Prolonged administration will result in PHYSICAL DEPENDENCE. The WITHDRAWAL SYMPTOMS are milder than those associated with morphine dependence but more severe than those of CODEINE dependence. Hydrocodone is primarily used as an antitussive (cough-reflex suppressant). A Schedule II drug under the CONTROLLED SUBSTANCES ACT. Compare HYCODAN, HYCOMINE.

hydromorphone. also called dihydromorphinone. A semisynthetic derivative of MORPHINE, hydromorphone is a more potent analgesic than morphine: an injection of 2 milligrams will give the analgesic effect of 10 milligrams of morphine. The analgesia lasts three to four hours. Not widely used among addicts, hydromorphone will produce PHYSICAL DEPENDENCE after prolonged administration, with WITHDRAWAL SYMPTOMS close to those of morphine dependence in severity. A Schedule II drug under the CONTROLLED SUBSTANCES ACT. Compare OPIUM, DILAUDID, DILOCOL.

hyoscine. SCOPOLAMINE.

hyoscyamine. active alkaloid found in jimsonweed, DATURA STROMONIUM, henbane, *Hyoscyamus niger,* and BELLADONNA, *Atropa belladonna,* among others. The action of hyoscyamine is similar to that of ATROPINE, although its effects on the peripheral nervous system are approximately twice as great. Difficult to obtain in its pure form, it is rarely used in medicine.

hype. [from *to hypo,* to inject with a needle, to prick; hence, to sting, and hence its meaning of shortchanging or swindling someone. Also, from *hypodermic,* a hypodermic user and hence a morphine or heroin addict; since the 1920s—*EP*] *1.* a phony story, a hoax, a put-on. *2.* to deceive someone with a phony story, hoax, put-on. *3.* a narcotics addict. *4.* a hard sell.

hyperventilate. see STEAMBOAT.

I i

iboga. the leaves of the plant *Tabernanthe iboga,* chewed in the Gabon Republic as a stimulant and antifatiguant. Poisonous alkaloids, IBOGAINE and iboganine, have been isolated from the leaves. No direct accounts of the drug have been published.

ibogaine. an alkaloid found in the root of the plant *Tabernanthe iboga,* which grows in West Africa. The natives there reportedly use it as a stimulant and antifatiguant. As such, its action is similar to that of the MONOAMINE OXIDASE INHIBITORS, which are used as antidepressants.

Ibogaine or IBOGA is given in dosages of 200 to 300 milligrams [3 to 5 milligrams per kilogram (2.2 pounds) of body weight]. It does not dilate the pupils or cause a rise in blood pressure as do other hallucinogenic drugs; it also tends to cause vomiting. The drug produces visions similar to those produced by HARMALINE, with images of animals and primitive men, sexual themes, and aggression predominating. The drug seems especially to release primitive instincts and innate aggressions, and to evoke, rather than past experiences, past fantasies buried in the subconscious.

> I am standing up. The doctor has asked me something. What was it? To dance? To tremble? To bring back the rhythm of the Negroes? Or that I imitate the cactus-animal? I don't know. Perhaps even then I didn't know. But I see myself standing in front of a giant drum. Beyond the drum I see many Negroes moving to a rhythm. They have thick lips, painted white, and skirts formed of white strips that hang from a red belt. Their legs and chests are bare. I beat the drum forcefully with my right hand, and then with my left. I have something like wooden hammers in my hands, and I beat with them. I stop drumming to carry the rhythm with my body. I want to dance. It does not come out right. I try again, and I cannot. Then I see, among the Negroes, Maria's white, smiling face. Her expression changes as I look at her, and she laughs aloud. She mocks me because I cannot dance. I feel so angry that I throw the hammer and kill somebody but I do not care. Something is interrupted. The doctor asks me to call the scene back to mind, but I find myself unable to do so. I sit down, and then I lie down. The doctor speaks, but I don't remember what he says. I only know that I cannot understand, I cannot understand. Something is going on.
>
> Then I suddenly become aware of having been sexually aroused for a long time. I say this. The doctor tells me: "Give in to your desire. Feel it." And then I feel as if somebody took my legs and moved them in such a way that it became like a sexual act. There is no orgasm—or thousands—it is difficult to explain. But nothing ends. Arousal continues. Again I see beautiful landscapes, sunsets, vegetation, the sea, great expanses of desert, and the sun as a marvelous fireball in the background. I say, "How beautiful!" The doctor has asked me not to judge whether what I see is beautiful or ugly, but just describe it. But how can I not say it, if it is so beautiful? The sensation of being, the sensation of coarse vibrations that beat on and sink into my flesh. I feel like saying a thousand times, I am I, I am I, I am. It is everything and too much.   —patient under ibogaine
>   in Claudio Naranjo, *The Healing Journey* (1974)

ice cream habit. irregular, moderate use of drugs. Compare CHIPPYING, WEEKEND HABIT.

idiot pills. BARBITURATE or other sedative pills.

in action. engaged in selling drugs, as in "Are you *in action* now?"

Indian hay. MARIJUANA.

Indian hemp. CANNABIS SATIVA.

infection. one of the major hazards of drug addiction is the risk of infection from unsterile needles or needle sores. Two diseases, frequently fatal, are common among addicts, tetanus and serum (or virus) hepatitis. Tetanus infections are almost always associated with the practice of SKIN POPPING, or subcutaneous injection. The tetanus bacillus enters the body through the open sores that cover the addict's body as a result of frequent injections. Older addicts, whose veins have collapsed, are particularly prone to this practice and to the resultant disease. Tetanus infections are relatively infrequent, but the majority of all cases occur in addicts; of these, over 50 percent are fatal.

Virus hepatitis, a contagious form of jaundice, is always associated with the practice of MAINLINING, or intravenous injections. Since addicts do not always own needles, and since they naturally associate with other addicts, they tend to borrow from their fellows or to rent out their needles as a source of money, thus exposing themselves to infection. The virus inhabits the bloodstream and is thus easily transmitted from one addict to another in a single injection. Virus hepatitis follows the needle, of course, rather than the drug. It has broken out among California HIPPIES and others who inject AMPHETAMINES or LSD-25.

Other infections associated with drug injection are phlebitis (infection of the vein), endocarditis (infection of the inside lining of the heart), abscesses, syphilis, and superficial venous thrombosis (collapsing)—swelling and blocking of veins—and (now rarely) malaria.

inhalants. DELIRIANTS.

inhalers. psychotoxic, DELIRIANT substances, such as airplane glue (see GLUE SNIFFING) or CLEANING FLUID, which are inhaled for their intoxicant effects.

in paper. method of smuggling narcotics into a penal institution, e.g., slitting a postcard lengthwise and inserting the drugs, wrapped in tinfoil.

into. *1.* to be using a kind of drug, as in "a lot of kids were *into* pot." *2.* deeply involved with something, as "*into* stamp collecting."

in transit. on an LSD TRIP.

intsaga. [Africa] CANNABIS.

intanfu. [Africa] CANNABIS.

iron cure. undergoing WITHDRAWAL SYMPTOMS in prison without drugs. Compare KICKING, COLD TURKEY.

IT-290. an indole analog of AMPHETAMINES which produces hallucinogenic effects.

J j

J. [from JAY SMOKE (?) or JOINT] a MARIJUANA cigarette.

jab. *1.* to inject a drug. *2.* to ambush someone.

jacking. stealing, as in "He was *jacking* from the methadone patients."

jag. [intoxication, whether from liquor or from a drug; slang since the 1930s—*EP*] a state of prolonged, agitated, intense stimulation caused by a drug, especially AMPHETAMINES or COCAINE; at the end of the jag one CRASHES, i.e., falls into an exhausted sleep.

jam. COCAINE.

jammed up. [since the 1950s] taken an overdose of drugs.

jay smoke. a MARIJUANA cigarette.

jduq jmel. [Arabic] small black DATURA seeds, sold in magic shops in Marrakesh, which have a hallucinogenic effect and probably contain SCOPOLAMINE.

jerk off. [from *jerked off,* masturbated; compare GET OFF] to inject a little HEROIN at a time, letting it flow back into the needle mixed with blood, reinjecting it, and so on. Supposed to prolong the initial RUSH; also, the first drawing of blood indicates that one has a HIT. Compare BOOTING.

. . . and after tying Gene's tie around her lower arm, [she] pricked a vein and *jerked off*—that is, pushed the stuff in and then brought it up with blood.   —Rabbi Joseph R. Rosenbloom, in *The Reporter* (June 25, 1959)

Over and over again one hears addicts describe the effects of their injection in sexual terms. One addict said that after a fix he felt as if he were coming from every pore. Another said that he used to inject the solution in a rhythmic fashion until it was all used up, and said that this was akin to masturbation albeit much better.
                         —M. Hoffman, *Comprehensive Psychology* (1964)

joint. [the narcotics user's (especially the opium smoker's) tool and eqiupment; since around 1920. A MARIJUANA cigarette; since around 1945—*EP.* Perhaps from the sense of *joint,* implying section, i.e., in rolling a cigarette one rolls a section, portion, of one's supply. Or perhaps *joint,* the penis. This latter theory is confirmed by Charles Winick in "Marijuana Use by Young People," included in *Drug Addiction in Youth,* edited by Ernest Harms (1965). He says that marijuana's "traditional association with sex" may be the reason a marijuana cigarette is referred to as a "joint" and a "root."] *1.* a marijuana cigarette, usually the roll-your-own kind. Compare STICK. *2.* (with *the*) prison.

jones. [since the 1950s, perhaps related to *the jakes,* a form of peripheral neuritis prevalent in the South in the 1920s, caused by bad homemade whiskey] drug dependence, a HABIT; the WITHDRAWAL SYMPTOMS arising out of this habit.

"He just beat me out of $5 and my *jones* is on me."
                —Claude Brown, *Manchild in the Promised Land* (1965)

joy juice. CHLORAL HYDRATE.

joypop. [a bout of OPIUM smoking; from *pop,* a shot, a hypodermic injection; since the 1930s—*EP;* and *joy,* i.e., just for pleasure] to inject HEROIN occasionally for pleasure, not motivated by the need to prevent WITHDRAWAL SYMPTOMS. Some heroin users continue to joypop on weekends for years without ever taking it frequently enough to become physically dependent. Many addicts, however, follow the classical route to addiction: SNIFFING to SKIN POPPING to MAINLINING. Usually, the joypopper injects the drug subcutaneously.

juanita. [Mexico] MARIJUANA.

juice. liquor.

"Juice is a down trip. Grass brings you up—up and away."
—"The Hippies," *Time* (July 7, 1967)

juice head. one who drinks liquor.

jungle drug, the. AYAHUASCA.

junk. [*junker,* drug user; since the 1920s; from *junker,* a pusher or peddler—*EP.* Since heroin was synthesized in 1898 and addicts were calling it *junk* in the early 1900s, either the name was taken from a word for opium or it was coined for heroin. If the latter, it apparently has the same invidious connotation of such synonyms as CRAP and SHIT, which *EP* says originated in the 1920s in addicts' expressions of contempt for diluted heroin. Another possibility is that, being readily available and a kind of patent medicine, heroin was considered inferior to opium and in this sense *junk*] *1.* HEROIN. *2.* any drugs. *3.* inferior, diluted heroin.

junkie. [from JUNK; also, perhaps the idea developed of the addict as "human junk." Veteran addicts sometimes apply it as a term of contempt to new addicts or those unable to support their habits] a HEROIN addict.

K k

kat. KHAT.

kava. a mild, soporific beverage made from the root of the plant *Piper methysticum,* a member of the pepper family. It is drunk by South Sea Islanders of New Guinea (where it is called *kavakava*) and Hawaii (where it is called *ava*). The beverage is served hot; it is aromatic, rather soapy in taste, and astringent. Kava is not addictive, and its action is sedative; if enough is drunk, the user will fall asleep. In Tonga the drink is prepared by young men or girls who chew the roots thoroughly, then expectorate the pulp into a bowl, where it is mixed with water and served.

key. also spelled ki,kee. A kilogram (2.2 pounds) of a drug, especially a pressed block of MARIJUANA of this weight.

khat. also qat, q'at. The buds or fresh leaves of *Catha edulis,* which are chewed or drunk as tea in East Africa and the Arabian peninsula (Yemen). It is a central nervous system stimulant very similar in chemical structure and effects to AMPHETAMINES. In Yemen it is used to banish sleepiness and hunger on long treks and also for its exhilarating effects. The drug's adverse effects include restlessness, insomnia, overstimulation of the heart, and loss of sexual desire. The usual mode of ingestion is to chew the leaves when they are from building up. However, PSYCHIC DEPENDENCE, without PHYSICAL DEPENDENCE, does occur: habitual khat users feel strongly impelled to use it once a day or more and will do so in preference to eating.

ki. KEY.

kick. [from the kicking the addict does while undergoing WITHDRAWAL SYMPTOMS] to break the (drug) habit, as in "I'm going into the hospital and *kick.*"

kickback. [a return to taking narcotics after kicking a habit; a relapse; since around 1930; from *kick back,* to return stolen property to the victim—*EP.* But also may be a pun on KICK THE HABIT] a relapse, a return to taking drugs after one has been withdrawn from them.

kick cold turkey. [from COLD TURKEY] *1.* to abruptly withdraw from drugs. *2.* to undergo full WITHDRAWAL SYMPTOMS unalleviated by any medicine. Compare A LA CANONA.

kicking. ridding oneself of addiction to narcotics.

kicks. [*kick,* a drug taking, since around 1945—*EP.* Probably from the jolt, the RUSH of the drug's initial onset; analogous to the *kick* in strong liquor. From that, any strong pleasure, as in "I get a *kick* out of you"] sheer pleasure, sheer hedonism, without any other redeeming qualities. To "take a drug for kicks" thus has a sharply ambivalent meaning in our society. Those who disapprove of drug taking cite the fact that users do so "just for kicks" as morally wrong; while the hedonists say that taking something for pleasure is a worthy motive in itself.

kick sticks. MARIJUANA cigarettes. Compare JOINT.

Joints are pulled out of the brims of hats and soon there's no noise

except the music and the steady hiss of cats blasting away on *kicksticks.*
                    —Piri Thomas, *Down These Mean Streets* (1967)

kick the habit. [from *kick it out,* suffer physically or mentally (withdrawal symptoms); since the 1920s—*EP.* Probably *kick it out* has its origin in the muscle spasms the addict endures during withdrawal, and so was extended from meaning withdrawal symptoms to ridding oneself of addiction by undergoing withdrawal. "I soon learned where the expression 'kick the habit' came from. When my drug quota was progressively cut down I got spasms in the muscles of my arms and my legs actually kicked."—Barney Ross and Martin Abramson, *No Man Stands Alone,* J. B. Lippincott, Philadelphia, © 1957 by Barney Ross and Martin Abramson] to break the drug habit, including undergoing WITHDRAWAL SYMPTOMS. Thus, to kick the habit is not the same as to KICK COLD TURKEY. Kick the habit also has a connotation of finality, i.e., one permanently stops using drugs.

kick the habit on the elevator. to undergo mild WITHDRAWAL SYMPTOMS. Modern addicts' HEROIN is often so heavily diluted that they develop only mild addiction, and when they go into the hospital for detoxification, their withdrawal symptoms are comparable to a case of flu.

I've seen guys go into jail, and like the expression goes, they *kicked their habit on the elevator.* In two or three days they're eating, sleeping, doing pushups.
                    —anonymous addict, James Mills, in *The Drug Takers* (1965)

kief. KIF.

kif. [Arabic, tranquillity, peace] name used in Northwest Africa, especially Morocco, for CANNABIS.

Kif is like fire; a little warms, a lot burns.   —Moroccan folk saying

killer. very good; strong, potent drugs.

killer weed. potent MARIJUANA.

kilo. a kilogram (2.2 pounds). Bulk sales of HEROIN and MARIJUANA are often made in kilo lots and the drugs shipped in kilo packages.

kilo connection. drug dealer next in line below the captain or major importer; he takes a kilo of relatively pure HEROIN, cuts it one to one, and sells it to the OUNCE MAN. Also called THE PEOPLE.

kilter. MARIJUANA.

King Kong. [from the giant movie ape] a very large, expensive HEROIN habit.

King Kong pills. BARBITURATES or other sedative pills. Compare GORILLA PILLS.

kit. equipment for injecting drugs; usually a hypodermic needle, eyedropper or pacifier, cotton, bottle cap or spoon, water, and a strap to use as a tourniquet to distend the vein. Compare GIMMICKS, WORKS, BIZ.

knockout drops. liquid CHLORAL HYDRATE, a hypnotic and sedative, mixed surreptitiously with alcohol (which POTENTIATES its effects) in order to render someone unconscious. BARBITURATES could be used just as well. The toxic oral dose of chloral hydrate is approximately 10 grams. Compare MICKEY FINN.

kratom. [Thailand] a plant, *Mitragyna speciosa,* which is believed to have a narcotic effect, although little is known about it. Compare BEINSA.

K.Y. U.S. Public Health Service (Narcotics) Hospital in Lexington, Kentucky, where addicts go voluntarily or by court sentence in order to be withdrawn from drugs.

L l

L. LSD-25.

lady snow. [from the resemblance of cocaine crystals to snow] COCAINE.

La Guardia Report. short title for a study of MARIJUANA ordered by Mayor Fiorello H. La Guardia in 1938, carried out by the New York Academy of Medicine, with the assistance of the New York Police Department. Finally published in 1944 under the official title *The Marihuana Problem in the City of New York, by The Mayor's Committee on*

Marihuana. The study was in two parts: a clinical study of the effects of marijuana and a sociological study of marijuana users in the city.

The clinical study was carried out under the supervision of doctors in Goldwater Memorial Hospital. Experimental subjects (prisoners) were given both natural and synthetic marijuana and subjected to a battery of physiological and mental tests to determine what the drug's pharmacodynamic effects were, whether it caused physical or mental deterioration, and if it possessed any possible therapeutic effects for the treatment of disease or for other drug addictions.

The sociological study was carried out by specially trained members of the police department, who visited places haunted by marijuana smokers in the city in an undercover capacity. The committee's conclusions were as follows:

> Marihuana, by virtue of its property of lowering inhibitions, accentuates all traits of personality, both those harmful and those beneficial. It does not impel its user to take spontaneous action but may make his response to stimuli more emphatic than it normally would be. Increasingly larger doses of marihuana are not necessary in order that the long-term user may capture the original degree of pleasure.
>
> Marihuana, like alcohol, does not alter the basic personality, but by relaxing inhibitions may permit antisocial tendencies formerly suppressed to come to the fore. Marihuana does not of itself give rise to antisocial behavior.
>
> There is no evidence to suggest that the continued use of marihuana is a stepping-stone to the use of opiates. Prolonged use of the drug does not lead to physical, mental or moral degeneration, nor have we observed any permanent deleterious effects from its continued use. Quite the contrary, marihuana and its derivatives and allied synthetics have potentially valuable therapeutic applications which merit future investigation.
>
> [Mayor La Guardia added this statement in his foreword to the report:] I am glad that the sociological, psychological and medical ills commonly attributed to marihuana have been found to be exaggerated insofar as the City of New York is concerned. I hasten to point out, however, that the findings are to be interpreted only as a reassuring report of progress and not as encouragement to indulgence, for I shall continue to enforce the laws prohibiting the use of marihuana until and if complete findings may justify an amendment of existing laws.
>
> —*The Marihuana Problem in the City of New York,*
> *by The Mayor's Committee on Marihuana* (1944)

Although it might be said that one of the main things the report proved was that prisoners given a holiday from jail and allowed to smoke marijuana will be happy, docile, and cooperative indeed under the influence of the drug, the La Guardia Report stands as a landmark study into the physiological effects of marijuana, and its conclusions, especially those about the relationship of marijuana to psychosis and crime, are still cited today. The book became a sort of underground bible among marijuana smokers who favored legalization of the drug. It has since been superseded by more contemporary studies, notably the report of the National Commission on Marijuana and Drug Abuse.

lame. a conventional person, a non–drug user. Compare SQUARE, STRAIGHT.

laudanum. [from Latin *ladanum,* a yellowish resin] a hydroalcoholic tincture containing 10 percent OPIUM; a solution of opium, first compounded by Paracelsus (1493?–1541). This, the first medicinal form of opium, was used widely for a variety of diseases up through the nineteenth century. It was sold without prescription, and its addictive liability was not clearly understood. As a result, many people who took laudanum for various indispositions became addicted, among them such well-known persons as Coleridge, Poe, Moussorgsky, Mrs. Browning, Swinburne, Chatterton, Francis Thompson, Dante Gabriel Rossetti, James Thomson, Wilberforce, Horace Day, John Randolph, and De Quincey.

> I possess a secret remedy which I call laudanum and which is superior to all other heroic remedies.   —Paracelsus, *Letter* (ca. 1530)

> But I took it; and in an hour, O heavens! What a revulsion! What a resurrection from the lowest depths, of the inner spirit! What an apocalypse of the world within me! That my pains had vanished was now a trifle in my eyes; this negative effect was swallowed up in the immensity of those positive effects which had opened up before me, in the abyss of divine enjoyment thus suddenly revealed. Here was a panacea for all human woes; here was the secret of happiness, about which the philosophers had disputed for so many ages, at once discovered; happiness might now be bought for a penny, and carried in the waist-coat-pocket; portable ecstasies might be had corked up in a pint-bottle; and peace of mind sent down by the mail.
> —Thomas De Quincey, *Confessions of an English Opium Eater* (1822)

laughing gas. NITROUS OXIDE.

lay. to smoke OPIUM. *Obsolete.*

lay down. [the price or fee for admission to an OPIUM den; since the 1920s—*EP;* but compare "to recline and smoke opium"—*MM,* 1946] to smoke opium in a reclining position, a practice which may decrease nausea and other undesirable side effects of the drug. *Obsolete.*

layout. [opium-smoking equipment since the 1880s—*EP*] *1.* opium-smoking equipment. *2.* equipment for injecting HEROIN; WORKS, KIT.

lay up. having acquired a large supply of drugs, to withdraw from hustling and lie about one's room using the drugs, as in "I used the money to buy a big stash of heroin and decided to just *lay up* for the next couple of weeks."

L.B. a pound. Compare O.Z., KEY.

L.B.J. [JB 336-N-Methyl-3 Piperidyl benzitate hydrochloride] a hallucinogenic substance.

leapers. AMPHETAMINES.

leaving-the-set walk. [from (?) *set,* a stage set] police term describing the characteristic demeanor of an addict after he has bought drugs from a pusher. See SET.

Lebanese. A brownish-red colored HASHISH from Lebanon.

legal high. generic term for a variety of substances that are not prohibited by law, can be obtained without prescription or are available as foods, and are supposed to alter the consciousness. Such substances include AMYL NITRITE, DILL, Sominex (see SCOPOLAMINE), ASTHMADOR, which contains BELLADONNA, cigarette tobacco dusted in aspirin powder, NUTMEG, MACE, cinnamon, CATNIP, lettuce juice, hydrangea leaves, niacin, green pepper, and dried banana pulp (see BANANA SMOKING). Compare NATCH TRIPS.

lemon. [from *lemon,* something that doesn't work] highly adulterated or worthless powder sold as narcotics.

lemonade. LEMON.

Leritine. [ANILERIDINE, Merck Sharp & Dohme] a SYNTHETIC OPIATE analgesic somewhat less potent than MORPHINE. Injections of 30 to 40 milligrams give analgesia equivalent to 10 milligrams of morphine. Prolonged administration will produce PHYSICAL DEPENDENCE. WITHDRAWAL SYMPTOMS are milder than those associated with morphine dependence and are more comparable to those of MEPERIDINE dependence. Manufacturer claims that Leritine is a more effective pain reliever than meperidine in equipotent dosages. The dosage is about half that of meperidine: about 50 milligrams initially; 75 milligrams in more severe pain; 100 milligrams in extremely severe pain, up to a total of 200 milligrams over three to four hours. An ungraduated, sudden intravenous injection of Leri-tine in excess of 10 milligrams is dangerous and may result in fatal respiratory depression. Manufacturer cautions that injection of un-diluted Leritine is to be avoided, except in grave emergencies. The product is sold in white tablets and in solution for injection. A Schedule II drug under the CONTROLLED SUBSTANCES ACT.

levallorphan. [1-3-hydroxy-N-allylmorphinan tartrate] a synthetic drug which reverses the action of MORPHINE and the synthetic mor-phine drugs and is used to counter acute respiratory depression resulting from overdosage. In persons addicted to narcotics, Leval-lorphan will trigger severe WITHDRAWAL SYMPTOMS. Compare LORFAN, NALLINE.

Levo-Dromoran. [LEVORPHANOL tartrate, Roche Laboratories] a SYNTHETIC OPIATE analgesic more potent than MORPHINE. Doses of 2 to 3 milligrams of Levo-Dromoran will produce analgesia equal to that produced by 10 milligrams of morphine, lasting four to five hours. After prolonged administration, PHYSICAL DEPENDENCE upon Levo-Dromoran will occur, with WITHDRAWAL SYMPTOMS equal to those of morphine in severity. The recommended clinical dose is 2 milligrams orally or injected subcutaneously. The product is sold in 2-milligram tablets or in solution. A Schedule II drug under the CONTROLLED SUBSTANCES ACT.

levorphanol. a SYNTHETIC OPIATE analgesic composed of the levo isomer of morphan. Dosages of 2 to 3 milligrams produce analgesia equal to that produced by 10 milligrams of MORPHINE, lasting four to five hours. Prolonged administration will result in PHYSICAL DEPEND-ENCE with WITHDRAWAL SYMPTOMS similar to those of morphine dependence in severity. A Schedule II drug under the CONTROLLED SUBSTANCES ACT. Compare LEVO-DROMORAN.

Lexington. also called K.Y., narco. U.S. Public Health Service (Nar-cotics) Hospital in Lexington, Kentucky.

Librium. [chlordiazepoxide hydrochloride, Roche Laboratories] a MINOR TRANQUILIZER of the BENZODIAZEPINE group that lies between CHLORPROMAZINE and MEPROBAMATE in potency, Librium is used to treat anxiety, to allay apprehension before surgery, and, in large doses, to alleviate acute panic psychoses, alcoholic anxiety, and paranoid and schizophrenic states. Usual recommended dosages are from 5 to 10 milligrams, three to four times daily up to 50- to 100-milligram injections totaling no more than 300 milligrams per day. Other depressant or stimulant drugs such as ALCOHOL,

BARBITURATES, phenothiazine derivatives, MONOAMINE OXIDASE (MAO) INHIBITORS, and imipraminelike compounds POTENTIATE Librium's effects, and the danger of fatal respiratory depression is increased. A number of suicides have employed Librium.

Prolonged, excessive use of Librium, i.e., 300 to 600 milligrams daily, or about ten times the normal therapeutic dose over a period of about five months, will result in PHYSICAL DEPENDENCE, in which case WITHDRAWAL SYMPTOMS will occur if the drug is abruptly stopped. Withdrawal symptoms are similar to those resulting from barbiturate dependence: loss of appetite, aggravation of existing psychopathological states, depression, agitation, insomnia, and convulsions. Since it is thought that Librium produces significantly less euphoria than meprobamate, OPIATE analgesics, or the barbiturates, the danger of PSYCHIC DEPENDENCE may be relatively less, but it does occur. In high doses its effects are indistinguishable from barbiturate intoxication. In some persons the drug will produce idiosyncratic or paradoxical reactions, i.e., inebriation, stimulation, loss of bodily coordination, delirium, drowsiness, rage, and confusion.

Librium is sold in capsules or solution for injection. The capsules contain 5 milligrams (green top, yellow bottom, both inscribed "ROCHE 5"); 10 milligrams (brown top, green bottom, both inscribed "ROCHE 10"); and 25 milligrams (green top, white bottom, both inscribed "ROCHE 25"). A Schedule III drug under the CONTROLLED SUBSTANCES ACT.

lid. [from the fact that MARIJUANA used to be sold in pipe-tobacco tins; see CAN] an amount approximately equal to 22 grams (0.77 to 1 ounce) of marijuana; a measure for purposes of sale. The price in 1967 ranged from $10 (West Coast) to $25 (New York City). The term is used mainly in the western United States. About forty marijuana cigarettes can be made from this amount. Compare TIN.

lid poppers. AMPHETAMINES.

life, the. the drug addict's characteristic life pattern, revolving around HUSTLING, copping (see COP), the FIX, interaction with fellow addicts, dealing with PUSHERS, and so on. When one is in the life, one is using drugs, of course, and committed to a whole complex of rituals, fraternalisms, lingo, etc., rather like joining a lodge. Compare STREET, ON THE.

light stuff. MARIJUANA or other nonopiate drugs, as opposed to HEAVY STUFF, i.e., HEROIN, COCAINE, other OPIATES. Compare HEAD DRUGS.

"When I came back, I started to hustle pot—*light stuff,* here and there a few bricks. But no mo' junk. I was gonna stay clean."
—Piri Thomas, *Down These Mean Streets* (1967)

light up. [since the 1930s] to smoke MARIJUANA. *Obsolete?* Compare BLAST.

Light up, Gates, Report Finds "Tea" a Good Kick.
—headline in *Downbeat,* after the publication of the LA GUARDIA REPORT (1944)

line. [from MAINLINE, to inject HEROIN into the large vein of the arm] the main vein in the arm; to "shoot in the *line*" is to inject heroin into this vein.

load. twenty-five to thirty DECKS (packets) of HEROIN, stacked and fastened together with a rubber band for delivery. Compare BUNDLE.

loaded. [from the sense of *load,* a heavy weight; one who is "carrying a load" is "burdened" by a heavy intoxication] in a state of drug intoxication (not limited to alcoholic intoxication).

loco. MARIJUANA. Compare MEXICAN LOCOWEED.

long con. a major, elaborately plotted confidence game. Compare SHORT CON.

lophophorine. one of the alkaloids found in the hallucinogenic PEYOTE cactus.

Lorfan. [LEVALLORPHAN tartrate, Roche Laboratories] a synthetic NARCOTIC antagonist which acts to reverse the effects of the OPIATE analgesics. Lorfan is customarily injected along with the opiate in order to lessen the danger of respiratory depression from the latter without impairing analgesia. Used alone, Lorfan may itself induce severe respiratory depression; hence, it is recommended that it be administered in conjunction with an opiate except in emergencies. It is also valuable in cases of accidental or deliberate narcotic overdosages resulting in respiratory depression (along with other medical measures). Lorfan is not effective against BARBITURATE-induced respiratory depression. Compare NALLINE.

LSD-25. [*d*-lysergic acid diethylamide tartrate 25] a hallucinogenic semisynthetic derivative of lysergic acid, an alkaloid found in the rye fungus ergot, *Claviceps purpurea.* The standard laboratory process for making the drug, developed in 1938 by Dr. Albert Hofmann at the Sandoz Laboratories in Switzerland, is to mix the lysergic acid with diethylamide, freeze the mixture, and extract the resulting LSD by fractional distillation with chloroform or benzine, or with a vacuum evaporator. The drug's hallucinogenic effects were first experienced by Dr. Hofmann in 1943, when he accidentally ingested some of it and experienced hallucinations.

The drug is one of the most potent known to man: 20 micrograms (1 microgram is one-millionth of a gram) or approximately 1/700,000,000 of the average man's body weight, will produce effects. In experiments the usual dose is 25 to 50 micrograms, though some doctors favor 100 micrograms. In treating alcoholics, when a more profound experience is considered desirable, doses of 300 micrograms are given. Illicit users customarily take amounts ranging from 100 to 700 micrograms, with 2,000 micrograms being the highest known dosage taken. The lethal dose in human beings is not known; rabbits have been given 120 times the average human dose and rats 2,000 without harm, but an elephant given 297 milligrams (297,000 micrograms) of the drug died.

In relation to the other HALLUCINOGENS, LSD is considered 5,000 times as potent as MESCALINE and 200 times as potent as PSILOCYBIN (this is arrived at by the comparative amounts needed to produce full effects in the average adult male weighing 150 pounds). It is said that 1 ounce of LSD will furnish enough for 300,000 individual doses on the illicit market. The drug is usually distributed as a soluble powder (a tartrate of lysergic acid diethylamide) packaged in capsules or as a liquid. In large quantities the liquid drug has a slight bluish or purplish cast; the powder is colorless, odorless, and crystalline.

Sometimes the liquid is soaked up into pieces of blotting paper, chewing gum, sugar cubes, tablets, animal crackers, and heart-shaped candies. The practice of dissolving doses in sugar cubes (a way to conceal them), once prevalent, gradually faded out, perhaps indicating that a more serious breed of drug takers, who wanted their drug in *drug form,* had made its appearance. It can also be injected, which induces a quicker HIGH but also involves the danger of INFECTION from unsterile needles.

The average price for a single dose (200 to 300 micrograms) on the illicit market in 1967 was between $2.50 and $10. The process of making LSD is fairly simple; however, certain items of laboratory equipment are needed, and the chemicals from which it is derived are difficult to obtain. Chief sources are the homemade LSD on the market, which is of unpredictable potency (due to inaccuracies in mixing the tiny amounts) or adulterated, and smuggled LSD, with Canada, England, Israel, Czechoslovakia, and Switzerland among the primary origins.

The effects of the drug vary widely among individuals and are in part related to the dosage, the mental state of the individual at the time it is taken (SET), and the circumstances in which it is taken (SETTING). The effects also vary with the same individual from time to time; one may have a series of pleasant experiences and then have an extremely unpleasant one. Because of its unpredictability, many HEROIN addicts, who are especially prone to experiment with other drugs, do not like LSD. The drug's effects occur within an hour after ingestion. The initial reaction is a vague anxiety and sometimes nausea. The anxiety may be unrelated to the drug; in one experiment a group of subjects was given an inert substance and told it was LSD; all of them experienced a heightened anxiety. Physiological alterations due to the drug's immediate action are relatively minor. The pupils dilate, the appetite is depressed, blood pressure and body temperature are increased, and insomnia follows upon the waning of its action. Sometimes there is restlessness, paralysis, or a suffocating sensation. The effects last from six to fourteen hours, tapering off into waves of alternating normality and abnormality. In a few cases they last for several days. An occasional postdrug experience, especially among long-time users, is *recurrence,* the phenomenon of some external or emotional stimulus setting off a more or less intense LSD experience even though the person has not taken the drug. This phenomenon has continued for periods of up to eighteen months.

Surprisingly, only a small percentage (about 0.01 percent) of the dose taken enters the brain, where it remains twenty minutes, then disappears; a much larger percentage goes to the liver and kidneys. The fact that the amount in the brain remains there only about twenty minutes suggests that LSD's action is indirect, i.e., it either releases or inhibits other substances naturally occurring in the brain, and this imbalance causes the subjective effects. (LSD can be detected in the bloodstream up to two hours after it is taken, but the amount is so tiny that especially sensitive laboratory tests are needed.)

The drug's subjective effects are spectacular if taken in large doses. They are similar to those produced by other hallucinogenic drugs but on a grander scale (if a large dose is taken) and include stimulation of the central and autonomic nervous systems, changes in mood (sometimes euphoric and megalomaniac, sometimes fearful, panicky, and anxiety-ridden), a sense of threat to the ego, an intensification of colors so that they seem brighter, intensification of the other senses so that inaudible sounds become magnified or food tastes better or normally unnoticed aspects of things (such as the pores in concrete) become strikingly vivid, merging of senses (synesthesia) so that sounds are seen as color patterns, a wavelike sense of time so that seconds seem like an eternity, distortions in the perception of space so that surrounding objects seem fluid and shifting, a sense of depersonalization, of being simultaneously both within and without oneself, a closely related feeling of merger (dissolving) with the external world and a loss of personality, a perception of ordinary things as if seen for the first time unstructured by perceptual "sets," hallucinations of flowers, snakes, animals, other people, etc., which subjects usually know to be hallucinations though they are powerless to stop them, a sense of closeness to, or merger with, other persons in the room as if barriers between individuals had been dissolved, enhanced sensuousness and sexual stimulation (the drug is neither an aphrodisiac nor an anaphrodisiac, but its overpowering mental effects tend to make it more of the latter), vivid swirling colors and shapes when the eyes are closed, an impairment in body coordination and in pain perception, impairment of performance on intelligence tests, sometimes voices commanding the user to do something, and the release from the subconscious of repressed material, sometimes in the form of terrifying, dreamlike, visual symbols, and breakdown of conscience and superego restraints.

Since some of these effects are similar to those of schizophrenia, LSD was first thought to produce an "imitation" psychosis and was called a PSYCHOTOMIMETIC drug. However, this term was found to be inaccurate because of many differences, notably that the subject is usually aware of undergoing the hallucinatory experiences, and generally responsive to others. Nevertheless, one of the chief dangers of the drug is that it will trigger a latent psychosis into activity. This may result from anxiety, panic, and the release of repressed material with which the subjects cannot cope, pushing them over the edge into an acute panic psychosis. Often such untoward effects can be headed off by the administration of a strong tranquilizer, such as CHLORPROMAZINE (THORAZINE), which reverses the drug's effects or calms the patient down sufficiently during the aftermath of the drug experience. Often no drug is necessary if companions reassure and persuade the user that it is a temporary experience caused by a drug. Such transient panic psychoses clear up more or less spontaneously in a day or so. But the drug has also induced chronic psychoses lasting several months or even longer. It also has induced severe depressions which are sometimes suicidal. (The suicide rate in a controlled group was 0.1 percent, which is low considering they were psychiatric patients.) Fatalities have also resulted from accidents occurring while individuals are under the drug, because their grandiose conception of themselves and loss of contact with reality impair their judgment. They may jump out of the window without realizing the hazardousness of their actions. Driving while under the influence of the drug is especially dangerous because of distorted perception.

Aggressive acts committed under the influence of LSD are comparatively rare, though there have been highly publicized cases alleging (but not proving) LSD use. Negative reactions to LSD generally occur among the following types of users: (1) unstable persons harboring a latent psychosis or severe neurosis (but who nevertheless may be functioning fairly successfully in everyday life), (2) persons who have been given the drug in large amounts without their knowledge (an extremely dangerous practice), (3) persons who take the drug in a strange or apparently hostile or nonsupportive environment or take it alone without any proper supervision (although negative reactions also occur among persons who have taken care to provide themselves with a congenial environment before using the drug or among persons who have taken the drug as many as 100 times without adverse effects), and (4) persons taking adulterated or poorly manufactured LSD.

Since the number of persons who have taken LSD outside of medical supervision in this country is not known (estimates range from 1 to 2 million), it is impossible to say what percentage have psychotic episodes. An analysis of medically supervised experiments with LSD revealed a very low psychosis rate of 0.8 per thousand. It may be that psychotic reactions among unsupervised users is considerably higher than that figure. Certainly, the number of admissions to hospitals for treatment of such psychoses increased as the drug became more widespread. In New York City, for example, the number of persons admitted to the psychiatric division of Bellevue Hospital with LSD-induced psychoses during the ten-month period from March 1, 1965, to December 31, 1965, numbered sixty-five; previous to that time there had only been a handful of such admissions. During the first six months of 1966, this admission rate roughly doubled (recent figures, however, show a decline in the admissions rate). Figures for California are similar.

The majority of users of LSD tend to be young, middle-class, and college-educated, or else from the bohemian fringe of society. The number of college students trying LSD has increased and a

Gallup Poll in 1970 found that 14 percent of the student sample queried had tried LSD. Motives for using the drug include expansion of consciousness; greater psychological insight into one's personality; a desire to change one's personality and become a more loving, "creative" individual; a religious or quasi-religious mystical experience; "kicks" (ranging from the novelty of the LSD state to enhanced experience of sex); improved creativity; solution of intellectual problems; a profound dissatisfaction with one's personality and way of life; and a desire to experience something more intense and beautiful than one's daily humdrum. In some individuals LSD does seem to induce profound changes in the personality—whether for the better or the worse is a complex question. Certainly it has proved dramatically effective in treating some alcoholics, with a lower relapse rate than any other treatment for this disease (compare the beneficial effects of PEYOTE on Indian alcoholics).

Whether creativity is enhanced by LSD is problematic; however, experiments with a group of architects suggested that they were better able to solve design problems while under the influence of the drug, but this capacity only exists while the subject is under the drug. For example, a physics major dropout said he could understand the theory of relativity only while under the drug. When asked to explain it when full of the drug, he could not. LSD has also been used with varying success in treating autistic schizophrenic children (it is not so effective with adult schizophrenics), as an adjunct to psychotherapy, in frigidity and homosexuality, and to ease the pains of terminal cancer and put patients in a state of mind in which they are better able to accept their imminent death. However, LSD is still a *highly unpredictable drug,* and its pharmacology and psychic potentialities are still only dimly understood. To explain its action is almost to explain the workings of the brain itself.

The adverse publicity inspired by the drug caused its only United States manufacturer, Sandoz Pharmaceuticals, to stop making it and withdraw it from the market. As a consequence, supplies on hand were transferred to the federal government, and the number of research projects with LSD dropped from seventy-two to twelve. Current projects are under the supervision of the National Institute for Mental Health and the Veterans Administration, both government agencies.

Modern authorities are still not certain as to the nature of the pharmacodynamic action of LSD. One theory postulates that it acts to block the production of SEROTONIN or some other neurohormone found in the brain, or replaces it. Apparently, its action causes the normal pattern of communication from various parts of the body to the brain to break down, so that instead of orderly, selective perception and analysis of incoming sensory data, the brain is deluged by a wide variety of undifferentiated external stimuli and subconscious material bubbling up in the consciousness at random and perceived in unstructured and startling ways—what Dr. Harold A. Abramson has called "an emotional storm." Experiments with animals have shown that LSD intensifies the electrical impulses sent along the optic nerve to the cortex, distorting them along the way; also impulses transmitted from both sight and auditory receptor nerves become confused, producing the effect of synesthesia.

LSD is nontoxic. It does not cause PHYSICAL DEPENDENCE and there are no WITHDRAWAL SYMPTOMS upon cessation of long-term use. TOLERANCE to the drug occurs very rapidly; usually within three days the original dose will have no effect. This tolerance just as rapidly abates, however. CROSS-TOLERANCE with psilocybin and mescaline also occurs, so a person who has built up a tolerance to one of these hallucinogens will also be tolerant to LSD, and vice versa. The nature of the drug itself seems to discourage long-term abuse, and this has been borne out in a survey of early LSD users who took the drug in the fifties. In fact, it differs in several ways from drugs of higher abuse liability, such as alcohol, the barbiturates and heroin, in that there is no physical dependence, complete tolerance comes on rapidly rather than gradually and up to large doses, the drug's intense emotional experience leads to a kind of psychological situation which makes users less desirous of repeating it, there is a lack of dependable effects—i.e., its effects, unlike depressant drugs, are unpredictable—and there is a point of diminishing returns in the LSD experience itself after which the new perceptions induced by the drug seem no longer new. There are a minority of cases of those who use the drug frequently over a period of years—finding the LSD dream world superior to the real one—and this often results in a change in lifestyle; the user may become more passive, more introspective, more pacific, less decisive, and more benign and euphoric. He usually gives up his career and becomes a dropout and thus by conventional standards a failure, although not, perhaps, by the user's own, new standards.

There have been warnings that LSD causes organic damage to the brain, but this has not been proven. Psychological tests administered to a group of LSD users showed little difference between them and the control group. Experiments in which LSD was applied to white blood cells seemed to indicate that it might cause chromosome breakage, but an equal number of experiments showed it did not, and this "danger" remains unproven. There is little evidence of genetic damage among babies born to LSD-using mothers, but the use of *any* drug during pregnancy should be strictly circumscribed.

In summary, supervised, directed, and goal-oriented use of LSD suggests some benefits in the areas of mental health, religion, and creative problem solving, but the drug is unpredictable in the small minority of cases. Certainly the setting and supervision under which it is administered and the user's expectations and underlying mental state go a long way towards shaping the LSD experience. The chief hazard lies in unsupervised use, without experienced standbys who can talk the user "down" from a "bad trip," in untoward circumstances which increase the risk of psychotic break under the influence of the drug, or use by latently psychotic individuals. Since LSD is colorless, odorless, powerful in minute quantities, soluble in any liquid, fairly easy to manufacture if one has the equipment, and quite easy to smuggle, it appears that the illicit traffic is difficult, if not impossible, to stop. Black market LSD carries the added hazard that it will contain some adulterant (AMPHETAMINES are a favorite), which will in turn increase the dangers of a bad trip.

As of now, research in LSD has been severly curtailed and harsh laws have been passed against it, without notable effect, although the use of the drug has fallen off from its high-water mark in the sixties when lurid publicity and the proselytizing of Timothy Leary and others gave it a powerful mystique. It was replaced by amphetamines, then depressants and heroin among the devotees —perhaps because of these drugs' more dependable effects, as already mentioned. Also potential users were frightened by reports that the drug caused chromosome breakage. Dedicated LSD users were, characteristically, almost compulsive proselyters in its heyday, but it is doubtful that their messianism had any lasting effects, and the LSD cult has cooled. The meditative, nonaggressive, inward orientation of the self, associated with the drug, runs counter to the values of an extroverted, aggressive, acquisitive society. In sum, LSD is still available, but the LSD fad seems to have run its course in a matter of five years. Compare DMT, DET, BUFOTENINE, MESCALINE, PSILOCYBIN, PEYOTE. Slang names: acid, deeda, Hofmann's bicycle, blue acid, sunshine acid. A Schedule I drug under the CONTROLLED SUBSTANCES ACT.

Here the notes in the laboratory journal stop. The last words were written down only with great effort. I asked my laboratory assistant to accompany me home, since I believed that events would take the same course as the disturbance on Friday [his first ingestion of LSD]. But even on the way home—by bicycle—it appeared that all the symptoms were more intense than the first time. Already I had the greatest difficulty in speaking clearly, and my field of vision wavered and was distorted like the image in a curved mirror. Also, I had the feeling that I was making no headway, although later my assistant told me that we were traveling at a fast pace. . . .

As far as I can remember, the following symptoms were strongly marked during the height of the crisis, which had already passed when the doctor arrived: dizziness and defective vision; the faces of those present seemed to me like colored masks; strong kinetic disturbances alternating with paralysis; my head, my whole body and limbs seemed at times very heavy, as if filled with lead; cramps in my legs, my hands sometimes cold and numb; a metallic taste on my tongue; my throat dry and contracted; a feeling of suffocation; I was alternately bewildered and in clear understanding of the situation, so that I sometimes stood outside myself as a neutral observer as I shrieked half madly or babbled unintelligible nonsense. . . .

The visual distortions were still pronounced. Everything seemed to waver and be out of proportion, like the reflection in an agitated sheet of water. Moreover, everything was soaked in changing, unpleasant, mostly poisonous shades of green and blue. With my eyes closed, colorful, ever-changing fantastic images invaded my mind continuously. It was especially remarkable how all sounds—for instance, the noise of a passing car—were transposed into visual sensations, so that with each tone and noise a corresponding colored image, changing in form and color like a kaleidoscope, was produced.

—Albert Hofmann, in "Mental Changes Experimentally Produced by LSD," *Psychiatric Quarterly* (1952).

A New Yorker made his first trip last November. It was a riot, a carnival of exquisite sensation, exploding color, visions so unspeakably beautiful that he sobbed with joy and said again and again, "Oh, my God, how lovely, how wonderful, how beautiful, how fair." Crystal palaces soared thousands of miles into a velvet void. His body dissolved in honey and quicksilver. He watched a bronze Buddha come alive and listened to a record of Ella Fitzgerald singing "My Ship" that he would give his soul to hear again. He went home and slept and the next day he was certain that the whole world was turned on. A month later he made his second trip. This is his account of how it ended:

"My guide's face changed. It became abstracted, reduced to a series of planes. His eyes were closed. In his expression there was absolute detachment, perfection, peace. An aura of silvery light flickered around his head. Then, between and slightly above the level of his eyes, I saw the third eye, the eye that gazes inward.

"The room darkened and the music faded. I was lying on my back on the floor. Then the room itself vanished and I was sinking, sinking, sinking. From far away I heard, very faintly, the word 'death.' I sank faster, turning and falling a million light years from the earth. The word got louder and more insistent. It took shape around me, closing me in. 'DEATH . . . DEATH . . . DEATH.' I thought of the dread in my father's eyes in his final hours. At the last instant before my own death I shouted, 'No.' Absolute terror, total horror. With immense effort I began to lift myself back to life. It seemed to take an eternity.

"Then the room reappeared and I was standing there shaking. My guide still sat in his chair, perfectly still. Suddenly I knew that he controlled me. There was no escape. No way to explain. I was his slave. His thoughts were my thoughts.

" 'Oh, you bastard!' I shouted. 'What have you done to me? What have you done?' From far away I heard another voice. It said, 'You are insane. Totally, finally, irrevocably insane.' My face got cold. I ran in circles in that little room. I scattered the bright stones that I had felt change and grow beneath my fingers a few hours earlier.

"I tried to be calm and think, but I couldn't. I could feel my brain splitting. I never pray, God knows, but I fell to my knees in that chamber of horrors. 'Jesus, help me!' I said. 'Help me! Help me!'

"My guide stood over me. 'Take it easy,' he said. 'You always knew it could end like this.' The way the words reverberated with menace, it was the most frightening thing I had ever heard. He held a white capsule in one hand and a glass of water in the other. 'Take this,' he said. 'It's Thorazine. It will calm you.'

"To me it looked like more LSD. 'Not on your life, you bastard,' I shouted. 'I'm getting out of here.' He stood in front of the door. I picked up a chair and went for him."

—Tom Buckley, *The New Republic* (May 14, 1966)

LSM. Lysergic acid morpholide, a chemical congener of LSD-25.

luding out. [from QUAALUDE] using METHAQUALONE.

Luminal. [phenobarbital, Winthrop Laboratories] a long-acting, slow-onset BARBITURATE hypnotic and sedative. Like all the phenobarbitals, Luminal is considered especially effective as an anticonvulsant, e.g., in epilepsy and delirium tremens. The hypnotic (sleep-inducing) dose is 100 milligrams; the sedative dose, 25 to 30 milligrams. The average daily intake over a long period of time should not exceed 0.6 grain (36 milligrams). Fatal overdoses of Luminal (ten to twelve times the hypnotic dose) occur, usually in suicides. Because it is a slow-onset, long-acting barbiturate, Luminal is perhaps more dangerous in such attempts. The coma induced is slower in taking effect, but deeper, longer lasting once it does take effect, and there is consequently less chance that the patient will be discovered in time to be saved.

Still the phenobarbitals, which have been in medical use since 1912, are among the most useful of the barbiturates. TOLERANCE to the drug's hypnotic effects builds up over time, so that there is a temptation to increase the dosage in order to continue getting the same effects. After prolonged use in excessive amounts, PHYSICAL DEPENDENCE will occur, with severe WITHDRAWAL SYMPTOMS if the drug is abruptly stopped.

Luminal is sold in sugar-coated, oval-shaped tablets of 16 and 32 milligrams. A Schedule III drug under the CONTROLLED SUBSTANCES ACT.

lush. [from an eighteenth-century English term for strong beer or from the German *loschen,* to quench flames or thirst—*EP*] *1.* a heavy drinker. *2.* an alcoholic. *3.* alcoholic beverages, as in "he was on *lush.*" *4.* to drink alcoholic beverages. Compare JUICE.

lysergic acid. a compound close in chemical structure to LSD-25 but without hallucinogenic effects; one of the direct chemical precursors of LSD-25. Sometimes LSD-25 is erroneously called by this name.

lysergide. LSD-25.

M m

M. [since around 1920—*EP*] MORPHINE.

mace. a common spice made from the integuments of NUTMEG and used, mixed with hot water, especially by prisoners, to produce stimulation and a light-headed HIGH.

macon. [West Africa] CANNABIS.

maconha. [Brazil] CANNABIS.

made. [from *make the man,* buy drugs—*EP.* Also *to make,* to obtain from by guile or cheating or by purchase; perhaps when one is *made,* one is "had," taken, seduced, beaten. But see MAKE] *1.* exposed; revealed for what you really are, as in "I *made* him as a narco." *2.* purchased narcotics, as in "I *made* him for a nickel bag." Compare COP.

magic mushrooms. see MUSHROOMS, SACRED.

mahjueme. concentrated HASHISH obtained by cooking the resin in butter.

mainline. [from *main line,* a major rail route or "a vein forms a line, and main rhymes with vein"—*EP;* since around 1925] *1.* the large arterial (ulnar or median cephalic) vein in the arm, the usual, because most convenient, place for the injection of HEROIN. *2.* to inject heroin or other drugs into this vein. *3.* to inject intravenously.

mainlining. injecting HEROIN into the main vein of the arm or other vein.

main stash. [home—*MM,* 1946] *Obsolete.* Compare STASH.

maintenance therapy. legally supplying addicts with a daily ration of drugs, either those to which they are addicted or those of the MORPHINE type, with the intention of preventing WITHDRAWAL SYMPTOMS, winning their confidence, and working with them to break their habits, transferring the addiction from HEROIN to another drug (see METHADONE) and thus weaning from the heroin addicts' life pattern, or simply enabling them to continue to function in the community as supervised drug addicts who do not have to acquire their drugs illegally.

In Great Britain addicts can register as such and receive daily dosages legally, under restricted conditions (BRITISH SYSTEM). Because of strict interpretations by the Supreme Court of the HARRISON NARCOTICS ACT in the 1920s, doctors were prohibited from giving narcotics to addicts for relief of withdrawal symptoms, and so in practice maintenance therapy by a private physician became impossible. More recent decisions have reversed those earlier interpretations, but most doctors are still reluctant to give narcotics to addicts on a long-term basis and have no knowledge of how to treat addicts or desire to become involved with them. Instead, medical efforts have been concentrated on maintenance with drugs like methadone or CYCLAZOCINE. The Federal Bureau of Narcotics was opposed to doctors' prescribing for addicts; thus the few doctors who did so as part of their treatment of an addicted patient experienced harassment and forfeiture of their licenses.

majoon. [Arabic *ma'jun,* jam; confection containing cannabis] also majoun. Greenish-black or brown confection of a gummy consistency containing powdered HASHISH or CANNABIS, honey, fruit, nuts, spices, and rancid butter, consumed in North Africa and the Middle

East for its hallucinogenic effects. Compare DAWAMESK, GOBLET OF JAM.

> The doctor stood by the side of a buffet on which lay a platter filled with small Japanese saucers. He spooned a morsel of paste or greenish jam about as large as the thumb from a crystal vase, and placed it next to the silver spoon on each saucer. . . . "This will be deducted from your share in Paradise," he said as he handed me my portion.
> —Théophile Gautier, *Revue des Deux Mondes* (1846)
> (Translation by Polly Kraft, *The Drug Experience*, 1961)

major tranquilizer. a pharmacological and chemical classification (compare MINOR TRANQUILIZER). The major tranquilizers are chemically of the phenothiazine type, which consists of three subgroups:

1. Dimethylaminopropyl compounds (CHLORPROMAZINE, promazine, triflupromazine)
2. Piperidyl compounds (mepazine, thioridazine)
3. Piperazine compounds (carphenazine, fluphenazine, perphenazine, prochlorperazine, trifluoperazine, thioprozate)

The major tranquilizers are unique in their effectiveness in treating acute and chronic psychotic states, specifically, by calming violent, hyperactive, hyperexcited, fearful patients without any soporific actions. Even large doses will not induce coma or anesthesia, and PHYSICAL DEPENDENCE and PSYCHIC DEPENDENCE are unlikely. Thus, psychotic patients can be calmed without the risk (present with BARBITURATES) of dangerous respiratory depression.

Major tranquilizers can be administered over a prolonged period without addiction, and the patient will be sufficiently alert mentally to respond to other psychotherapeutical measures. It is also possible to return the patient to the community sooner, substituting outpatient for institutional care. The major tranquilizers also lessen the patient's hallucinations and delusions, or at least the fears and anxieties about them. Once the patient is calmed and the mental tortures and delusions brought under control, the possibility of achieving rapport with others and especially with a psychiatrist is greatly increased; further, if maintenance doses of the tranquilizer are continued after the patient leaves the institution, there is less chance of rehospitalization.

Some TOLERANCE develops to several effects of the major tranquilizers. Their main danger lies in such untoward side effects as loss of control over muscles of the head, arms, and hands; tremors, shuffling gait, drooling, etc.; skin and liver disorders (jaundice); drowsiness, dizziness, and fatigue, which are usually produced by large doses; and various anticholinergic reactions (see ATROPINE), such as fall in blood pressure or ocular pressure.

majoun. MAJOON.

make. [from *make*, to detect or recognize, since around 1900—*EP*. Also *make*, to steal, burgle, or sell things to a person or at a house, or *make it*, to arrive, to succeed, which is related to a specialization of the convicts' *make it*, to get a parole or pardon, since around 1900; and also the colloquial sense of "to gain a desired point," since the 1880s—*EP*.] *1.* to detect or recognize someone for what they really are. *2.* to purchase drugs from a peddler, as in "I tried to *make* him for some junk." *3.* to flee, leave, "beat it." Compare MADE.

make it. [see MAKE] to do, achieve, accomplish something; specifically, to inject a narcotic and experience a HIGH or to have sexual intercourse.

making a croaker for a reader. [from CROAKER, a doctor, and READER, prescription] bribing a doctor to write an illegal prescription for a NARCOTIC. Compare BRODY.

man, the. [in Harlem during the 1930s *the man* was the law—*EP*. Also probably taken from *to make the man*, to purchase narcotics from a peddler—*EP*. Current usage among blacks has extended *the man* to mean the boss, i.e., the white man] *1.* police, detective, or parole officer. *2.* a connection, a PUSHER, a drug peddler. Compare BIG MAN, the high-level seller, wholesaler, or importer of narcotics.

M and C. [from *Marmon* and *Cadillac,* the motor cars; in turn, from the drugs' initials; the 1920s—*EP*. Also connoting the high prices of the drugs and their relative value to the addict, i.e., the equivalent of a Cadillac to a nonaddict] a mixture of MORPHINE and COCAINE ("usually four parts morphine to one part cocaine"—*EP*). *Obsolete.* Compare SPEEDBALL.

manicure. to clean MARIJUANA for smoking.

manita. [from (?) Spanish transliteration of *mannite*] MILK SUGAR.

mannite. a mild laxative used to adulterate HEROIN, it counters the drug's constipative effects.

MAO inhibitors. MONOAMINE OXIDASE INHIBITORS.

marijuana. [probably a mutilation of Portuguese, *maran guango,* intoxication; first applied to CANNABIS SATIVA in Brazil. Pablo Oswaldo Wolff posits a possible (Mexican) Indian derivation, which is dubious and too complex etymologically to go into here] the flowering tops, stems, and leaves of the female Indian hemp plant, *Cannabis sativa,* dried, shredded, and cleaned of twigs and seeds and ingested for the low-level hallucinogenic effects. Sometimes the name is applied to the plant itself, but hemp or Indian hemp is the correct name, and marijuana more precisely refers to the portions of the plant prepared and used for their hallucinogenic effects.

The name refers to the variety of *Cannabis sativa* grown in the Western Hemisphere and to the manner in which it is customarily taken, i.e., smoked in a pipe or cigarette (occasional users brew a tea from the seeds and twig waste, or bake them into cakes or cookies; the untreated seeds contain the ACTIVE PRINCIPLE of the plant). Unlike CANNABIS consumed in other countries, the Western marijuana is relatively mild from the standpoint of hallucinogenic potency. For example, it is considered about one-tenth as potent as CHARAS or HASHISH (the pure resin of the plant, which contains the active principle, TETRAHYDROCANNABINOL or THC, in concentration), which are used in India, North Africa, and the Middle East, respectively. Ordinarily marijuana is not specially cultivated, as it is in the Far East (see GHANJA), where methods of cultivation induce a more copious exudation of the resin when the female plant is mature. (Geographical origin and variety of *Cannabis sativa* are also closely related to potency. Hence, Tunisian cannabis is three times as potent as American varieties. Mexican marijuana contains 1 percent THC; American, 0.2 percent; Jamaican and Southeast Asian, 2–4 percent; Jamaican ganja, 4–8 percent; and hashish, 8–12 percent.) It is most comparable to the BHANG used in India. The resin contains the most potent concentration of THC, followed by the flowers and the leaves.

The quality of marijuana sold in the illicit market also varies widely: sometimes the male plant (which has a higher percentage of THC) is sold along with the female (which produces a high amount of the resin), with no effort made to separate the flowering tops of the female plant (where the resin is exuded at maturity) and with immature plants of both sexes being sold along with mature plants, which, again, contain the most resin. A hot, dry, upland climate is also considered to produce a more potent plant, and most marijuana consumed in North America is not grown in such a climate. Most American marijuana is grown in Mexico, within the United States—especially the southwest, Iowa, Kentucky, and Pennsylvania, although it grows wild as a weed (see WEED MARIJUANA) in most parts of the country, even in vacant lots and window boxes in large cities (the New York City Sanitation Department has destroyed over

100,000 pounds of the plant growing within the city), Jamaica, Colombia, Panama, and Canada.

Marijuana varies in potency according to informal, ill-defined "grades," ranging from MEXICAN GREEN or Kentucky blue up to ACAPULCO GOLD. Because of the difficulty in finding sufficient quantities of marijuana of uniform potency, controlled research with the plant is difficult. More reliable for research purposes are the eighty-odd preparations of marijuana synthesized from the oil of the plant, e.g., PYRAHEXYL, or the recently synthesized active principle of the plant, tetrahydrocannabinol. Some experiments were conducted with the semisynthetic derivatives of marijuana in the late 1930s and 1940s in the treatment of severe depression and drug-addiction WITHDRAWAL SYMPTOMS, but professional interest in these clinical applications has declined, and the drugs are not employed now. (It should be added that experiments with the synthetic derivatives of marijuana are only useful as tests of derivatives themselves and do not constitute a study of the effects of marijuana, as used in its traditional form; the synthetics have different, though related, effects. In devising, say, a urine or blood test to detect whether a person involved in an accident has smoked marijuana, the drug proper must be used, for that is the form in which it is used most frequently.) What effects synthetic tetrahydrocannabinol (first synthesized at Princeton University in 1966 and in Israel in 1967) will have on marijuana research is difficult to say.

Marijuana smoking was probably introduced into the United States by Mexican laborers in the early twentieth century and by merchant seamen of Latin American descent into New Orleans in the 1920s, although it was known by the Indians before Columbus. The practice was largely ignored by state authorities (although several states had laws against it) until the mid-thirties, when reports of a "crime wave" in New Orleans involving schoolchildren high on "muggles" received much publicity. In 1937, goaded by lurid publicity about marijuana-induced crimes and the testimony by the then Commissioner of Narcotics, Harry Anslinger, that marijuana was criminogenic, Congress passed the Marijuana Tax Act modeled after the HARRISON NARCOTICS ACT. Hearings on the bill produced only one witness opposed to the bill (aside from representatives from the birdseed industry—marijuana seeds were used to feed pigeons—who succeeded in having sterilized marijuana seeds excluded from the ambit of the statute), and Commissioner Anslinger's testimony was controlling. The assertion that marijuana use caused criminal activity was later dropped, and in 1951, during the hearings on amendments to United States narcotics laws, Commissioner Anslinger testified that the real danger of marijuana was that its users inevitably proceeded to HEROIN addiction (in 1937 he had said that marijuana users and heroin addicts were entirely different classes).

Despite efforts of the Federal Bureau of Narcotics, use of marijuana steadily increased, spreading from Latin American, black, and musician subcultures to middle-class users, especially college youths from urban areas. Meanwhile the legitimate cultivation of marijuana in the country rapidly declined from its peak during World War II, when Japanese conquests cut off Asian sources of hemp and stimulated domestic cultivation of *Cannabis sativa* for the fibers obtained exclusively from the male plant. The return of Manila hemp to the domestic market after the war and the increasing use of substitutes such as nylon has displaced the use of *Cannabis sativa* for this purpose, and the plant is no longer legally cultivated. Difficult to kill, it grows wild in several states, however.

In the 1950s marijuana use was given a literary boost in the writings of the "beat generation," which effected a sort of literary bridge between marijuana use among the lower classes and jazz musicians and among intellectual, student, and middle-class circles. The use in colleges, and later high schools, increased in the 1960s, becoming a fad, and current estimates are that 40 percent of the student body has experimented with the drug at least once. An estimated 24 million people have tried marijuana in the United States, and 8.3 million continue to use it. These numbers are heavily concentrated in the 18–25 age group. Concomitant with this increase in the number of middle-class users (some of whom have been sent to prison for violation of federal or state marijuana laws), a growing body of opinion has urged that the nation's marijuana laws be made less harsh. Chief target of these efforts was the state and federal narcotics laws which placed sale, transfer, or possession of marijuana in the same category as that of OPIATES and COCAINE. (Parallel to this, federal arrests on marijuana possession charges declined, although efforts against traffickers presumably continued unabated.)

Proponents of changes in the laws argued that marijuana could more properly be classified as a HALLUCINOGEN—although this is somewhat inaccurate, for only high doses cause usually brief hallucinations. Other arguments for outright repeal (in the extremist wing) or modifications of the law included assertions that marijuana was less dangerous to health than alcohol and cigarettes—and perhaps less habit-forming than the latter; that Commissioner Anslinger's characterization of marijuana use as inevitably leading to heroin addiction was belied by the large percentage of marijuana

smokers who do not go on to heroin (24 million marijuana experimenters compared with 250,000 or so heroin addicts); that
falsely exaggerating the dangers of marijuana makes youths skepti-
cal of warnings about other drugs, which may be more dangerous;
that prohibition encourages the illicit traffic and gives the drug a
"forbidden fruit" allure; and that marijuana smoking is a harmless
private pleasure in the pursuit of which the government has no
business interfering.

Arguments against changing the laws include the Bureau of
Narcotics' stubborn claim that 75 to 80 percent of the heroin addicts
began their drug use with marijuana; that marijuana is still an
intoxicant whose effects are more unpredictable and uncontrollable
than alcohol; that our society is already too obsessed with "escape"
drugs, whether prescription pills or alcohol, and does not need
another intoxicant; that marijuana is not completely innocuous and
that habituation (PSYCHIC DEPENDENCE) occurs and heavy usage may
be physically harmful; that if marijuana were sold commercially,
Madison Avenue advertising techniques like those employed with
cigarettes and alcoholic beverages would increase use of marijuana
until it reached the scale of a national problem; and, finally, that this
country is a signatory to United Nations treaties discouraging the
export and import of cannabis and, further, that the World Health
Organization is opposed to the use of cannabis and American pres-
tige, if nothing else, would suffer, aside from the demands of
international comity.

In the CONTROLLED SUBSTANCES ACT of 1970 Congress made
simple possession of marijuana a misdemeanor; sale and transfer or
possession with intent to sell remained a felony. A report by the
President's National Commission on Marijuana and Drug Abuse
issued in 1972 made an exhaustive study of the drug and concluded
that both federal and state penalties should be ameliorated even
more (and state laws made uniform throughout the country). Specifically, the Commission recommended that simple possession or
transfer when no money was involved should no longer be a crime,
although public possession made users liable to confiscation of their
supplies. It should be pointed out that the Commission was not
advocating "legalization" of marijuana; indeed it advocated curbing
of the traffic in the drug and warned of possible harmful organic
and psychological effects of very heavy use. What it did was merely
to ratify the practice of most federal and state narcotics police who
no longer direct their efforts against possession. President Nixon
decided to reject the Commission's findings.

A Canadian commission studying marijuana concluded that enforcement of anti-marijuana laws did more harm than good. Only a tiny percentage of users were ever prosecuted, leading to a selective enforcement of the law, which could be directed at unpopular political and social groups, especially among the young who are the heaviest users, and which engendered disrespect for the law. The commission also pointed out the high cost of enforcement of such laws, their lack of deterrence, the fact that they impinged primarily upon the young, thus blighting lives by exposing them to the criminal population in the jails, that there was an unjust disparity of sentencing, leading to further disrespect for the law, and that by its very nature, since it involved private transactions between individuals, marijuana use could only be stamped out by repressive laws—as witness the "no knock" provisions introduced into America's drug law, enabling police to enter a home without a search warrant. Since only 2 percent of the marijuana users in the United States are sufficiently heavy users to be considered harmful to themselves or society, it would seem that this country should face up to the question of whether the costs of enforcing strict marijuana laws do not indeed exceed the benefits.

Marijuana's effects are on the near end of a continuum with LSD as its opposite end. Physiological alterations induced by the drug include (within a few minutes of consumption) dizziness, buzzing and cottony sounds, a lightness in the head; followed by dryness of the mouth and throat (probably due to the harshness of the marijuana smoke); unsteadiness in movement, loss of bodily coordination, and a feeling of heaviness in the extremities; hunger and/or a craving for sweets; nausea and vomiting occasionally; sensations of warmth around the head and the body; burning irritation of the eyes; blurring of vision; tightness in the chest; palpitations or rapid beating of the heart; ringing or pressure in the ears; and occasionally an urge to urinate or defecate.

Psychologically, marijuana's effects include vague dread or anxiety or fear of bodily harm, especially among inexperienced users, at the outset, followed by disorientation of thinking, which includes fragmentation of thought patterns, disturbance of memory so that things thought or said immediately slip out of one's mind, and frequent and sudden interruptions in the flow of thoughts—blanks or gaps lasting a few seconds (similar to the "epileptic absence"); a wavelike aspect to the flow of perceptions; euphoria; giggling and hilarity ("fatuous euphoria"); perception of some parts of one's body as distorted; depersonalization (double consciousness), the sense that one is both within and outside oneself; spatial and temporal distortion, i.e., far objects seem near, a minute seems to stretch elastically; feelings of grandiosity (megalopsia) and mystical insight into the true meaning of life, as well as a detached, amused view of cares and suffering; a heightened sensuousness and perception of colors, music, pictures; a more favorable sense of one's worth and an increased sociability; and sometimes, fear, anxiety, or panic. (Such subjective experiences are not common to all users of marijuana and vary also with the amount taken; indeed, some persons get no pleasant reaction to initial amounts of marijuana at all, or else find it unpleasantly dulling and stupefying.) Because marijuana distorts depth perception and sometimes impairs bodily coordination, driving under its influence can be dangerous.

PHYSICAL DEPENDENCE on the drug, it is agreed, does not occur, and there are no withdrawal symptoms. Most of the small samples of users interviewed through the years say that they easily stopped using the drug without any physical symptoms and usually without any strong craving to resume. However, psychic dependence can develop among certain users, usually passive, dependent, perhaps latent schizophrenic types, who seek the mental escape the drug provides in preference to their normal state of consciousness. Such heavy users tend to become indolent, dreamy, and negligent of their jobs and personal appearance. (Such types are more often seen among cannabis users in Morocco and India, where, among certain social groups, use is widespread and accepted.) Dr. P. Kielholz, of the Psychiatric University, Basel, Switzerland, termed the habitual heavy marijuana user a "disinhibiting decrement seeker." The increment seeker, e.g., user of alcohol or AMPHETAMINES, seeks to do more; the decrement seeker seeks to do less.

Marijuana users, then, enjoy the release the drug gives to their thoughts and the breakdown of normal patterns of perception, as well as the intensified sensuousness, relaxation, and release from social inhibitions. At the same time, they usually sit quietly saying little and prefer their introspective flights to seeking out new experiences. Hence, persons whose personality structures were withdrawn and introverted might find in marijuana the mental state and well-being that would be vastly superior to the "real world," in which they were chronically dislocated and ill at ease, and become heavy users.

Such heavy users of the drug generally smoke from six to ten marijuana cigarettes daily, enough to keep them permanently in a state of HIGH. Probably they could stop the habit with relatively little discomfort, although the result might initially be mental unease or perhaps the activation of a latent psychosis. Only a tiny percentage of marijuana users in this country use the drug so heavily (the Presidential Commission estimates that 2 percent—about 166,000 people—of the current users of marijuana use the drug heavily), although such use has been observed in Morocco and India. Marijuana causes no bodily damage (occasional cases of conjunctivitis with heavy use have been reported; chronic, long-term use may cause asthma, chronic bronchitis, or other pulmonary disorders and one experiment has indicated a decrease in white corpuscle production among users), and there is no known lethal dose. When smoked, marijuana has a kind of built-in safety factor, for the smoker regulates his intake ("titration"), finds too much unpleasant, or, after taking large amounts, sinks into a deep sleep. To a large degree, pleasurable use of marijuana is a learned technique. Not only is the novice instructed in inhaling the smoke and holding it in his lungs, he "learns" what he should feel; hence, many novices who experience no feeling at all or feel anxiety and dysphoria may pretend to be high until they have learned to recognize and enjoy the drug's pleasurable effects. The mystique associated with the drug, the experiences recounted by users face to face or in literature, and the desire to be at one with an admired ingroup are usually sufficient for the novice to desire and achieve a positive experience. Perhaps mainly for this reason (rather than any physiological changes induced by continuous use of the drug), only a slight TOLERANCE develops; which is to say that the veteran user will not get so high on so little as the novice will because he is thoroughly familiar with the drug's effects (see DRAGGED).

In this country, acute or chronic psychoses and panic reactions triggered by smoking marijuana appear to be relatively rare, probably at a much lower percentage of incidence than among users of LSD and other of the stronger hallucinogens. Perhaps an indication of their rarity is that no sensational cases have been reported in the press, unlike LSD. When the number of LSD-induced chronic psychoses observed at Bellevue Hospital in New York was increasing during 1966, there were no cases of marijuana psychoses. Again, this factor probably reflects the relatively mild nature of marijuana's effects and also that it is not a new and strange drug (stimulating underlying uneasiness in some users). The customary ingestion by smoking also enables users to control their intake (while they swallow LSD and experience its effects in a sudden onrush); if they smoke a large amount, they will probably fall asleep. Then, too, the socioeconomic level of the majority of users is high, and they perhaps tend to be more educated, stable individuals. Also, the large majority are experimenters and infrequent users. This is not to say that chronic psychoses do not or have not occurred. The studies leading to the La Guardia Report in New York in the early 1940s recorded nine psychotic breaks, of varying duration, among a sample of 200 studied intensely. Most of these were found to be cases of already psychotic personalities, and one of the psychiatrists involved in the study wrote, in 1942, "Marijuana will not produce a psychosis *de novo* in a well-integrated stable person." The team who observed New York's marijuana smokers of the period found them to be a rather passive, peaceful, and friendly group, distinctly not prone to violence (though above average perpetrators of petty crimes).

In countries where the use of cannabis, and especially hashish, is more widespread, clinical studies have shown the occurrence of psychotic breaks, sometimes accompanied by acts of violence and usually associated with a toxic overdose, among a relatively small minority of users. Similarly, criminal acts attributed to cannabis use have been reported in several countries over the years, but most authorities (the Federal Bureau of Narcotics excepted) agree that marijuana plays a very minor role as a cause of major crimes, both in this country and abroad. As for long-term psychoses attributed to marijuana use, again there is little evidence of this in the United States, although investigators in Morocco have identified, among mental patients, a "KIF psychosis." A survey made in 1963 concluded, "The prevalence of *major* mental disorder among cannabis users appears to be little, if any, higher than that in the general population."

Finally, the contention that marijuana smoking in some mysterious fashion "leads" to addiction to opiate drugs is at best a partial truth. The large majority of marijuana users do not use narcotics, either because they have no desire or no opportunity. Younger marijuana smokers often have a contempt for narcotics users or fear of the well-known dangers of ADDICTION and look upon it as "square" or sick. Marijuana is the most readily available drug on campus, followed by the other hallucinogens, pep pills, and miscellaneous drugs. After college the students lose their connections and probably their interest. The general prognosis for heavy marijuana users is that after about twelve years, if they do not get involved with stronger drugs, and otherwise survive the emotional turmoil of adolescence and young adulthood, they will no longer desire marijuana. However, the slackening of motivation attendant to regular use might rarely cause the loss of twelve years out of their lives —enough to blight their entire careers. A more complex relationship between marijuana and narcotics addiction is related to the way of life that use of marijuana introduces the young user into—a life where a variety of illegal drugs are acceptable (why not the ultimate, the BOSS drug, heroin?) and available, or else, especially in slum areas, where use of drugs is related to a need to escape from one's environment and the heroin pusher stands always available on the nearest corner. Such slum users apparently are initiated to drugs with marijuana (though it often is glue sniffing) at a very young age (perhaps because it is cheaper: around 50¢ a cigarette as opposed to $5 for a bag of heroin). Then, in the classic sense, they "graduate" to heroin when they are older, when marijuana seems an inadequate escape mechanism, and heroin promises a stronger—a boss—high, and many of their contemporaries are similarly disposed or already using. Perhaps this is analogous to the "good child" who begins reading comic books, finds them inadequate, and "graduates" to adventure novels, and finally to works of literature—instead of a set of WORKS. For the middle-class child it would be the world of reading, for the slum child the world of HARD NARCOTICS. Both worlds have gradations of pleasure and demands. When that middle-class child who reads has deep personality problems, when drugs become available and an "in" thing, when an obsession with them in all their varieties comes to dominate life so that the various kinds become almost interchangeable, and to be really sophisticated one leaves the "kid stuff" and goes on to heroin, the ultimate super-drug, *then* marijuana is usually a link in the chain clipped at its nether end to the plummeting weight of addiction. Slang names: pot, righteous bush, grass, grifa, gauge, kif, muggles, muta, V., tea, snop, twist, hemp, wheat, hay, juanita weed, herb, yerba.

About 4:30 PM, September 23, I took most of this extract [a tincture of the powdered leaves of male hemp plants grown in the vicinity of Lexington, Kentucky, and "obtained for me by R. B. Hamilton, Esq. to whom my thanks are due for the trouble taken by him to aid my investigation"] which a druggist estimated to contain from 20 to 30 grains [an enormous dose, the effects of which would be more drastic when taken by swallowing—*RRL*]. No immediate symptoms were produced. About 7 PM a professional call was requested and forgetting all about the hemp, I went out and saw my patient. Whilst writing the prescription, I became perfectly oblivious to surrounding objects but went on writing, without any check to or deviation from the ordinary series of mental acts, connected with the process, at least that I am aware of. When the recipe was finished, I suddenly recollected where I was and looking up, saw my patient sitting quietly before me. The conviction was irresistible that I had sat there many minutes, perhaps hours and directly the idea fastened itself that the hemp had commenced to act and had thrown me into a trance-like state of considerable duration, during which I had been stupidly sitting before my wondering patient.

I hastily rose and apologized for remaining so long, but was assured I had only been a very few minutes. About 7:30 PM I returned home. I was by this time quite excited, and the feeling of hilarity now rapidly increased. It was not a sensuous feeling, in the ordinary meaning of the term; it was not merely an intellectual excitation, it was a sort of *bien-être*—the very opposite of *malaise*. It did not come from without; it was not connected with any passion or sense. It was simply a feeling of inner joyousness; the heart seemed buoyant beyond all trouble; the whole system felt as though all sense of fatigue were ever banished; the mind gladly ran riot, free constantly to leap from one idea to another, apparently unbound from its ordinary laws. I was disposed to laugh; to make comic gestures—one very frequent recurrent fancy, was to imitate with the arms the motions of the fiddler and with the lips the tune he was supposed to be playing. There was nothing like wild delirium nor any hallucinations I can remember. At no time had I any visions, or at least any that I can now call to mind; but a person, who was with me at that time, states that once I raised my hand and exclaimed, "Oh the mountains! The Mountains!" Whilst I was performing the various antics, already alluded to, I knew very well I was acting exceedingly foolishly but couldn't control myself. . . . [About 8] my skin to myself was warm, in fact the whole surface felt flushed; my mouth and throat were very dry; my legs put on a strange foreign feeling as though they were not a part of my body. . . . A foreboding, an undefined, horrible fear, as of impending death now commenced to creep over me. . . . [There were] periods when all connection seemed to be severed between the external world and myself. . . wild reveries. . . . The mind seemed freed from all its ordinary laws of association so that it passed from idea to idea, as it were, perfectly at random. . . . I now entirely lost my power of measuring time. Seconds seemed hours; minutes seemed days; hours seemed infinite. . . . The oppressive feeling of impending death became more intense. It was horrible. Each paroxysm would seem to have been the longest I had suffered: as I came out of it, a voice seemed constantly saying, "You are getting worse—your paroxysms are growing longer and deeper—they will overmaster you—you will die."

I felt as if some evil spirit had control of the whole of me, except the will power, and was in determined conflict with that, the last citadel of my being. I have never experienced anything like the fearful sense of almost hopeless anguish and utter weariness which was upon me. Once or twice during a paroxysm, I had what might be called nightmare sensations; I felt myself mounting upwards, expanding, dilating, dissolving into the wide confines of space, overwhelmed by a horrible, rending, unutterable despair. Then with tremendous effort I seemed

to shake this off and to start up with the shuddering thought "next time, you will not be able to throw this off, and what then!"
—Dr. Horatio C. Wood, *"On the Medical Activity of the Hemp Plant as Grown in North America,"* American Philosophical Society Prize Essay (1869)

After I finished the weed I went back to the bandstand. Everything seemed normal and I began to play as usual. I passed a stick of gauge around for the other boys to smoke, and we started a set.

The first thing I noticed was that I began to hear my saxophone as though it was inside my head, but I couldn't hear much of the band in back of me, although I knew they were there. All the other instruments sounded like they were way off in the distance; I got the same sensations you'd get if you stuffed your ears with cotton and talked out loud. Then I began to feel the vibrations of the reed much more pronounced against my lip, and my head buzzed like a loud speaker. I found I was slurring much better and putting just the right feeling into my phrases—I was really coming on. All the notes came easing out of my horn like they'd already been made up, greased and stuffed into the ball, so all I had to do was blow a little and send them on their way, one right after the other, never missing, never behind time, all without an ounce of effort. The phrases seemed to have more continuity to them and I was sticking to the theme without ever going tangent. I felt I could go on playing for years without running out of ideas and energy. There wasn't any struggle; it was all made-to-order and suddenly there wasn't a sour note or a discord in the world that could bother me. . . .

It's a funny thing about marijuana—when you first begin smoking it you see things in a wonderful soothing, easygoing new light. All of a sudden the world is stripped of its dirty gray shrouds and becomes one big bellyful of giggles, a special laugh, bathed in brilliant, sparkling colors that hit you like a heat-wave. Nothing leaves you cold any more; there's a humorous tickle and great meaning in the least little thing, the twitch of somebody's little finger or the click of a beer glass. All your pores open like funnels, your nerve ends stretch their mouths wide, hungry and thirsty for new sights and sounds and sensations; and every sensation, when it comes, is the most exciting one you've ever had. You can't get enough of anything—you want to gobble up the whole goddamned universe just for an appetizer. Them first kicks are a killer, Jim. . . . You know how jittery, got-to-be-moving people in the city always get up in the subway train two minutes before they arrive at the station? Their nerves are on edge; they're watching the clock, thinking about schedules, full of that high-powered mile-a-minute jive. Well, when you've picked up on some gauge that clock just stretches its arms, yawns, dozes off. The whole world slows down and gets drowsy. You wait until the train stops dead and the doors slide open, then you get up and stroll out in slow motion, like a sleep walker with a long night ahead of him and no appointments to keep. You've got all the time in the world. What's the rush, buddy? Take-it-easy, that's the play, it's bound to sweeten that way. . . .

(Before I go any further I want to make one thing clear: I never advocated that anybody should use marijuana, and I sure don't mean to start now. Even during the years I sold the stuff . . . I sold it to grown-up friends of mine who had got to using it on their own, just like I did. . . . Sort of everybody to their own notion, that was the whole spirit. I laid off five years ago, and if anybody asks my advice today, I tell them straight to steer clear of it because it carries a rap. That's my final word to all the cats: today I know of one very bad thing the tea can do to you—it can put you in jail. 'Nuff said.)

—Mezz Mezzrow and Bernard Wolfe, *Really the Blues* (1946)

mary. MORPHINE. *Obsolete.*

mary ann. [variation of MARY JANE. Since the 1920s—*EP*] MARIJUANA. *Obsolete.*

mary jane. [the English of the folklore interpretation of marijuana; since the 1920s—*EP;* i.e., marijuana was sometimes mispronounced with a hard *j,* from which mary *jane.*] MARIJUANA. *Obsolete.*

mary warner. [also from the phonetic resemblance to marijuana, soft *j*] MARIJUANA. *Obsolete.*

mary weaver. [compare MARY WARNER] MARIJUANA. *Obsolete.*

mash Allah. [Arabic, gift of God] OPIUM. Called by this name by eighteenth-century Tartars who used it to sustain themselves and their horses over long journeys.

matchbox. [probably from the use of a large, empty kitchen matchbox to measure lots of MARIJUANA for sale; penny matchboxes were also used.

". . . he gave us a cut-rate price, a tobacco tin full-up with muta for two dollars or a Diamond *matchbox* full for four or five"—*MM.* 1946]

a measure of marijuana for sale; about 1/5 ounce, enough for rolling five to eight cigarettes. Compare CAN, LID, NICKEL BAG.

MDA. [methylenedioxyamphetamine] an amination product of safrol, a psychoactive oil found in NUTMEG and related to the AMPHETAMINES. The effects of MDA were accidentally discovered by G. Alles, the discoverer of amphetamine, who took 1.5 milligrams and saw illusionary smoke rings. Present-day researchers do not regard the drug as a HALLUCINOGEN, since subjects do not report hallucinations, visual distortions, color enhancement, or mental imagery. Instead they experience intensification of feelings, greater desire to communicate, and heightened reflectiveness. The drug has been used in psychotherapy because it also induces age regression—a sense of reliving specific childhood experiences while remaining aware of one's present self. This effect has been induced with other hallucinogens, but with MDA it recurs so regularly and without prompting that it appears to be related to the pharmacology of the drug.

Usual dosages are 150 to 200 milligrams and the effects wear off after seven or eight hours. MDA can be toxic, in dosages of varying amounts, depending upon the individual's sensitivity to it. A regular dose for some may be fatal to others. Deaths have occurred after ingestion of MDA. Experimenters start with a low dose—e.g., 10 milligrams—and gradually increase it until toxic symptoms (skin reactions, profuse sweating, and confusion) appear.

medical hype. [from *hypodermic,* and HYPE, a drug addict] *1.* one who has become accidentally addicted to MORPHINE during medical treatment. *2.* one who obtains drugs, through a legal prescription, from a doctor or a hospital.

meet. [shortening(?) of *meeting*] the appointment between an addict and his PUSHER, always used as a noun, as in "I made a *meet* with him for six."

megahallucinogen. [journalese] STP.

Mepergan. [MEPERIDINE hydrochloride and promethazine hydrochloride, Wyeth Laboratories] a synthetic narcotic analgesic containing meperidine. Manufacturer's rationale for the combination with promethazine is that the latter strengthens the analgesia of the meperidine and consequently a smaller dosage is needed. Thus, addiction is less likely. Whether this is true or not, PHYSICAL DEPENDENCE upon the meperidine will occur if Mepergan is used continuously over a prolonged period. Manufacturer's recommended dose: one capsule every four to six hours. Capsules contain 50 milligrams of meperidine hydrochloride and 12.5 milligrams of promethazine, or, as Mepergan Fortis, 50 milligrams of meperidine and 25 milligrams of promethazine. A Schedule II drug under the CONTROLLED SUBSTANCES ACT. Compare SYNTHETIC OPIATES.

meperidine. [ethyl-*l*-methyl-4 phenylpiperidine-4-carboxylate] a synthetic narcotic analgesic which, despite its structural dissimilarity to MORPHINE, has many similar pharmacological effects when given in equipotent doses. Meperidine was introduced in 1939 and first employed as a substitute for ATROPINE; however, it was soon discovered that the two drugs were unlike in their actions, and meperidine's chief medical use is as an analgesic. Dosages of 80 to 100 milligrams injected intramuscularly give analgesia equivalent to that of 10 milligrams of morphine. The duration of the action is two to four hours, as compared with four to five hours for morphine. Most therapeutic doses range between 50 and 200 milligrams.

The drug has several advantages over morphine which account for its frequent medical use, especially in obstetrics. It does not usually produce constipation or urinary retention and does not induce respiratory depression. The danger of ADDICTION is also considered less, for reasons discussed below. Meperidine occasionally produces undesirable side effects, such as nausea and vomiting (probably less than morphine), giddiness, vertigo, and faintness. In toxic doses meperidine causes excitement of the central nervous system, resulting in tremors, muscle twitches, disorientation, hallucinations, palpitating heart, and convulsive movements.

Large doses of the drug can be taken safely; although the lethal dose is not specified, in one case a dose of 2,000 milligrams was survived, while in another a dose of 1,200 milligrams was fatal. The drug also has a sedative action, although this is apparently brief, the sleep marred by dreams, and large doses are necessary. Meperidine does not produce so much euphoria as morphine and in a painfree patient may produce dysphoria.

PHYSICAL DEPENDENCE and PSYCHIC DEPENDENCE upon meperidine do occur, however, although most addicts vastly prefer morphine or HEROIN and most subjectively cannot differentiate among them. Addiction is most common among hospital personnel (some of whom erroneously believe it to be nonaddictive), and though some may have a euphoric reaction to the drug, many seem to use it for analgesic—sedative effects or simply because it has no "dope addict" stigma.

TOLERANCE to meperidine's analgesic action develops slowly, so patients can be kept on the same dosage for months; however, tolerance to its sedative and other effects occurs more rapidly. Tolerance developing to the excitatory effects of the drug also induces addicts to increase their dosage. On the other hand, tolerance to side effects of meperidine, such as muscle twitching and tremors, may be incomplete, and users will continue to experience them, with the result that their efficiency is impaired. Some meperidine addicts are able to take 3,000 to 4,000 milligrams of the drug a day, although the usual amount is less. One reason meperidine was not at first thought to be addictive is that WITHDRAWAL SYMPTOMS, resulting from abrupt cessation of the drug after physical dependence has developed, are much less severe than those of morphine. Though dissimilar in degree, however, these symptoms are similar in kind to those of morphine dependence. The symptoms reach their peak eight to twelve hours after the last dose, then subside and are completely gone in four to five days. Meperidine addiction also differs from morphine addiction in that the pupils are not pinpointed. Also, meperidine addicts will not respond to the NALLINE TEST, which indicates addiction by inducing withdrawal symptoms in addicts, unless they are using over 1,600 milligrams per day. Ketbemidone, a derivative of meperidine, is thirty times as potent; hence, the addiction liability is much greater, and ketbemidone is not used in medicine. Meperidine is usually known as DEMEROL in the United States; it is called pethidine in Great Britain. Compare ALPHAPRODINE.

Demerol [meperidine] is probably less addicting than morphine. It is also less satisfying to the addict, and less effective as a pain killer. While a demerol habit is easier to break than a morphine habit, demerol is certainly more injurious to the health and specifically the nervous system. I once used demerol for three months and developed a number of distressing symptoms: trembling hands (with morphine my hands are always steady), progressive loss of coordination, muscular contractions, paranoid obsessions, fear of insanity. Finally I contracted an opportune intolerance for demerol—no doubt a measure of self preservation—and switched to methadone. Immediately all my symptoms disappeared. I may add that demerol is quite as constipating as morphine, that it exerts an even more depressing effect on the appetite and the sexual functions, does not, however, contract the pupils. I have given myself thousands of injections over a period of years with unsterilized, in fact dirty, needles and never sustained an infection until I used demerol. Then I came down with a series of abscesses one of which had to be lanced and drained. In short demerol seems to me a more dangerous drug than morphine.

—William Burroughs, *Naked Lunch* (1965)

meprobamate. [2-methyl-2-*n*-propyl-l, 3-propanediol dicarbamate] a nonbarbiturate sedative classified as a MINOR TRANQUILIZER. Meprobamate, under a variety of commercial names (the most prominent of which is MILTOWN), is used with varying effectiveness in the treatment of tension and anxiety states and insomnia resulting from these. As with other TRANQUILIZERS, PSYCHIC DEPENDENCE, or habituation, to meprobamate occurs, especially among patients to whom it becomes a psychic "crutch," producing a state of lethargy and indifference to the stresses endemic in their lives without touching the underlying neurosis. When the daily dosage is stopped —especially if the drug has been used excessively—these patients may suffer a reemergence in magnified degree of symptoms formerly masked by the drug, such as insomnia, anxiety, and loss of appetite.

TOLERANCE to meprobamate's calming effects can occur and prolonged heavy use can result in PHYSICAL DEPENDENCE with physical WITHDRAWAL SYMPTOMS if the drug is withdrawn suddenly, rather than being tapered off. These symptoms resemble BARBITURATE withdrawal symptoms, including tremors, insomnia, gastrointestinal upset, hallucinations, serious epilepticlike convulsions, and sometimes death. The usual daily dosage is 1,200 to 1,600 milligrams; daily dosages above 2,400 milligrams are not recommended by manufacturer.

As with the other depressants, overdose of meprobamate can result in respiratory depression, coma, and death. It has been used in a number of suicide attempts, although fatalities have been rare. Amounts of 20,000 to 40,000 milligrams have been survived; however, alcohol in combination with it may POTENTIATE meprobamate's effects, and the danger of death from respiratory depression is correspondingly increased. Meprobamate is a Schedule IV drug under the CONTROLLED SUBSTANCES ACT of 1970, although experts agree that it has a potential for abuse. Some people become addicted to meprobamate while using it to combat withdrawal symptoms from other drugs, especially alcohol. The drug produces euphoria in some, and this, along with the fact of tolerance and physical dependence, give it a high addiction liability, although manufacturers dispute this. Diversions of the drug into the black market have been reported, and it might well serve as a substitute for barbiturates if controls on the latter are strengthened. At any rate, meprobamate intoxication resembles barbiturate intoxication (there is also CROSS-TOLERANCE between the two drugs)—the user exhibits slurred speech, loss of coordination and muscular control. Users are cautioned not to drive or use machinery. The following are brand names for meprobamate preparations:

Apascil	Calmiren	Cyrpon
Atraxin	Casil	Ecuanil
Biobamat	Cirpon	Equanil

Equanil L-A	Nervonus	Probamyl
Harmonin	Neuramate	Quanil
Mepavlon	Pameco	Quilate
Meproleaf	Panediol	Sedabamate
Meprosin	Perequil	Sedazil
Meprospan	Perquietil	Urbil
Meprotabs	Pertranquil	Viobamate
Miltown	Placidon	

Compare LIBRIUM, VALIUM.

merck. [from Merck, the drug manufacturers] the real thing; quality, high-grade drugs. Compare PHARMACEUTICALS.

mesc. MESCALINE.

mescal. *1.* PEYOTE (compare MESCALINE). *2.* an intoxicating beverage distilled from the maguey plants.

mescaline. [from *mescal,* the surface tops (mescal buttons) of the PEYOTE cactus] the hallucinogenic alkaloid (3,4,5,-trimethoxy-phenylethylamine) extracted from the peyote cactus, *Lophophora williamsii,* or synthesized in the laboratory. The alkaloids in the cactus were first identified in 1886 by Louis Lewin, a German pharmacologist. Like the AMPHETAMINES, mescaline belongs to the amine group. Its chemical structure distantly resembles norepinephrine, which is, in turn, a close relation of adrenalin (epinephrine). Both are mind-altering chemicals which are manufactured in the body and which have activating effects upon certain tissues and organs.

Mescaline induces a variety of alterations of consciousness, sense distortions, and hallucinations rather like in kind to those produced by LSD. Because it generates less nausea, vomiting, and other unpleasant side effects than the peyote cactus, it is preferred, both by illegal drug users and researchers. (Other hallucinogenic drugs which produce no nausea are available.) It is usually ingested in the form of a soluble crystalline powder, which is dissolved, or in a capsule. The standard human dosage of mescaline (producing full effects in a person weighing 150 pounds) is 500 milligrams; the effects appear within two to three hours and last for four to twelve hours or more. (Doses above 1,000 milligrams may provoke toxic reactions.)

TOLERANCE develops to the drug, although more slowly than to LSD. There is also CROSS-TOLERANCE between LSD, mescaline, and PSILOCYBIN; i.e., one who has developed a tolerance to one of those drugs will be tolerant to the others. PHYSICAL DEPENDENCE with WITHDRAWAL SYMPTOMS does not occur. PSYCHIC DEPENDENCE may develop, with the user craving a repetition of the drug's mental effects in a pattern similar to that of the habitual user of LSD. Other dangers of the drug to the individual's mental health are similar to those of LSD, but it is not known what, if any, organic damage the drug may cause.

STP, a close chemical relative of mescaline said to produce more violent and prolonged psychic effects, has been reported in use, while illicit mescaline use is relatively rare; other drugs are frequently falsely represented as mescaline in the illicit market. Mescaline and its derivatives are Schedule I drugs under the CONTROLLED SUBSTANCES ACT.

My ideas of space were very unusual [under the influence of mescaline]. I could see myself from head to foot as well as the sofa on which I was lying. All else was nothing, absolutely empty space. I was on a solitary island floating in the ether. No part of my body was subject to the laws of gravitation. On the other side of the vacuum—the room seemed to be unlimited in space—extremely fantastic figures appeared before my eyes. I was very excited, perspired and shivered, and was kept in a state of ceaseless wonder. I saw endless passages with beautiful pointed arches, delightfully colored arabesques, grotesque decorations, divine, sublime and enchanting in their fantastic splendour. These visions changed in waves and billows, were built, destroyed and appeared again in endless variations, first on one plane and then in three dimensions, at last disappearing in infinity. The sofa-island disappeared; I did not feel my physical self; an ever-increasing feeling of dissolution set in. I was seized with passionate curiosity, great things were about to be unveiled before me. I would perceive the essence of all things, the problems of creation would be unravelled. I was dematerialized.

Then the dark room once more. The visions of fantastic architecture again took hold of me, endless passages in Moorish style moving like waves alternated with astonishing pictures of curious figures. A design in the form of a cross was very frequent and present in unceasing variety. Incessantly the central lines of the ornament emanated, creeping like serpents or shooting forth like tongues towards the sides, but always in straight lines. Crystals appeared again and again, changing in form and colour and in the rapidity with which they came before my eyes. Then the pictures grew more steady, and slowly two immense cosmic systems were created, divided by a kind of line into an upper and a lower half. Shining with their own light, they appeared in unlimited space. From the interior new rays appeared in more luminescent colours, and, gradually becoming perfect, they assumed the form of oblong prisms. At the same time they began to move. The systems approaching each other were attracted and repelled. Their rays were broken into infinitely fine molecules along the middle line. This line was imaginary. This image was produced by the regular collision of the rays against one another. I saw two cosmic systems both equally powerful in appearance and the difference of their structure, and in perpetual combat. Everything that happened in them was in an eternal flux. At the beginning they moved at a giddy speed which gradually changed to a quiet rhythm. I was possessed with a growing feeling of liberation. This is the solution of the mystery, it is on rhythm that the evolution of the world is finally founded. The rhythm became more and more slow and solemn and at the same time more strange and indescribable. The moment drew near when both the polar systems would be able to oscillate together, when their nuclei would combine in a tremendous construction. Then everything would become visible to my eyes. I would experience everything, understand all, no limits would bind my perceptions. A disagreeable trismus tore me away in this moment from the supreme tension. I gnashed my teeth, my hands perspired and eyes burnt with seeing. I experienced a very queer muscular sensation. I could have detached separately every single muscle from my body. I felt great unhappiness and profound discontent. Why had physical sensations torn me from the supremacy of my soaring soul?

However, I had one unshakable conviction: Everything was ruled by rhythm, the ultimate essence of all things is buried in rhythm, rhythm was for me a medium of metaphysical expression. Again the visions appeared, again the two cosmic systems, but at the same time I heard music. The sounds came from infinity, the music of the spheres, slowly rising and falling, and everything followed its rhythm. Dr. B. played music, but it did not harmonize with my pictures and disturbed them. It came again and again, that mighty tension of the soul, that desire of solution, and then each time at the decisive moment the painful cramping of the muscles of the jaw. Crystals in a magic light with shining facets, abstract details of the theory of knowledge appeared behind a misty vaporous veil which the eyes sought to pierce in vain. Again forms appeared fighting one another; in concentric circles, from the middle Gothic, from the outside Romanesque forms. With an increasing jubilation and daring the Gothic pointed arches penetrated between the Romanesque round arches and crushed them together. And again, shortly before the decision, the gnashing of teeth. I was not to penetrate the mystery. I was standing in the midst of the evolution of the universe, I experienced cosmic life just before its solution. The impossibility of understanding the end, this refusal of knowledge was exasperating. I was tired and experienced bodily suffering.

—"an unprejudiced physician who was under the influence of the substance [mescaline]," in Louis Lewin, *Phantastica: Narcotic and Stimulating Drugs* (1964)

meserole. [corruption or misspelling of *mezzrole,* from *Mezz's roll;* Mezz Mezzrow, jazz musician and Harlem MARIJUANA peddler in the 1940s, gave his name to the type of marijuana cigarettes he sold, which were supposed to contain highly potent marijuana in generous amounts] a fat marijuana cigarette. *Obsolete?*

messerole. MESEROLE.

methadone. [4,4-diphenyl-6-dimethylamino-3-heptanone] a SYNTHETIC OPIATE analgesic completely dissimilar in chemical structure to MORPHINE but having similar actions. The drug was synthesized by German chemists (and called DOLOPHINE after Adolph Hitler) and made available in the United States after World War II. It is used in medicine as an analgesic, to suppress the cough reflex, in treatment of heroin or morphine WITHDRAWAL SYMPTOMS, and in maintenance therapy with addicts (the "methadone treatment"; see below).

As an analgesic, methadone is slightly more potent than morphine; doses of 7.5 to 10 milligrams produce relief of pain equal to that of 10 milligrams of morphine, lasting for three to five hours. Methadone produces somewhat less respiratory depression than morphine and, unlike morphine, is nearly as effective in oral doses as in injections. It does not produce so much sedation or euphoria as morphine; however, in pain-free individuals, the drug does have a pronounced euphoric effect in intravenous injections of 10 to 20 milligrams. This effect lasts longer than morphine-induced euphoria and is potentially just as significant in producing PSYCHIC DEPENDENCE. Consequently, addicts sometimes use methadone, especially to forestall heroin withdrawal symptoms, producing a nodding, dozing state akin to a HEROIN NOD; widespread cases of diversion of legal methadone to addicts were reported in New York, and it remains a cheap, available, and effective substitute if heroin is scarce. In New York City in 1973, methadone-connected deaths outnumbered heroin-connected deaths for the first time, reflecting an increase in street methadone (in all cases the user was not in a program) and the decrease in the heroin supply. Some users report unpleasant side effects, including pains in the bones and muscles, nausea, constipation, mental sluggishness, hallucinations, and impotence.

PHYSICAL DEPENDENCE upon methadone occurs after continuous administration, with withdrawal symptoms less severe than those of morphine dependence but more prolonged. When methadone is substituted for heroin and addicts gradually withdrawn from the drug, they will undergo withdrawal symptoms of methadone, rather than those of heroin. For this reason methadone is used in hospitals to withdraw addicts. Addicts also use it, usually in the form of pills ("dollies") as self-medication for withdrawal symptoms, e.g., when they are unable to obtain heroin, or their heroin habit has grown too expensive to support. However, withdrawal symptoms can be severe and include diarrhea and pains in the stomach, hot and cold flashes, insomnia, and sweating. One addict reported: "The pain was excruciating. The marrow of my bones screamed." After the physical symptoms have passed (after about two weeks), the addict may continue to experience lethargy, insomnia, and loss of appetite for months. Narcotic antagonists such as NALLINE will induce more severe withdrawal symptoms in the methadone addict than simple gradual withdrawal of the drug does.

TOLERANCE to methadone's effects develops through continued usage. Because methadone is effective orally and long-lasting (so that patients can be maintained on one dose a day and do not go from extremes of incipient withdrawal symptoms to the excess tranquilization of the "nod"—thus they function better), it is given in this form in maintenance therapy—the so-called methadone treatment. The purpose is to wean patients from heroin by substituting another addiction under medical supervision, thus enabling them to break out of the conditioned life pattern of the heroin addict. Addicts in the program report once daily for their dosage, usually 100 to 180 milligrams in orange juice. Taking it orally, addicts subsequently can inject heroin without any effects since there is a CROSS-TOLERANCE between the two; their dose is also stabilized and they avoid the needle with its risk of infection and whole magical ritual of a FIX. The methadone assuages the addict's subjective craving for heroin and serves as a reasonably satisfactory substitute for it. (Addicts report that the subjective effects of 300 to 900 milligrams of methadone orally equal those of 5 to 9 grains, or 300 to 540 milligrams, of morphine.) Thus methadone taken in large doses creates a tolerance to other opiate drugs, lasting twenty-four to thirty-six hours. If addicts are tempted to take a shot of heroin, they will experience none of the customary euphoria or other pleasurable sensations they used to associate with the drug. The heroin-conditioned response pattern is broken and there is no reinforcement of the habit by any pleasurable effects; thus they have no further motive for taking heroin. (Methadone addicts do, however, sometimes use other depressant drugs, with alcohol being the favorite and BARBITURATES second.) Likewise, addicts are motivated to continue taking methadone, because it is addictive, in the same way they were motivated to take heroin; thus they will continue going to the methadone maintenance center for their daily dose, or be given several days' supply to take by themselves. After they have functioned free of heroin for a sufficiently long time, undergone counseling at the methadone center (if it is available), secured steady employment (if they can overcome society's reluctance to hire methadone patients), and otherwise readjusted their lives away from the addict's characteristic heroin-seeking lifestyle, they theoretically can ultimately be withdrawn from methadone and go on to lead a drug-free life. But, since another benefit of taking methadone is that it quells the post-abstinence syndrome—the depression, anxiety, and hunger for drugs all ex-addicts feel—it may be that such complete abstinence is difficult to achieve, and may not even be desirable. Certainly methadone patients are quite capable of functioning normally on the job and in their families while taking the drug.

How successful is methadone maintenance? The most comprehensive study of such a program was made in New York City covering the years 1965 through 1970. A total of 3,485 patients in the Dole-Nyswander program were studied and it was concluded that the dropout rate was 20 percent, of whom only 3 percent were voluntary dropouts; that 15 percent of the patients continued to use heroin intermittently (even though they presumably got no effect from it); that the crime rate among the patients was dramatically reversed in comparison to their crime rate before methadone—only 5.6 percent were found guilty of criminal offenses; and that the number of patients who held regular jobs—nearly 75 percent-—showed a marked rise. Compared to the 90 percent failure rate of most other drug programs, then, methadone must be counted an almost unqualified success.

Criticisms of the methadone program range from the moralistic belief that addicts should make themselves drug-free by "will power," that the continued administration of an addictive drug merely substitutes one "immorality" for another; other critics say that methadone addicts do not function normally, feel that they are in a drugged state, and complain about various side difficulties such as sexual impotence (but the Nyswander-Dole studies showed most methadone patients became more potent than they were on heroin). Activist groups in the ghetto also contend that methadone keeps the ex-addict in a state of drugged dependence and is thus a subtle form of racism, aimed at blacks and the poor. Since narcotics addicts in poverty areas prey on their fellow poor this argument seems emotional. Lastly, advocates of the various group-therapy and encounter-group programs sometimes say that methadone therapy does not attack the roots of the addicts' problems, which lie in basic defects of character; hence, they have no chance to change themselves and are condemned to a perpetual life on drugs, which, these critics hold, is both psychically and morally an abnormal life, inferior to a life without drugs. Proponents of methadone therapy answer that they do not rule out a multidiscipline approach to drug addiction and that other forms of therapy can also be useful. In sum, the methadone treatment is primarily a chemical therapy that posits a physiological cause for drug addition, which is best treated by a drug that satisfies the addicts' craving and conditions and motivates them off a destructive drug such as heroin and into a more positive program of controlled methadone addiction, coupled with counseling and other services. If the only alternative to drug addiction is total abstinence from all drugs, then methadone maintenance might be considered a failure. But if the aim is to rehabilitate addicts and enable them to hold jobs and function in society, then it has been very successful.

There are efforts to find a chemical alternative to methadone—notably nonaddicting heroin-blocking drugs such as CYCLAZOCINE, naloxone, and naltrexone. These drugs are heroin antagonists, do not produce any euphoria, and if addicts take them daily they will not achieve any effects from heroin. Critics of the drugs point out that it is precisely methadone's addictive qualities and its ability to quell the post-abstinence syndrome that makes it effective, for the other drugs do not assuage the craving and the patient is tempted to skip a dose and go back to heroin. However, if a nonaddicting drug with the other effects of methadone could be found, it would indeed be more desirable.

> We got shots four times a day and an additional barbiturate sedative at night. They gave us a synthetic horror called Dolophine [*methadone*], which was invented in Germany under the Nazis and named after the great Adolph! The ward physician, another polite and good-natured young man, who visited us every morning, told me that it was easier to get off Dolophine than regular opiates. I'm sure he was convinced of it. Everybody not addicted to drugs was convinced of it.
>
> Day by day my dosages were decreased. I felt real discomfort and anxiety only about half an hour before each shot was administered. Sometimes the hack was late in dealing out the medications, and this caused real suffering—pain in the knee joints, eyes out of focus, shortness of breath, palpitation, sweat gushing out of every pore, and too many other calamities to list properly. . . .
>
> After seven days they stopped giving me even Dolophine and I instantly caught a cold. This is a standard development, as is vomiting, diarrhea and sleeplessness.
>
> I stayed thirty days in Lexington and I never slept more than half an hour a night. The nights of the recently weaned drug addict are a special horror, because even after a few minutes' sleep his pajamas and his sheets are soaked with cold sweat. . . .

After vomiting for about ten days I was so dehydrated that I passed out in our room one day, so I was shipped back to the infirmary and . . . I was put to bed and given intravenous glucose, and I was sure that nobody in the whole world had ever been so deathly sick.

—Alexander King, *Mine Enemy Grows Older* (1958)

Methadone is completely satisfying to the addict, an excellent pain killer, at least as addicting as morphine.

—William Burroughs, *Naked Lunch* (1959)

methamphetamine. METHEDRINE, DESOXYN

methaqualone. [2-methyl-3-ortho-tolyl-4-quinzalonone) a nonbarbiturate hypnotic–sedative first synthesized in India in 1951 as an antimalarial drug. When it was observed that it made rats drowsy, it was developed as a soporific. Manufacturers recommend it for people who are allergic to BARBITURATES or CHLORAL HYDRATE —especially elderly people. Although medical usage of methaqualone would thus seem small, the drug became widely prescribed in Great Britain after its introduction in 1965. It was combined with an antihistamine, dephenhydramine, and marketed as Mandrax; by 1968 it was the most widely prescribed hypnotic (doctors believed that, unlike the barbiturates, it was nonaddicting) and over 2.5 million prescriptions were issued. In the United States sales of $3.4 million in 1970 nearly doubled the following year.

Soon after the drug appeared in Great Britain there were reports of poisonings, suicide attempts, and street abuse. Heroin addicts were among the first to appreciate the drug because of the "buzz" it gave them. By 1972 in the United States methaqualone was becoming widely used among illicit users. Advertised as the "love drug" because it allegedly enhanced sexual pleasure, it was especially popular among the young on campuses and in New York City, where its popularity became part of the "juice bar" scene—hangouts that featured music and dancing and sold only nonalcoholic beverages (thus not being required to conform to legal standards for a liquor license). In a survey of drug use among New York City students, it was the most frequently mentioned prescription-type drug.

Methaqualone thus rode in on the tide of increased use of downers (see DOWNIE) in the early 1970s—sedative drugs such as the barbiturates. Typically, users resisted the drug's sedative effects and achieved a mellow, dissociative HIGH: if they took too many, their behavior resembled alcohol intoxication; they would stagger about (in Britain the drugs were called "wallbangers") and ultimately would fall asleep. Although users touted the superiority of methaqualone, it is doubtful that its effects were markedly different from those of barbiturates (like AMYTAL and SECONAL, it is a fast-acting sedative; effects occur within 15 minutes). As a "love drug" it is probably no different from alcohol or other drugs which act on the central cortex of the brain and thus release inhibitions while freeing the more primitive functions of the brain.

Although as late as 1972 manufacturers of the drug claimed that it did not produce PSYCHIC or PHYSICAL DEPENDENCE, this in fact is not true. TOLERANCE to the drug's euphoric effects does develop, causing a tendency to increase the dose. Where physical dependence has developed, there are distinctive WITHDRAWAL SYMPTOMS, similar to those associated with barbiturate dependence. These may be fatal if detoxification is not done under medical supervision. An American expert described the symptoms as follows: "Initial withdrawal signs are headaches and severe cramps, followed by convulsions and possibly stomach hemorrhaging three to five days after discontinuing the drug. Addiction symptoms include irritability, sleeplessness, delirium tremens, mania, and convulsions. If convulsions are not treated, status epilepticus usually develops. To avoid risk of convulsions during withdrawal, patients should be detoxified in a hospital." A British health official warned that one pill a day for two months would result in at least some physical dependence. Perhaps implicitly recognizing this fact, manufacturers sometimes state that the drug should not be used for periods longer than 4 weeks to 3 months. Recommended dosages range from 75 milligrams (for sedation) to 150 to 300 milligrams for sleep. Pills come in 150, 200, 300, and 400 milligrams (the last being PAREST 400, which is highly regarded among users, who call it "super Quaalude" or "super Sopor").

A number of suicides employing methaqualone have been reported. The lethal dose per 150 pounds body-weight is estimated at around 8,000 milligrams, though a dose of 22,000 milligrams has been survived. Dosages of 2,400 to 3,000 milligrams will probably result in dangerous poisoning and coma. Severe poisoning is accompanied by convulsions and vomiting; the former may be so severe as to require treatment with other depressant drugs—a dangerous measure—while the latter could conceivably result in an unconscious persons strangling on their own vomit. Death is frequently caused by acute heart failure. Tolerance to the drug's euphoric effects develops faster than tolerance to its respiratory-depressant effects, which increases the danger of overdose. The frequent practice of combining the drug with alcohol is also dangerous, since alcohol POTENTIATES methaqualone's effects.

In view of the drug's limited medical use and its high potentiality for abuse, strict controls would seem to be the answer. Since the methaqualone in illicit circulation is invariably of the brand-name type, it is obvious that manufacturers' supplies are being diverted into the black market. Federal government drug authorities have already asked that the drug be placed in Schedule II of the CONTROLLED SUBSTANCES ACT, but the manufacturers have been contesting this.

Brand names of methaqualone include: QUAALUDE, OPTIMIL, SOPOR, PAREST, SOMNAFAX, and BIPHETAMINE T. Slang names: sopers, ludes.

"It makes me feel friendly, open and receptive. Other downs just bring me too down. I just fall out, so I have to fight them and by the time I stop fighting them, I'm not high anymore."

"Most people are into speed *or* downs but Quaaludes are a great in-between. They calm me and make me mellow but I can still stay loose and agile. I can also make love on them nicely."

"When I first discovered it, I thought it was the antidote to New York. But I gave it up after I started taking three 150 mg. pills a day and got really jangled. I had incredible muscular tensions, it was as if everything was rubbed raw. When I started throwing things, I decided it wasn't such a good scene after all."

—methaqualone users, quoted in *The New York Post,* August 17, 1972

Methedrine. [methamphetamine hydrochloride (*d*-desoxyephedrine hydrochloride), Burroughs Wellcome & Co.] a central nervous system stimulant, methamphetamine, of which Methedrine is a brand name, was first used widely during World War II by the German army to counter fatigue among the troops engaged in prolonged missions with little sleep possible.

Chemically, methamphetamine is closely related to AMPHETAMINE and norephedrine. It is considered a more potent central nervous system stimulant than amphetamine sulfate (BENZEDRINE) and *d*-amphetamine sulfate (DEXEDRINE). The manufacturer recommends Methedrine as a short-term appetite depressant for loss of weight, in cases of depression, as an analeptic (awakener) in BARBITURATE overdose, and to raise abnormally low blood pressure, e.g., in anesthetized patients. Recommended doses range from 2.5 milligrams three times a day, working up, over a period of weeks, to 30 milligrams a day (for cases of chronic depression). The drug produces euphoria, excitability, feelings of power, aggressiveness, and insomnia. Excessive doses can cause talkativeness, pupil dilation, nervousness, hyperexcitability, insomnia, dryness of the mouth, rapid heartbeat, violent actions, or paranoid delusions. The drug is considered dangerous for patients with high blood pressure, irregular heartbeat, and various cardiac disorders.

Methedrine is a favored drug among habitual amphetamine users, who frequently take it by intravenous injection, which produces an almost instantaneous onset of the drug's euphoric properties (the FLASH or RUSH), which many Methedrine users compare to a sexual orgasm (the drug also acts to delay orgasm in sexual intercourse). Such use can produce a particularly persistent form of PSYCHIC DEPENDENCE: users keep injecting until, after several days without sleep (the RUN), they sink into an exhausted coma (FALLING OUT or CRASH) lasting three to six days. After recovery, they tend to return to using the drug for its euphoric properties; apparently, they do not require sedation from barbiturates to damp down the excitative effects of the Methedrine. Nor do they seek the lulling, narcotizing follow-up effects of HEROIN, like heroin addicts who inject amphetamines mixed with heroin for a heightened initial thrill followed by a NOD (though they may take them at the end of the run in order to sleep). Compare BOMBITA, SPEEDBALL.

Amounts taken range from 1,200 to 3,600 milligrams a day over three to six days and may engender acute or chronic psychoses, paranoia, loss of memory and powers of concentration, or possibly brain damage in the habitual user. Other adverse effects are loss of weight and malnutrition (due to the drug's appetite-depressant effects), and various INFECTIONS from unsterile needles. The user may also engage in violent or self-destructive acts. TOLERANCE to the drug also develops, so that the dose must be markedly increased to achieve euphoria.

Methedrine is sold as 5-milligram scored tablets and ampuls for injection containing 20 milligrams each. A Schedule II drug, CONTROLLED SUBSTANCES ACT. Slang names: meth, speed.

Speed kills   —hippie slogan (1967)

meth freak. [from FREAK, *freakish,* bizarre, unpredictable behavior which the drug induces] a frequent, habitual user of METHEDRINE.

methyldihydromorphinone. also known as Metopon. A semisynthetic analgesic derived from MORPHINE, methyldihydromorphinone is considerably more potent than morphine: 3.5 milligrams produce analgesia equivalent to that produced by 10 milligrams of morphine, lasting four to five hours. Hence, it is of the same potency as HEROIN, but its use among addicts is rare (heroin dominates the illicit market, and the illicit market supplies most addicts). Prolonged use will result in TOLERANCE, PSYCHIC DEPENDENCE, and PHYSICAL DEPENDENCE, with WITHDRAWAL SYMPTOMS at least as severe as those produced by morphine dependence. A Schedule II drug under the CONTROLLED SUBSTANCES ACT.

methyprylon. a nonbarbiturate hypnotic and sedative derived from piperidinedione and chemically similar to GLUTETHIMIDE (DORIDEN), methyprylon is used as a daytime sedative or a hypnotic to induce sleep in insomnia, especially when the patient is allergic to BARBITURATES. Since it is less potent than the barbiturates, larger amounts must be taken, but large doses can cause respiratory depression and death. The drug has been used in suicide attempts. Similarly, prolonged usage can result in TOLERANCE and PHYSICAL DEPENDENCE, with severe WITHDRAWAL SYMPTOMS (major epileptic, or grand mal, convulsions and delirium) upon abrupt cessation of the drug. Chronic intoxication, similar to alcoholic intoxication, can also result from heavy use. A Schedule III drug under the CONTROLLED SUBSTANCES ACT of 1965. Compare NOLUDAR 300.

metopon. METHYLDIHYDROMORPHINONE.

Mexican brown. [from the color; presumably indicating a more mature or longer cured plant than MEXICAN GREEN] a grade of MARIJUANA.

Mexican green. [from the color; presumably indicating low resin content] perhaps the commonest grade of MARIJUANA, emanating from Mexico.

Mexican locoweed. [term prevalent in the southwestern United States; the locoweeds proper, e.g., *Astragalus mollissimus*, cause intoxication in animals] MARIJUANA.

Mexican mushroom. hallucinogenic mushroom, *Psilocybe mexicana*. See MUSHROOMS, SACRED.

Mexican red. [the pills are imported from Mexico and are red in color] Sodium secobarbital, or SECONAL.

mickey. MICKEY FINN.

mickey finn. [from a notorious saloonkeeper in Chicago, circa 1896, a synonym for a double drink; a drink containing KNOCKOUT DROPS or drugged liquor—*EP*] liquid chloral, often in capsule form, mixed with alcohol and given to an unwitting drinker to cause unconsciousness. Compare CHLORAL HYDRATE.

Mighty Joe Young. [from the movie ape] See KING KONG.

mike. a microgram (one-millionth gram), usually as a measure of LSD for purposes of sale or consumption.

> [LSD] sells for between a half-cent to as much as two cents a microgram and you usually take anywhere from 250 to a 1,000 *mikes* a trip.
> —"Ric," "Confessions of a Campus Pot Dealer,"
> *Esquire* (September, 1967)

milk sugar. Crystals of lactose with a sweetish taste, closely resembling HEROIN in appearance and hence used for CUTTING it prior to sale to addicts. Quinine is also often added to imitate heroin's bitter taste, so addicts, who know the drug is diluted, are still unable to estimate how much heroin they are actually getting.

Miltown. [MEPROBAMATE, Wallace Laboratories] a MINOR TRANQUILIZER used in alleviating nonpsychotic anxiety and tension states, as a muscle relaxant, and as an anticonvulsant. Manufacturer's recommended dose is one to two 400-milligram tablets three times daily; total dosages above 2,400 milligrams a day are not recommended, though they have been administered by researchers in cases of severe convulsions, spasm, or anxiety.

Miltown's main action is to depress the central nervous system, hence its calming effects. Like other minor tranquilizers, Miltown does not produce drowsiness or significant respiratory depression in small doses. Massive overdosages, while sometimes resulting in coma, shock, respiratory depression, and death, are less likely to be fatal than those of the BARBITURATES.

PSYCHIC DEPENDENCE upon Miltown can develop among patients who seek its sedative effects, both as an adjunct to sleep and to blur the stresses and strains of normal living. Excessive (1,600–2,400 mg. daily), prolonged use results in PHYSICAL DEPENDENCE, accompanied by WITHDRAWAL SYMPTOMS when the drug is abruptly discontinued, including vomiting, tremors, muscle twitching, and epilepticlike seizures. They can be as serious as those produced by barbiturate dependence.

Miltown is sold as a white scored 400-milligram tablet inscribed with a "W," as a white 200-milligram sugar-coated tablet, and as 400-milligram white coated tablets called Meprotabs. A Schedule IV drug under the CONTROLLED SUBSTANCES ACT. Compare EQUANIL.

minor tranquilizer. A pharmacological and chemical classification (compare MAJOR TRANQUILIZER). The minor tranquilizers are generally not effective in serious psychoses and are used mainly in treating mild to moderate anxiety and tension and undue stress in response to outside pressures. They are commonly divided into three types, determined by their effects (other than the common one of depressing the central nervous system without causing sleep):

1. Those which act mainly on the central nervous system but also relax the skeletal muscles and have anticonvulsant actions (chlordiazepoxide, chlormezanone, diazepam, emylcamate, hydroxyphenamate, mephenoxalone, meprobamate, oxanamide)
2. Those which have antihistaminic and antinausea action (hydroxyzine, buclizine) and are useful in allergy and motion sickness
3. Those which do not belong in type 1 or type 2, have a calming effect, but differ widely in both chemistry and pharmacological action.

The first category, which includes such well-known commercial preparations as LIBRIUM, VALIUM, EQUANIL, and MILTOWN, is the most widely used, with varying degrees of success, both in treating anxiety and as skeletal–muscle relaxants in a variety of therapeutic situations. Often a BARBITURATE will give better results in small "daytime sedative" doses than the minor tranquilizers. Further, experiments have shown that often a placebo is just as effective as the tranquilizer, creating the suspicion that the drug's effectiveness is often due to the patient's faith in what the doctor says it will do.

Nevertheless, the minor tranquilizers are somewhat safer than the barbiturates in that deep coma and fatal respiratory collapse, an ever-present hazard with hypnotics and sedatives, come only after much larger doses. Undesirable side effects include drowsiness, loss of coordination, dizziness, stomach upset, rash, chills, fever, etc. Taken in excessive amounts over long periods of time, the tranquilizers of types 1 and 2 induce PHYSICAL DEPENDENCE with WITHDRAWAL SYMPTOMS equal in severity to those associated with barbiturate dependence, including convulsions and delirium.

PSYCHIC DEPENDENCE upon their mildly euphoric and sedative effects (roughly similar to psychic dependence upon alcohol) also occurs, leading to habitual excessive use. Although they are safer than the barbiturates, large doses can lead to death, and suicide attempts with them have been successful. The minor tranquilizers POTENTIATE the effects of other central nervous system depressants such as alcohol and barbiturates and when used in conjunction with them magnify the dangers of fatal respiratory collapse; i.e., the lethal dose of alcohol and barbiturates is lowered. Compare RESERPINE.

miss emma. [from morphine. M, em, emma, Miss Emma; since around 1925—*EP*] MORPHINE.

M.J. [from MARY JANE] MARIJUANA. *Obsolete?*

MMDA. [3-methoxy-4, 5-methylene dioxyphenyl isopropylamine] an amination product of MYRISTICIN, a psychoactive oil in NUTMEG. MMDA differs from MDA only in that it has a methoxyl group in its chemical formula. Researchers claim that while MDA stimulates the reexperiencing of incidents in one's past, MMDA intensifies pleasant or unpleasant feelings in the present. The effects of MMDA have been analyzed by Claudio Naranjo, a Chilean psychiatrist who has used them both with patients:

> Broadly speaking . . . I will consider the effects of MMDA as belonging to five possible states or syndromes: one which is subjectively very gratifying and may be regarded as a particular kind of peak experience; another where habitual feelings and conflicts are magnified; a third and fourth in which feelings are not enhanced but physical symptoms or visual imagery are prominent; and, lastly, one of lethargy or sleep. . . .
> The MMDA peak experience is typically one in which the moment that is being lived becomes intensely gratifying in all its circumstantial reality, yet the dominant feeling is not one of euphoria but of calm and serenity. It could be described as a joyful indifference, or, as one subject has put it, "an impersonal sort of compassion"; for love is embedded, as it were, in calm. . . .
> While awaiting the first effects of MMDA, the patient felt uneasy and somewhat afraid of looking ridiculous, but to his own surprise, he gradually entered into the state of calm enjoyment which is typical of the more pleasant experiences with the drug: "like not needing anything, like not wanting to move, even; like being tranquil in the deepest and most absolute sense, like being near the ocean, but even beyond; as if life and death did not matter, and everything had meaning; everything had an explanation, and nobody had given it or asked for it—like being simply a dot, a drop of honey—pleasure radiating in a pleasurable space."   —Claudio Naranjo, *The Healing Journey* (1974)

mojo. [from a "disguise" or codeword for morphine, a play with *morph,* which is more obscure; since around 1930—*EP;* another theory has it that *mojo* is a voodoo word for magic; drugs are magic] HEROIN, COCAINE, or MORPHINE.

monkey. [from MONKEY ON (MY) BACK, addicted to a drug] an addict's drug dependence, regarded as so independent of his will as to be a separate person living inside him.

The addict needs more and more junk to maintain a human form . . .
buy off the *Monkey.*   —William Burroughs, *Evergreen Review* (1960)

monkey on (my) back. [from *monkey,* a Chinaman, since around 1912—*EP;* and perhaps a variation of the phrase *have a Chinaman on one's back,* meaning to have a drug habit, have WITHDRAWAL SYMPTOMS. Chinese immigrants to the United States in the nineteenth century frequently used opium and became associated with the opium habit] *1.* to be physically dependent upon OPIUM, MORPHINE, or HEROIN. *2.* to undergo OPIATE WITHDRAWAL SYMPTOMS. Compare KING KONG, MIGHTY JOE YOUNG.

monoamine oxidase (MAO) inhibitors. central nervous system stimulants, related chemically to the AMPHETAMINES and used as psychic mood elevators. The stimulation these drugs produce is indirect and thought to arise from their inhibitory action on the flow of monoamine enzymes (compare SEROTONIN). There are four main types of MAO inhibitors in current medical use: isocarboxazid (Marplan), mialamide (Niamid), phenelzine dihydrogen sulfate (Nardil), tranylcypromine (Parnate), and pargyline hydrochloride (Eutonyl).

The drugs are employed in psychotic depressive states where other drugs and electric-shock treatments have not proved effective. The MAO inhibitors are potent, unpredictable drugs, capable of producing a variety of side effects. They are particularly dangerous, and deaths have resulted from administration in conjunction with the following drugs, whose effects they POTENTIATE: ALCOHOL, AMPHETAMINES and other stimulant drugs, NARCOTIC and other depressant drugs, antihistamines, sedatives, anesthetic drugs, and insulin. Also, deaths have been caused by eating cheese while taking MAO inhibitors. They may also have toxic effects on the liver, brain, and cardiovascular system. Other complications include cerebral hemorrhage, convulsions, tremors, insomnia, excessive perspiration, hallucinations (rare), confusion (rare), and high blood pressure, sometime followed by death. Because of their myriad dangers, the MAO inhibitors are administered only under conditions of constant medical supervision. Compare IBOGAINE.

moocah. [variation of (?) MUTA or (?) MU] MARIJUANA. *Obsolete?*

moon. *1.* PEYOTE; the circle of lumps, or buttons, making up the top of the peyote cactus. *2.* a cake of HASHISH, the form in which hashish is sold in bulk on the illicit market.

moota. [variant spelling (?) of MUTA] MARIJUANA. *Obsolete?*

mooters. [from MUTA] MARIJUANA cigarettes. *Obsolete?*

mootie. [from MUTA] MARIJUANA; a marijuana cigarette. *Obsolete?*

morning glory seeds. the seeds of certain members of the large bindweed family *(Convolvulaceae)* have been used for centuries in America for their hallucinogenic effects. The Aztecs called the active varieties OLOLIUQUI or TLITLILTZEN. The former is believed to be the morning glory *Rivea corymbosa,* and the latter a morning glory of the genus *Ipomoea.* Both species are still used by Mexican Indians.

The seeds, which are either brown or black, are ground until reduced to a flour, which is soaked in cold water for a set period of time. Then the water containing the drug is strained through a cloth and drunk. Like their forebears, the Indians use the drug for divination, religious ceremonies, and healing (the content of the visions is analyzed and the cure determined). In the United States the seeds are available commercially, and trade names include HEAVENLY BLUES, FLYING SAUCERS, and Pearly Gates.

Analysis (by Albert Hofmann, discoverer of LSD-25) has shown the seeds to contain amides of lysergic acid, *d*-isolysergic acid amide, chanoclavine, and clymoclavine, all of which are also found in the fungus ergot, *Claviceps purpurea,* from which Hofmann first synthesized LSD. Hence, the ACTIVE PRINCIPLE in the seeds is quite similar to LSD and about 1/10 as potent; 300 Heavenly Blue seeds give the effects of about 200 to 300 micrograms of LSD-25.

The seeds are ingested after grinding them up more or less as the Indians did; by eating the seeds whole (seedsmen claim to have added a nauseating ingredient to the seeds, which makes this method extremely unpleasant; even without the ingredient, some nausea is produced); or by extracting the active principle chemically, using such highly toxic chemicals as wood alcohol. The seeds have also been used as the source of lysergic acid in the illicit manufacture of LSD-25 in home laboratories, along with other chemicals.

Cases of acute, chronic psychotic reactions, similar to those caused by LSD, following ingestion of morning glory seeds have been reported, although their use among illicit drug users is probably relatively rare, since LSD or MARIJUANA is preferred.

A suicide related to the morning glory seed psychosis was studied by Dr. Sidney Cohen. A student chewed 300 Heavenly Blue seeds and experienced the characteristic depersonalization, pseudo hallucinations, feelings of wonderment and self-transcendence, and grandiose fantasies for about twenty-four hours; then, for the next three weeks, he found himself sliding into a dissociation state at frequent intervals. These states were very unpleasant, and he feared he was going crazy. Despite sedation the condition persisted. One morning, feeling himself going off balance again, he became over-wrought, dressed, got into his car, and drove down a hill at a speed estimated at 90 to 100 miles an hour, crashing to his death into a house at the bottom.

> When it is drunk, it provokes lasciviousness. . . . The priests of the idols used to eat of this plant when they wanted to deal with the devil and to have answers to their doubts. They became mad and saw a thousand phantoms that appeared to their eyes. . . . It is not a great mistake to leave unsaid where it grows because it is not important . . . that the Spaniards know the plant.
>
> —Hernandez on the use of morning glory seeds
> among the Indians, *Historia plantar.*
> *Novae Hispaniae* (1721)

This patient first learned of the hallucinogenic effects of *morning glory seed* ingestion through a newspaper article cautioning against the use of the seeds. He first tried the Heavenly Blue variety *(Rivea corymbosa)*, but later preferred the Pearly Gates variety *(Ipomea [sic] violacea)* because they provided more dramatic effects. After finding that four inges-tions (using approximately 200 to 300 seeds) did not produce a "high" quickly enough, he prepared an injectable dose. By boiling 200 seeds in water, he developed a brown, oily fluid containing many small parti-cles. Using a 10 cc. syringe, he drew the fluid up through a wad of cotton which he used as a filter. Frightened by the appearance of the liquid, he used only 0.5 cc. instead of the 10 cc. he had originally intended.

The results were dramatic. Within seconds he was stiffened and "jolted back" in his chair. He experienced a feeling of "nothing-ness" and "negate thought." He repeatedly asked himself, "Am I high?" but could not decide. He became fascinated with his bodily movements and desired to move very slowly, imagining himself doing a primitive African tribal dance. There seemed to be "more substance" to his head than to the rest of his body, and his head seemed detached from his shoulders. He moved the rest of his body carefully under his head to prevent it from falling on the floor.

He said he felt "very human," i.e., no longer estranged from others; "very compassionate," i.e., optimistic and loving everyone and everything. About ten minutes after injection of the solution, he de-veloped a "catatonic feeling" and desired to remain completely still. He felt pain if he moved rapidly. While in this state he noticed that shadows on a marble wall about 60 feet away seemed to be "undulat-ing" or "creeping across the wall."

He thought that he could make a darkened doorway light up as if a searchlight had been turned on it, and he began to experiment with this, believing himself to be very powerful. Within a few moments, the light fixtures in the ceiling and one end of a balcony began to droop. He could make them bend but only to a certain point, after which they reassumed their "reality positions."

During this time, he was not frightened, because he knew that the changes in perception and sensation were not real and would not occur unless he made himself "receptive" to them. One half hour after the injection, he suddenly developed nausea, vomiting, diarrhea, and chills. He craved sugar, and obtained a soft drink which nauseated him. He was unable to see clearly. Subsequently, he developed frank shock with a drop in blood pressure to 60/40 mm. Hg.

He was taken to an accident ward. After supportive treatment for shock, his condition improved promptly, except for blurring of vision, which persisted for several hours.

One month later the patient reported that the perceptual distortions recurred when he was fatigued or distracted. He believed he had permanently damaged his brain. Four months following the original injection, the patient reported that he was powerfully attracted to the drug, that the sensations could be made to return at will, that at times the sensations returned against his will, and that despite this, he planned to continue the use of psychotomimetic drugs.

—P. J. Fink, M. J. Goldman, and I. Lyons,
Archives of General Psychiatry (1966)

morning shot. WAKE-UP. Compare EYE OPENER.

morph. MORPHINE.

morphine. [from Morpheus, god of dreams] a natural alkaloid in OPIUM, occuring in proportions of about 10 percent of the total weight, with analgesic properties. Morphine was first isolated from opium in 1803 by Sertürner, who named it (and whose wife died from an overdose of it), and first received widespread use in this country during the Civil War (see ARMY DISEASE). It was used in Hong Kong as a "cure" for opium addiction, until it was discovered that morphine was even more addictive. It is still considered one of the most useful drugs in the medical armamentarium for the relief of nearly all kinds of pain (in sufficient doses), especially continuing, dull pain. Morphine acts directly on the central nervous system and also on the bowel muscles (hence its constipating effect).

The usual dosage in mild to moderate pain is 5 to 10 milligrams, producing an analgesia that lasts four to five hours, and no sedation. In severe pain doses of 15 to 20 milligrams, sometimes higher, are given. Injected intravenously, morphine reaches its peak within twenty minutes, but the analgesia is shorter in duration. The preferred method of administration is by subcutaneous injection, with analgesia occurring after sixty to ninety minutes and lasting the maximum amount of time. Taken orally, morphine is not so potent, though the analgesia lasts longer; 60 milligrams orally produces a peak analgesia somewhat inferior to 8 milligrams injected.

Physiological effects produced by the drug include constipation, nausea, sometimes vomiting, constriction of the pupils, heaviness of the limbs, itchiness of the face and nose, yawning, warmth in the stomach, respiratory depression, sweating, flushing of the skin, and fall in body temperature (occurrence of these effects varies with the individual). The drug's psychological effects include analgesia, drowsiness, impairment of mental and physical performance, especially complex learned behavior, reduced sex and hunger drives, changes in mood, mental clouding, sometimes excitation, inability to concentrate, sometimes apathy, and euphoria. This last effect is attributed to the drug's action in dramatically relieving pain, discomfort, worry, and anxiety. (Given to a person free of pain, the drug's effect may be unpleasant.) Although morphine's precise pharmacological action within the body to relieve pain is not known, the drug does seem to depress a pain center in the cortex and does so without affecting the other senses of touch, taste, hearing, etc. Psychologically, it seems to operate to raise the perceived threshold of pain (especially if given before the pain, or preoperatively); i.e., patients cannot feel a degree of pain they would have perceived without morphine. Second, the drug relieves the anxiety and fear associated with pain, so that while the pain is known to be there, it can be regarded with equanimity and detachment. Although in small doses morphine does not induce sleep, in larger doses it will; this, in turn, can operate as an effective antidote to pain. Hence, morphine differs from general anesthetics in that it (1) produces analgesia without inducing sleep and (2) depresses the respiratory center, while anesthetics stimulate it. It differs from hypnotics and sedatives in that (1) it has no anticonvulsant action and (2) it does have an analgesic action, which sedatives do not have.

As the dosage increases to the 15- to 20-milligram range, drowsiness increases, followed in time by a deep sleep; the euphoria is also intensified, as is the vomiting reaction. Respiratory depression becomes more marked, and indeed death from respiratory failure is the chief hazard of morphine, aside from addiction. An overdose of morphine, then, results in a magnification of the symptoms seen in lesser doses: profound coma, very slight respiration, markedly constricted pupils, marked fall in body temperature, cold and clammy skin, shock, and flaccid skeletal muscles. The lethal dose of the drug varies from individual to individual; in the pain-free, nonaddicted adult, however, an oral dose of less than 120 milligrams or an injected dose of less than 30 milligrams will not cause any serious toxic reactions. Where TOLERANCE has developed, this allowable dosage will of course go much higher.

Tolerance develops specifically to the depressant effects of the drug on the nervous system but not to some of its other effects, such as constipation, constriction of the pupils, and excitation. Tolerance to the depressant effects usually develops after two to three weeks of daily dosages; it develops more rapidly if a clockwork regularity of dosage is followed or if relatively large doses are administered. (As an interesting sidelight to the development of tolerance, it has been shown that the morphine antagonist NALLINE will precipitate WITHDRAWAL SYMPTOMS in a person who has been taking 15 milligrams of morphine three or four times a day after only three days, which indicates that the mechanisms of PHYSICAL DEPENDENCE are already at work, even though the addict will not be aware of them for weeks or months.)

Once tolerance has set in, the user can take rapidly increasing doses without adverse effects, and cases of addicts taking 4,000 to 5,000 milligrams a day, or nearly 200 times the dose that is dangerous to the normal, pain-free adult, have been reported. This tolerance is not unlimited, however, and as a general rule, the longer the time and the greater the amount of the drug used, the more severe the physical dependence and resultant withdrawal symptoms when the drug is discontinued.

Since the advent of HEROIN, a semisynthetic derivative of morphine, the use of morphine among the addict underworld has declined. The subjective effects of the two drugs in equipotent doses are almost identical. The differences seem to be in potency, mode of ingestion, and what the addict is used to. Heroin is more potent —three or four times as potent as morphine, analgesically, i.e., less is needed to produce analgesia. It also produces more euphoria and excitation than any other OPIATE drug. Also, heroin is more potent when it is injected intravenously (the favored mode of addicts because it produces the quickest effect and thus the way they habitually experience the drug) than when it is injected subcutaneously (although, paradoxically, it produces less euphoria). Just the opposite is true with morphine, which may explain why addicts offered a choice between the two with which they have been injected intravenously, without knowing which drug they are getting, tend to choose heroin even when both drugs are given in equipotent doses.

The total amount of illegal morphine seized by the Bureau of Narcotics in 1964 was 140 grams, compared to 45 kilograms of heroin. When used by addicts, morphine is most commonly in the form of a salt, e.g., morphine sulfate (the origin of M.S., a slang term for morphine), which is soluble in water and hence injectable. Pure morphine is only slightly soluble in water. The drug is also swallowed in capsules, taken through the rectum in suppositories, drunk in solution, or heated and inhaled.

Experiments have shown that *d*-AMPHETAMINE injected with morphine counteracts the depression, weakness, and dizziness usually caused by morphine while enhancing its analgesic action; addicts have discovered this medical fact for themselves and hence the frequent combination of the two drugs (also amphetamines with heroin or COCAINE with morphine or heroin). Morphine is a Schedule II drug under the CONTROLLED SUBSTANCES ACT. Slang names: M, morph, dreamer, Miss Emma, M.S.

morpholinylethylmorphine. PHOLOCODINE.

mota. [Mexican, MUTA] MARIJUANA.

mother. *1.* a drug peddler, or PUSHER. *2.* MARIJUANA.

M.S. MORPHINE sulfate. *Obsolete?*

mu. [from (?) MUTA] MARIJUANA.

muchamor. [Siberian Indian] FLY AGARIC.

muggles. [from (?) smuggle—*EP; since around* 1930] MARIJUANA cigarettes. *Obsolete.*

multihabituation. also called panaddiction; poly-drug use. Using two or more drugs interchangeably or simultaneously in an attempt to counteract the adverse effects of one with the other or to POTENTIATE the effects of one with the other or both, so that an interdependent habit is formed. The heavy drinker who habitually uses BARBITURATES or TRANQUILIZERS to relieve his hangover, so that he becomes dependent upon both, has a multihabituation. More common is the combined use of AMPHETAMINES and barbiturates or the two with alcohol. The barbiturate-dependent person may begin increasing his dose as tolerance builds up, in order to sleep; this increased dose leads to a morning-after barbiturate hangover, and so he begins taking amphetamines to counteract the morning drowsiness and enable him to function in society. The increased use of amphetamines may in turn so overstimulate him that he requires more barbiturates to sleep, increasing the morning-after hangover, and so on in a vicious circle. Methamphetamine (METHEDRINE) addiction has become common. The addict tries to correct every defect in his life with this and sedative drugs—a "lift" in the morning, a sedative during the day, another lift, another sedative, etc. The HEROIN user may become multihabituated—or addicted—to barbiturates because the weak doses of heroin on the market do not give him the NOD he wants, and he supplements it with barbiturates, with the result that he develops a PHYSICAL DEPENDENCE on barbiturates that may have graver WITHDRAWAL SYMPTOMS than those caused by his heroin dependence. Patients in METHADONE treatment programs sometimes resort to barbiturates, amphetamines, or alcohol to replace the heroin high they can no longer achieve.

muscarine. an alkaloid found in the hallucinogenic mushroom FLY AGARIC, *Amanita muscaria*. Muscarine may be the hallucinogenic ACTIVE PRINCIPLE in the mushroom; other authorities claim that it is BUFOTENINE, which in turn is closely related to the hallucinogen dimethyltryptamine (DMT) and PSILOCYBIN.

Muscarine is a deadly poison which acts to slow the heartbeat and dilate the blood vessels. In lethal amounts (usually as a result of eating the mushroom), death ensues within a few hours; toxic symptoms (weeping, salivation, sweating, constriction of the pupils, severe abdominal pain, vertigo, watery and painful bowel movements, coma, occasionally convulsions, etc.) occur within two minutes to two hours. ATROPINE is an effective antidote to muscarine poisoning if administered in time and is effective in the majority of cases. More deadly is the related mushroom *Amanita phalloides,* which contains a different, slower-acting, yet more uniformly fatal alkaloid.

mushrooms, sacred. various species of fungi growing in the Western Hemisphere with hallucinogenic actions. The mushrooms were used by the Aztecs for visions and hallucinations and as a sacrament in religious ceremonies (they called it *teonanactl,* God's flesh) and are still used today by Mexican Indians for divination and religious worship. Several species of mushrooms with hallucinogenic properties were identified by R. Gordon Wasson and Roger Heim, in 1953, and there are probably others still unclassified. The most widely used and studied of all these is *Psilocybe mexicana,* a small tawny mushroom which grows in marshy pastures, often in cow pats. Other species include *Conocybe siliginoides, Psilocybe aztecorum, P. zapotecorum, P. caerulescens,* and *Stropharia cubensis.* Albert Hofmann, discoverer of LSD-25, analyzed *P. mexicana* and in 1958 isolated its hallucinogenic alkaloid, PSILOCYBIN (the phosphoric acid ester of 4-hydroxydimethyltryptamine, a close relative of

BUFOTENINE and SEROTONIN and with an indole position identical with LSD-25). Hofmann also synthesized psilocybin. The alkaloid has since been found in *Stropharia cubensis* and in other species of *Psilocybe*.

Indians who use the mushroom in religious rites usually ingest (by eating) twelve of the mushrooms, which have an unpleasant bitter taste and an acrid odor. The initial reactions are nausea, muscular relaxation, coldness of the limbs, dilation of the pupils, and then abrupt mood changes, often characterized by wild hilarity. After this come the visions—brilliant colors, shapes, geometric patterns, and myriad scenes sometimes perceived as if from a lofty height, as well as aural hallucinations. They last four to five hours and are followed by lassitude, mental and physical depression, and a loss of time and space perception.

> [The visions] were in vivid color, always harmonious. They began with angular art motifs, such as might decorate carpets or wallpaper or the drawing board of an architect. Then they evolved into palaces with courts, arcades, gardens—resplendent palaces all laid over with semi-precious stones. Then I saw a mythological beast drawing a regal chariot.
>
> Later it was as though the walls of our house had dissolved and my spirit had flown forth, and I was suspended in mid-air viewing towering landscapes of mountains, with camel caravans advancing slowly across wide slopes, the mountains rising tier above tier to the very heavens. . . . They were sharply focused, the lines and colors so sharp that they seemed more real to me than anything I had ever seen with my own eyes. . . .
>
> The Senora stood up in the darkness where there was an open space in our room and began a rhythmic dance with clapping or slapping. . . . The claps or slaps were always resonant and true. So far as we know she used no device, only her hands against each other or possibly against different parts of her body. . . . We think the Senora faced successively the four points of the compass, rotating clockwise, but we are not sure. One thing is certain: this mysterious percussive utterance was ventriloquistic, each slap coming from an unpredictable direction and distance, now close to our ears, now distant, above, below, here and yonder, like Hamlet's ghost.
>
> —R. Gordon Wasson, in *The Drug Takers* (1965)

muta. [from (?) Spanish *mudar,* to change—*EP*] MARIJUANA.

myristicin. also called ELEMICIN. Hallucinogenic substance in NUTMEG. See MMDA.

N n

nab. an arresting officer, policeman.

nail. [variant of SPIKE] hypodermic needle; addicts usually affix it to a medicine dropper and use the rubber bulb to inject the drug.

nail-polish remover. adolescents sometimes inhale the fumes for their intoxicatory effects. Compare BENZINE, CARBON TETRA-CHLORIDE, CLEANING FLUID, GLUE SNIFFING, DELIRIANTS.

Nalline. [nalorphine hydrochloride (*N*-allylnormorphine hydrochloride), Merck, Sharp & Dohme] a semisynthetic derivative of MORPHINE, first synthesized in 1941, which has no analgesic action and which acts to reverse the effects of morphine and other synthetic and semisynthetic opiates. Its primary action is as a narcotics antagonist which counters the depression of the central nervous system and especially that of the respiratory system induced by OPIATE drugs. Hence, it is valuable in cases of opiate OVERDOSE (but not in BARBITURATE or other drug-induced respiratory depressions). In conjunction with morphine or opiates, Nalline acts to prevent respiratory depression and promptly abolishes already existing respiratory depression. Usually respiration is restored to normal in two to three minutes. Dosages of 5 to 10 milligrams are usually effective; larger doses (30 to 40 milligrams) more completely reverse the action of the narcotic drug.

In persons who have not taken any narcotics, small doses of Nalline produce relaxation and drowsiness, similar to that from whiskey or MARIJUANA; larger doses cause slurred speech, racing thoughts, panic, anxiety, lethargy, hallucinations, pallor, nausea, heaviness of the limbs, and respiratory depression. Thus, Nalline is a depressant drug itself, yet it acts to antagonize other depressant drugs of the opiate type. In addicts Nalline precipitates WITHDRAWAL SYMPTOMS, which is the basis for the NALLINE TEST. Nalline does not cause PHYSICAL DEPENDENCE or withdrawal symptoms upon discontinuance after long-term administration. A Schedule III drug under the CONTROLLED SUBSTANCES ACT. Compare LEVALLORPHAN.

Nalline test. a test using NALLINE to ascertain whether a paroled addict who has been withdrawn from narcotics has returned to using them. Since it is a narcotic antagonist, Nalline reverses the effects of any narcotic present in the system; hence it precipitates WITH-DRAWAL SYMPTOMS by reversing the depressant action of the narcotic. This serves to unleash the symptoms of PHYSICAL DEPENDENCE just as if the addict had abruptly stopped taking the drug.

The severity of the withdrawal symptoms is directly proportional to the amount of Nalline administered (and also varies somewhat with the drug addicted to). Hence, to avoid precipitating severe withdrawal distress, the Nalline test is begun with a small dose (3 milligrams), which usually precipitates a minor syndrome; if none is observed, the dosage may gradually be increased. The California Department of Correction uses a circumscribed form of the Nalline test on all paroled or outpatient addicts. A dosage of 3 milligrams is injected, and if the pupil dilates (the addict's pupils will be constricted before the injection) by 1/2 millimeter, the patient is presumed to have become readdicted. (In nonusers Nalline constricts the pupils.) If the California test is positive, urine tests are made to establish the actual presence of the narcotic in the system. Nalline precipitates unusually strong withdrawal symptoms in METHADONE addicts, stronger than the normal symptom; it has no effect on MEPERIDINE addicts unless they are taking more than 1,600 milligrams of the drug a day (sixteen to twenty times the usual analgesic dose). Its effectiveness in detecting CODEINE or other OPIATE addiction is not known. Compare LEVALLORPHAN.

nalorphine. NALLINE.

naloxone. a synthetic narcotics antagonist similar in chemical structure to OXYMORPHONE. Naloxone is used in the treatment of narcotics OVERDOSE because it reverses the respiratory–depressive action of opiate drugs. It is not effective in nonopiate overdose, such as those that are BARBITURATE-induced. There is no evidence thus far that naloxone causes PSYCHIC or PHYSICAL DEPENDENCE; TOLERANCE does not develop. Nor does naloxone produce any of the analgesic or euphoric actions of the opiate drugs, and indeed the manufacturer states that it exhibits no pharmacological actions, in the absence of narcotic drugs. If the patient is physically dependent upon narcotics, however, naloxone will produce withdrawal symptoms. To combat narcotics-induced respiratory depression, naloxone is injected in doses of 0.4 milligram (1 milliliter); this dose can be repeated as necessary. See METHADONE.

narc. a federal, state, or local narcotics officer.

Narcan. NALOXONE hydrochloride, Endo Laboratories.

narco. *1.* U.S. Public Health Service (Narcotics) Hospital, Lexington, Kentucky. *2.* any narcotics treatment center to which the addict may be committed. *3.* a federal, state, or city narcotics policeman.

narco fuzz. a federal, state, or city narcotics officer.

narcotic. [from Greek *narkotikos,* benumbing.] *1.* any drug that numbs the senses, induces lethargy and drowsiness or coma in large doses, and relieves pain. As defined by United States narcotics laws: addictive drugs, including OPIUM, MORPHINE, and CODEINE; their derivatives; SYNTHETIC OPIATES; and COCAINE and ECOGNINE (although the last are not addictive in the sense of causing PHYSICAL DEPENDENCE and are stimulant rather than narcotic in their action). Compare ADDICTION.

narghile. [Turkish] a water pipe used for smoking tobacco or CANNABIS, especially HASHISH. The smoke is bubbled through the water, thus cooling it and alleviating the harshness characteristic of cannabis smoke. Compare HOOKAH.

nark. NARC.

natch, on the. [from *natch,* natural] not using drugs; leading a natural life as opposed to a life centered around chemicals.

natch trips. [from *natural*] HIGHS, produced by natural substances such as NUTMEG, banana pulp, MACE, cinnamon, green peppers, wild rice, or peanut skins. Smoking or drinking in hot water are the preferred modes of consumption. These substances are of dubious psychopotency.

natéma. [South American Indian] BANISTERIOPSIS CAAPI.

nebbie. NEMBUTAL capsule.

needle. hypodermic needle used for injecting drugs.

needle freak. one who will inject almost anything, reputedly getting part of his pleasure from the needle itself.

needle park. a traffic island at Sherman Square, corner of West 71st Street, junction of Broadway and Amsterdam Avenue, that was a meeting place and hangout for drug addicts in New York City.

negative. a BUMMER, a BAD TRIP.

Nembutal. [pentobarbital sodium, Abbott Laboratories] a short-acting BARBITURATE hypnotic and sedative. The sedative dosage is 30 to 50 milligrams two to three times a day; the recommended hypnotic dose is 100 milligrams. TOLERANCE to the drug's action, especially its hypnotic action, builds up over a period of continuous use. PSYCHIC DEPENDENCE upon the drug's hypnotic and sedative (and sometimes euphoric or excitatory) effects can occur. PHYSICAL DEPENDENCE occurs after prolonged usage in amounts several times the hypnotic dose.

Since pentobarbital is metabolized through the liver, taking it when the liver is impaired means danger of acute intoxication and possibly fatal respiratory depression. Nembutal is sold in 30-milligram all-yellow capsules bearing a symbol representing a lowercase *a;* 50-milligram capsules with yellow cap and white bottom, *a* symbol on the white part; and 100-milligram all-yellow capsules bearing the *a* and the word "Abbott" on the cap. A Schedule II drug under the CONTROLLED SUBSTANCES ACT. Slang names:nebbies, nemmies, nemish, yellow jackets, yellows.

nemish. NEMBUTAL capsules.

nemmies. [since around 1938—*EP*] NEMBUTAL capsules.

Neurosine. [sodium, potassium, ammonium, and zinc bromides in combination with other ingredients, including hyoscyamus and BELLADONNA, Dios Chemical Company] a nonbarbiturate hypnotic, sedative, and anticonvulsant. Recommended dosage is 1 to 2 teaspoonfuls a day, which manufacturer says is 33 3/4 grains of bromides, equal in combination to 45 grains of any bromide separately. Overdosages or prolonged use can result in bromism (rash and mental disturbances).

nickel. *1.* five dollars. *2.* a NICKEL ($5) BAG. *3.* five-year sentence, as in "the judge gave me a *nickel* at K.Y." Compare DIME, QUARTER, CENT.

nickel bag. *1.* a $5 measure of heroin diluted to roughly 3 percent with quinine and/or MILK SUGAR; total weight is roughly 1/100 ounce, or 310 milligrams, or 5 grains. The average nickel bag contains 5–10 milligrams of heroin, or the equivalent of 15–30 milligrams of MORPHINE, the dose for medium to severe pain. In times of heroin shortage (PANIC) a nickel bag may sell for $10 or more. *2.* a $5 package of MARIJUANA, roughly 1/5 to 1/7 ounce and yielding five to eight marijuana cigarettes depending upon how CLEAN it is, i.e., how free it is of waste material (seeds, twigs, stems). Compare CAN, DECK, DIME, LID, MATCHBOX, PAPER, FIVE-DOLLAR BAG.

nimby. NEMBUTAL, a BARBITURATE.

nitrous oxide. also called nitrogen monoxide. A general-acting inhalant anesthetic. It was discovered in 1776 by Priestley, but use as an anesthetic did not come until the mid-nineteenth century. The gas's primary action is on the central nervous system to effectively obliterate the perception of pain. Nitrous oxide does not depress the central respiratory center, however, like MORPHINE; in fact, it stimulates it. Its action is clearly anesthetic and does not arise from asphyxiation. It is most effective analgesically as a general anesthetic in medical practice. Because it does not induce sufficient muscle relaxation for major surgery, has a low anesthetic potency, plus danger of anoxia, it is often used in minor surgery, in childbirth, as a preinduction anesthetic (followed by ether), or in conjunction with other analgesic drugs.

Nitrous oxide is sometimes used nonmedically for its consciousness-altering effects; it produces giddiness, hilarity and hallucinations. Such use, or abuse, suggests the possibility of PSYCHIC DEPENDENCE (see the quotation below), but occasional use is probably the rule, and undoubtedly harmless. The chief danger of nitrous oxide and its harmful effects arise from the anoxia produced by sustained inhalation unaccompanied by adequate oxygen. When the pure gas is inhaled, anoxia will set in after about two minutes and can result in death from oxygen deprivation, from heart failure, or pulmonary edema ("drowning" due to bodily fluid accumulating in the lungs), or in organic brain damage resulting in personality change and psychosis. Anoxia is usually accompanied by cyanosis (blueness of the skin), although not in anemic persons. Cyanosis is accompanied by slow pulse, rise in blood pressure, twitching of the muscles, and violent respiration; then respiration becomes shallow and irregular and finally ceases altogether. The heart continues to beat after respiration has stopped, so that resuscitative measures are usually successful, although permanent brain damage may occur. Reawakening from normal anesthesia is rapid—within one to three minutes—and the gas is completely out of the system within five to ten minutes. Nitrous oxide alone is not considered useful as an anesthetic.

> A Grand Exhibition of the Effects Produced by Inhaling Nitrous Oxide, Exhilarating or Laughing Gas!
>
> Men will be invited from the audience, to protect those under the influence of the Gas from injuring themselves or others. This course is adopted so that no apprehension of danger may be entertained. Probably no one will attempt to fight. The effect of the gas is to make those

who inhale it either: Laugh, Sing, Dance, Swear or Fight—according to
the leading trait of their character. They seem to retain consciousness
enough not to say or do that which they would have occasion to regret.
   N.B. The Gas will be administered only to gentlemen of the first
respectability. The object is to make the entertainment in every respect
a genteel affair.   —broadside, dated 1845

High on Laughing Gas
I've been here before
the odd vibration of
the same old universe

the nasal whine of the dentist's drill
     singing against the nostalgic
     piano Muzak in the wall
insistent, familiar, penetrating
     the teeth, where've I heard that
     asshole jazz before?

The universe is a void
in which there is a dreamhold
The dream disappears
     the hole closes

It's the instant of going
into or coming out of
existence that is
important—to catch on
to the secret of the magic
     box

Stepping outside the universe
     by means of Nitrous Oxide
anesthesizing mind-consciousness
     the chilicosm was an impersonal dream—
one of many, being mere dreams,
     the sadness of birth
     and death, the sadness of
changing from dream to dream,
     the constant farewell
     of forms . . .
          saying ungoodby to what
didn't exist
The many worlds that don't exist
all which seem real
all joke
all lost cartoon   —Allen Ginsberg, "Laughing Gas,"
                                 Kaddish and Other Poems (1961)

A chemist gradually acquired the habit of inhaling every day a small quantity of nitrous oxide (laughing gas). At the beginning the sweetish smell of the gas was very unpleasant, but he slowly became used to it. In order to be able to inhale the gas at all times he fitted a small apparatus to the reservoir from which he could easily take a whiff. This gave rise to a permanent state of inebriety, the source of extremely pleasant sensations. He had wonderful dreams in which he saw beautiful landscapes, marvellous figures and scenes. The young man soon began to neglect his duties, but could not renounce his passion. He went mad and ended in an asylum.

—Louis Lewin, *Phantastica: Narcotic and Stimulating Drugs* (1964)

Nixon. low-potency narcotics.

Noctec. [CHLORAL HYDRATE, E.R. Squibb and Sons] a nonbarbiturate hypnotic and sedative. Recommended dose for sleep is 500 to 1,000 milligrams. Sold in red 250- and 500-milligram capsules, and as a syrup. Noctec is apparently the form in which chloral hydrate appears in the illicit market.

nod. [from the characteristic lolling of the head] a drowsy, dreamy dozing state following the injection of an opiate drug and due to its sedative action. Most HEROIN addicts seek this effect and take enough to achieve it if possible. Compare GOOFING.

It is, first of all, useful to see that there are three levels of the *nod* corresponding to the unconscious, pre-conscious, and conscious levels in the Freudian topography of the mind. In the very deep nod there is true oblivion; then, moving up, there is the less intense nod in which a man is vaguely aware of the life both inside and outside himself; finally, there is the superficial nod in which he is fitfully awake and asleep, and often falsely conscious of what is happening around him. In the deep nod the man loses touch with the reality outside, and in the superficial nod he is easily irritated into angry awareness.

There is no doubt that the nod is valued as such by addicts. They prefer to nod rather than to sleep. Sleeping, they say, keeps a man from enjoying the nod.

The nod is therefore the culmination of the shot and represents the narcotization and apparent stimulation which the addict craves. It represents the end of striving, the cessation in varying degrees of all troubled reflection as well as the abandonment of all other projects except that of the quest for apparent euphoria and homeostasis.

The nod produces anguish because its standards are ever escalating beyond the capacity of the addict to be satisfied. In the nod, at any of its levels, the addict experiences an expectation of a certain stimulus, and it is in the nature of heroin addiction that as time goes on the nod becomes harder and harder to achieve. This is a Sisyphian task, doomed to failure and anguish, this attempt to meet the internalized expectations of the nod.

—Seymour Fiddle, *Portraits from a Shooting Gallery* (1967)

nodding. In a state of NOD, the head lolling forward, slowly jerking up and down.

nod, on the. going off into a NOD.

Noludar 300. [METHYPRYLON, a piperidine derivative (3,3-diethyl-5-methyl-2,4-piperidinedione), Roche Laboratories] a nonbarbiturate hypnotic and sedative. Manufacturer recommends for insomnia in doses of 200 to 400 milligrams, with 400 milligrams per day the maximum taken. In conjunction with alcohol, Noludar may lower resistance to the latter and POTENTIATE its effects. It also dulls mental alertness, so driving a car or operating machinery should be avoided after taking it. As with the BARBITURATES, PSYCHIC DEPENDENCE upon the sedative effects of the drug can occur. PHYSICAL DEPENDENCE with WITHDRAWAL SYMPTOMS similar in severity to those associated with barbiturate dependence can occur after prolonged, excessive use. Death has occurred from overdoses of Noludar. Sold as 300-milligram capsules, with an amethyst top and white bottom bearing the word "ROCHE," and also as 50- and 200-milligram scored tablets bearing the word "ROCHE." A Schedule III drug under the CONTROLLED SUBSTANCES ACT.

noscapine. a natural alkaloid of OPIUM in the benzylisoquinoline group, similar to PAPAVERINE. It is nonaddictive and unlike members of the phenanthrene group (MORPHINE, CODEINE, etc.), has no analgesic, gastrointestinal, or central nervous system depressant actions. Because of its mild suppressive action on the cough reflex, it is used in cough medicines. A Schedule IV drug under the CONTROLLED SUBSTANCES ACT.

number two sale, the. [narcotics police term] the second conviction for narcotic sales, which carries a much severer penalty (under federal law it is ten to forty years, compared to five to fifteen for the first sale).

Numorphan. [OXYMORPHONE (dihydrohydroxymorphinone) hydrochloride, Endo Laboratories] a semisynthetic derivative of MORPHINE with analgesic action. Oxymorphone has a more potent analgesic effect action than morphine. A dose of 1 to 1.5 milligrams results in equivalent analgesia to that produced by 10 milligrams of morphine. PHYSICAL DEPENDENCE occurs after continuous, frequent use. WITHDRAWAL SYMPTOMS are similar to those associated with morphine dependence in severity. Numorphan is sold in solution for injection, rectal suppositories, and in 10-milligram tablets. A Schedule II drug under the CONTROLLED SUBSTANCES ACT.

nutmeg. the dried seeds of the East Indian evergreen tree, *Myristica fragrans,* family *Myristicaceae,* to which the hallucinogenic snuff-producing genus VIROLA also belongs. Taken in powdered form, nutmeg has mind-altering properties. A dose of 10 grams (1/3 ounce) can produce a mild, brief euphoria, accompanied by light-headedness, floating feelings, and central nervous system stimulation—an effect very roughly akin to that produced by one MARIJUANA cigarette. Sometimes tension and fear are also experienced. Over 10 grams will often produce unpleasant results, including rapid heartbeat, excessive thirst, agitation, anxiety, and sometimes acute panic. Hallucinations are rare.

The ACTIVE PRINCIPLE is believed to be ELEMICIN (MYRISTICIN), which is chemically close to the HALLUCINOGEN TMA. Other authorities state that nutmeg contains a compound of the dimethoxy group related to STP and MESCALINE. Nutmeg is commonly used as a drug substitute by prisoners (perhaps because it can be stolen from the kitchen), who drink it or MACE in hot water, and by teen-agers seeking a substitute for illegal drugs. See MMDA.

> I recently got a visit from a "beatnik" acquaintance who smokes marijuana frequently and has tried other drugs. I asked him if he had heard that *nutmeg* was a narcotic, and he replied, "We've known about that for years!" He explained that he and many of his friends had tried nutmeg several times, taking it both as snuff and by mouth. They didn't think it was very good, however, because "you either get very sick or have a horrible experience." He said that people who blow pot sometimes take nutmeg when they can't get marijuana.
> —student, quoted by Dr. Andrews T. Weil, "The Use of Nutmeg as a Psychotropic Agent," *Bulletin on Narcotics* (1967)

> Well, it [nutmeg] is peculiar, it's a kind of drunkeness, I suppose, in a way you would call it a hallucinatory experience, but mostly it is just being wacked out of your head, sort of. It's really not a specially pleasant high. There are certainly wild distortions of perception and the brain functions, sort of in spirts and spasms. It's interesting, you mix it with hot beverages or so, and then it takes some time to come on. It can take one hour or two before you really feel it . . . . You take it in coffee or hot chocolate, then it tastes better; in hot chocolate it tastes quite nice. But you really have to take a lot. You have to take at least a teaspoon of that powder. And you will get sick as well as high, more or

less simultaneously. And you will not feel right the next day either. It is not exactly a hangover, but you will not feel quite right. Maybe we took too much when we took it. But it is pretty violent. Sort of disrupting the mental processes.

—ex-addict, interview with Haidi Kuhn, September, 1973

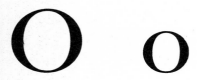

O. OPIUM in raw form.

Op. OPIUM.

O.D. OVERDOSE, whether fatal or nonfatal, of an opiate or other depressant drug, producing a coma, respiratory depression, and sometimes death, unless appropriate medical supportive measures are taken.

O.D.-ing. exhibiting symptoms of an OVERDOSE.

off. *1.* to kill. *2.* HIGH on a drug. *3.* get rid of.

off artist. a TAKE-OFF ARTIST, a thief.

oil. liquid extracted from HASHISH resin, high in TETRAHYDROCANNIBINOL.

ololiuqui. [Nahuatl, round thing, pellet] Aztec name for the hallucinogenic seeds of *Rivea corymbosa.* See MORNING GLORY SEEDS.

on. [from *turned on;* or, simply, *on drugs*] using drugs.

"I wish I had me some stuff."
"You *on* man?"   —Piri Thomas, *Down These Mean Streets* (1967)

one and one. using both nostrils, as in "she blew the coke *one and one.*"

on the needle. injecting narcotics.

opiate. a natural or semisynthetic derivative of the juice in the unripe seed pods of the OPIUM poppy, *Papaver somniferum,* such as MORPHINE, HEROIN, CODEINE. Compare SYNTHETIC OPIATES.

opioid. synthetic substance with pharmacological action similar to that of MORPHINE. Compare SYNTHETIC OPIATES.

opium. [from Greek *opion,* poppy juice] the milky exudate of the incised, unripe seed pods of a poppy, *Papaver somniferum,* which is dried in the air to form a brownish gummy substance. The effects of opium (dulling of pain, euphoria, detachment from the anxieties of existence) have been known to man since prehistoric times. The opium poppy was probably first cultivated in Asia Minor and used medically in Egypt, whence its use spread to Greece. The first reference to its pharmacology occurs in the writings of Theophrastus in the third century B.C. In the *Odyssey* Homer may have meant it by "the drug of Sleep and forgetfulness" (our word *nepenthe*). Arab traders carried it to India and China, where it was used medicinally (to suppress dysentery) and for pleasure. Opium addiction spread rapidly in China, while in Turkey soldiers commonly used it before going into battle in the belief that it gave them added courage and endurance.

In the eighteenth century the Chinese government attempted to prohibit the importation, sale, and use of opium, so harmful had the habit become. The British, however, who were conducting a profitable trade in opium grown in India, opposed the ban, an action which led to the Opium War (1839–1842). One result was the legalization of opium in China and its cultivation by the Chinese government. Many Chinese emigrants carried the opium habit with them wherever they settled and introduced the practice of opium smoking into the United States.

Meanwhile, the medical use of opium to relieve pain, suppress coughing, act as sedative, and counter diarrhea grew apace. In the early part of the sixteenth century the physician Paracelsus had compounded a tincture of opium called LAUDANUM, which became a standard drug. Dover's Powder, concocted by the English physician Thomas Dover as a remedy for gout in 1732, and the "brown mixture" (opium and licorice), compounded by the American Dr. Barton, in 1814, two other staple remedies containing opium, followed, and by the end of the nineteenth century it was estimated that 1 in 400 Americans (mainly housewives) were addicted to it.

Doctors awoke to the problems of ADDICTION, and laws were passed making opium available only through a doctor's prescription. In 1914 the HARRISON NARCOTICS ACT placed opium under federal regulation. With the advent of MORPHINE (1803) and HEROIN (1897), opium smoking in the addict underground gave way to consumption of these more powerful alkaloids and semisynthetic derivatives. Opium smoking is practiced mainly in China, Hong Kong, and

Southeast Asia, where American soldiers were introduced to it during the Vietnam War. Crude opium becomes much more valuable when it is converted to heroin, and hence its movements in the illicit drug traffic are mainly to this end. Opium is grown in Burma, Turkey, Mexico, Communist China, Thailand, Lebanon, Laos, and Cambodia. The raw opium gum is converted to smoking opium by a simple heating process. It is sometimes eaten but mainly smoked, the smoker characteristically lying down (to lessen nausea and stupor) on a pallet furnished by the owner of the establishment—the "opium den" of lurid journalism.

In the United States the illicit use of opium is mainly confined to such standard remedies as PAREGORIC (opium and camphor) and opium tincture (laudanum), which addicts use when they cannot obtain heroin. (Nonaddicts sometimes mix opium with HASHISH or smoke ordinary cigarettes which have been soaked in paregoric and dried out.) Since opium's chief actions on the central nervous system and the bowel muscles are caused by its natural alkaloid morphine, the latter is most widely used in medical practice because it can be standardized and made soluble for injection. In medical opium, morphine must make up 10 percent of the total weight; consequently, 60 milligrams of opium will give analgesic effects equivalent to 6 milligrams of morphine. The PHYSICAL DEPENDENCE which results from long-term use of opium of course results from the actions of morphine. Other alkaloids found in opium are as follows:

class	alkaloid	average percent weight in opium
phenanthrene	morphine	10.0
	codeine	0.5
	thebaine	0.2
benzylisoquinoline	papaverine	1.0
	narcotine (noscapine)	6.0
	narceine	0.3

Only the phenanthrene class of alkaloids is significant in producing opium's characteristic narcotic actions and in inducing addiction. Opium addiction produces WITHDRAWAL SYMPTOMS comparable to those produced by morphine dependence in severity; an addict's inexorably increasing TOLERANCE to opium, necessitating inexorably increasing doses, means that one will take anywhere from 20 to 40 grams of the drug a day, or 200 to 400 milligrams of morphine, enough for a very severe habit. On the other hand, opium smoking carries a much lower addiction liability than intravenous injection of heroin. A Schedule II drug under the CONTROLLED SUBSTANCES ACT.

Optimil. [METHAQUALONE hydrochloride, Wallace Pharmaceuticals] a nonbarbiturate hypnotic and sedative. Manufacturer recommends doses of 200 or 400 milligrams one-half hour before bedtime to induce sleep. Optimil is sold in 200-milligram capsules with an opaque pink cap and clear pink body and 400-milligram capsules with an opaque powder, blue cap, and clear pink body.

ounce man. a HEROIN distributor on the upper level, next in line to the KILO CONNECTION or the PEOPLE; the ounce man buys kilos of heroin from the kilo connection, who has cut it once; the ounce man cuts it again and sells to the DEALER.

outfit. addict's equipment for injecting drugs, especially HEROIN, i.e., needle, syringe or medicine dropper, COOKER, strap, etc. Compare COOKING, FIX, GIMMICKS, WORKS, KIT.

overcharged. in a state of drowsiness or semicoma from a heavy ingestion of a drug.

overdose. ingestion of an OPIATE, stimulant, or hypnotic–sedative drug in larger amounts than the system has acquired TOLERANCE to. Since such drugs act to depress the central nervous system, the result of an overdose is often coma and death from heart failure, respiratory depression, and cessation of breathing, or such complications as pneumonia, pulmonary edema (fluid in the lungs), or heart failure. Deliberate BARBITURATE overdose is one of the leading methods of suicide in the United States; other related hypnotic–sedatives such as DORIDEN, LIBRIUM, VALIUM, METHAQUALONE, CHLORAL HYDRATE, etc., are also used. Accidental overdose through DRUG AUTOMATISM or combination of a sedative drug with alcohol, which will POTENTIATE the depressant effects of the sedative, are also significant causes of fatalities. Although the lethal doses of barbiturates for the prolonged user who has acquired tolerance and for the nonaddict are similar in quantity, the HEROIN, METHADONE, or MORPHINE addict acquires a tolerance to the respiratory depressant effects of those drugs to a much greater degree, so that the addict is taking without ill effects ten to twenty times what would be a lethal dose for a nontolerant person. Nevertheless, fatal heroin or morphine overdose is the leading hazard of the addict's life.

Sometimes addicts do indeed find themselves at a point where their tolerance is low; perhaps they have been withdrawn from heroin. Then, too, pushers sometimes sell addicts suspected of being informers relatively uncut heroin, or, to escape arrest, "dump" their uncut heroin on the market. The amount of heroin in bags can vary widely, and any mixture containing more than 20 percent heroin presents the likelihood of an overdosage. Lastly, of course, the addict may be a beginner, imitating a veteran addict. But all these cases are relatively rare.

Instead, it is more likely that deaths listed as due to overdoses are misnomers; they are simply deaths associated with heroin usage which do not have a determinable cause. Addicts have been found with needles in their arms, indicating death was instantaneous, yet death from respiratory failure caused by an overdose of an opiate drug takes from one to twelve hours. Further the bags and syringes found in the vicinity of those who die from such causes have been analyzed and found not to contain more than the usual amount of heroin. Since the usual amount of heroin in one bag is 5–10 milligrams and the addict with tolerance can take many times this amount without harm, death from an overdose would be impossible. Finally, pulmonary edema has been found in a number of these deaths —something that is not present in a simple overdose.

As a result of these findings, medical examiners now prefer the term "acute reaction" (which of course does not explain the cause of death). They note indications of a severe shock or perhaps allergic reaction to the fatal injection. It has been hypothesized that the quinine that is mixed in with the heroin might be the instigating agent of such a reaction. Further, when a number of cases were analyzed it was learned that many of them had been drinking alcohol. The possibility is that the use of alcohol or barbiturates among addicts when heroin supplies are low may thus be the real contributing factor. Whatever the cause, the implication is clear: the hazards of heroin use—especially adulterated "street" heroin accompanied by MULTIHABITUATION—are greater than they would be if the cause of death was simply administration of more heroin than the system could tolerate. Certainly the death rate from overdose—or acute reaction, or whatever—has shot up in the last few years. There were over 1,200 such deaths in New York City alone in 1971; overdose is the cause of more than 80 percent of addict deaths and is the leading cause of death of *all* persons between the ages of fifteen to thirty-five in New York City. (The number of such deaths showed a gradual decline between 1972 and 1973, however, while methadone deaths rose.)

Symptoms of simple heroin overdose include extreme sleepiness, frequent yawning, coma, pinpointed pupils, cyanosis (blue skin), gasping as if something were caught in the throat, shock, and either deep, extremely slow respiration or very rapid shallow respiration. Overdosage can be immediately reversed by the use of a narcotics antagonist such as NALLINE, LEVALLORPHAN, or NALOXONE. Addicts, to whom such drugs are not available, resort to a variety of home remedies such as icy baths, placing snow on the genitals, walking the victim around, and the injection of milk or salt solutions. In view of the efficacy of the narcotics antagonists, such home remedies would seem illusory, if not dangerous. There is no known treatment for the overdoses of the acute reaction type, and indeed death is so nearly instantaneous that none could be administered in time.

overjolt. OVERDOSE.

over the hump (go). [since around 1930—*EP*. Sometimes meaning, in women, achieving orgasm] to feel the full exhilaration of a narcotic. *Obsolete?*

oxycodone. also called dihydrohydroxycodeinone. A semisynthetic derivative of MORPHINE, oxycodone is close to it in potency: an injection of 10 to 15 milligrams will produce analgesia equal to that of 10 milligrams of morphine and lasting four to five hours. Prolonged use will produce PHYSICAL DEPENDENCE, with WITHDRAWAL SYMPTOMS comparable to those of morphine dependence in severity. A Schedule II drug under the CONTROLLED SUBSTANCES ACT. Compare EUCODAL, PERCOBARB, PERCODAN.

oxymorphone. also called dihydrohydroxymorphinone. A semisynthetic derivative of MORPHINE which is a much more potent analgesic than the latter. A dose of 1.0 to 1.5 milligrams injected subcutaneously produces analgesia equal to that produced by 10 milligrams of morphine, lasting four to five hours. Oral doses of 10 milligrams and intravenous doses of 0.5 milligram produce similar results. Oxymorphone has 100 times the analgesic potency of MEPERIDINE (DEMEROL). PHYSICAL DEPENDENCE occurs after prolonged use, with WITHDRAWAL SYMPTOMS equal to those of morphine dependence in severity.

oz. an ounce of a drug.

O.Z. an ounce.

P p

P. PEYOTE.

packed up. HIGH on a drug.

pad. [from the mats upon which OPIUM smokers lie, since around 1930—*EP;* also, perhaps from similar pads used by MARIJUANA smokers in the Harlem tea pads of the 1940s] room used for taking narcotics or marijuana, usually in a private residence. (Now, of course, the specialized drug-taking meaning has been replaced by the more general slang sense of one's room, house, or apartment.)

Palfium. [DEXTROMORAMIDE bitartrate or hydrochloride] a SYNTHETIC OPIATE.

Pall Mall and paregoric. cigarettes soaked in PAREGORIC, dried out, and then smoked, producing a mild OPIATE euphoria. (Not to be identified with any one brand of cigarette.)

panaddiction. MULTIHABITUATION.

Panama. PANAMA GOLD.

Panama (Panamanian) gold. [from origin and color] local variety of MARIJUANA grown in Panama and highly valued by marijuana users, who consider it more potent than varieties grown in the United States.

Panama red. also called P.R., red. Local variety of MARIJUANA, grown in Panama and considered more potent than varieties grown in the United States.

panatella. [from its size, i.e., a large cigarette, like a cigar compared with a cigarette; since the 1930s] bigger, fatter, more potent MARIJUANA cigarette made of Central or South American marijuana. *Obsolete.*

panic. [connoting a state of anxiety, as WITHDRAWAL SYMPTOMS begin to occur, and addicts do not know where their next supply of drugs will come from] a shortage of HEROIN in a general area, due, usually, to arrests of key suppliers and/or interception of a large supply being smuggled into the country.

panic man. an addict who cannot obtain drugs.

Pantopon. [hydrochlorides of alkaloids of OPIUM, Roche Laboratories] an opium preparation containing all its alkaloids in their natural percentages but with inert gums and resins removed. Manufacturer recommends as an analgesic in place of MORPHINE on the theory that 20 milligrams of Pantopon, thanks to the synergistic action of the several alkaloids in combination, gives analgesia equal to 15 milligrams of morphine (Pantopon is one-half morphine; hence 20 milligrams would contain only 10 milligrams of morphine). Goodman and Gilman, however, report in their book *The Pharmacological Basis of Therapeutics* that the analgesia is not greater than would be expected for the amount of morphine. The usual dosage is 20 milligrams. Pantopon is sold in ampuls or hypodermic tablets and administered only by subcutaneous or intramuscular injection. A Schedule II drug under the CONTROLLED SUBSTANCES ACT.

papaverine. a naturally occurring alkaloid of OPIUM of the benzylisoquinoline class, which acts mainly to depress the heart and smooth muscles. Unlike MORPHINE and CODEINE, alkaloids of the phenanthrene class, it has no analgesic, euphoric, or other central nervous system effect, and PHYSICAL DEPENDENCE is not produced by prolonged administration. Papaverine has limited use in medicine in treating cardiovascular system diseases and as a cough suppressant. A Schedule III drug under the CONTROLLED SUBSTANCES ACT. Compare NOSCAPINE.

paper. folded piece of paper containing narcotics; has been superseded by BAGS. Compare DECK.

> He opened his fly and extracted a rectangular paper packet—the junkie fold, with one end fitting into another. Inside the packet were two smaller packets, each similarly folded. He placed the *papers* on the table.   —William Burroughs, *Junkie* (1953)

papers. *1.* cigarette papers used for rolling MARIJUANA cigarettes. *2.* measures of HEROIN in folded paper sold for $10.

paracki. PARALDEHYDE.

parahexyl. PYRAHEXYL.

Paral. [PARALDEHYDE, Fellows Testagar] a nonbarbiturate hypnotic and sedative. Paraldehyde can produce PSYCHIC DEPENDENCE and PHYSICAL DEPENDENCE, with WITHDRAWAL SYMPTOMS similar to delirium tremens. Sold in 15-grain (1-gram) capsules. In the liquid form 1 cubic centimeter (1/5 teaspoonful) contains 15 grains of paraldehyde. Manufacturer's recommended dosage is one to two capsules or, by injection, one to four cubic centimeters.

paraldehyde. [a polymer, i.e., fusion of molecules, of acetaldehyde] a fast-acting, nonbarbiturate hypnotic and sedative, somewhat less potent and toxic than CHLORAL HYDRATE and somewhat more potent and toxic than ethyl ALCOHOL. Discovered in 1829 and first introduced into medicine in 1882, paraldehyde has been largely replaced today by the BARBITURATES, although it is considered quite as effective as a hypnotic.

Paraldehyde is a colorless, inflammable liquid with a strong odor and a bitter, burning, unpleasant taste, which has made its use unpopular, although it is often masked with various flavoring agents. On the other hand, this unpleasant flavor makes the drug less habit-forming than the barbiturates, which are tasteless and easy to administer, and for this reason authorities recommend its more widespread use. It is frequently given to alcoholics in a state of delirium tremens to induce sleep; and, of course, it may be used as a substitute for barbiturates when a patient is allergic to them.

When 4 to 8 milliliters (1/7 to 2/7 ounce) are taken, sleep ensues within ten to fifteen minutes. Larger doses of 15 to 30 milliliters are frequently given to calm psychiatric patients. The lethal dose is not known, and the drug has a wide margin of safety when taken orally (injected, it is much more dangerous); doses of 150 and 240 milliliters have been survived. However, fatalities have occurred due to respiratory depression and collapse of the cardiovascular system. Sometimes these fatalities have been related to liver damage or hepatitis in the patient.

Despite its unpleasant taste and its capacity to burn the mucous membranes when swallowed, PSYCHIC DEPENDENCE upon paraldehyde has occurred—frequently among former alcoholics treated with the drug who acquired a liking for it. Chronic paraldehyde intoxication resembles chronic alcoholism, including WITHDRAWAL SYMPTOMS similar to those of alcohol dependence, i.e., delirium tremens, auditory and visual hallucinations, convulsions, psychoses, etc. A Schedule IV drug under the CONTROLLED SUBSTANCES ACT.

paranoia. drug users' pervasive, perhaps exaggerated fear that the police have them under watch and may arrest them at any time. Drug users' paranoia implies taking elaborate precautions (see STASH, HOLDING) so as not to be caught possessing or dealing in drugs. The term also connotes that their fears, though possibly imaginary, like those of the paranoid psychotic, may well be based on fact; certainly, they arise out of the central fact that their drug use involved breaking the law, and so they are theoretically subject to arrest at any time. Thus, though the term is half ironic, it refers to a real and oppressive state of fear which drug users sometimes experience.

> Even Paranoids Have Real Enemies   —Hippie slogan (1967)

paregoric. tincture of OPIUM in combination with camphor, first prepared in the early eighteenth century and used medicinally ever since, largely in the control of diarrhea (from the constipating action of the opium). The usual mixture contains 4 percent tincture of opium, of which one-tenth (0.4 percent) is MORPHINE. The usual dose is 4 milliliters (about 1/7 ounce), which is equivalent to 16 milligrams of opium or 1.6 milligrams of morphine. Addicts often resort to paregoric (obtainable in some locales without a prescription) if HEROIN is not available. They either drink it (usually around a quart per day is taken for the desired effects; this would contain roughly 350 milligrams of morphine) or inject it, after first boiling it to remove the camphor, which causes abscesses when injected. Paregoric is considered a rather old-fashioned preparation today, containing several superfluous ingredients. A Schedule III drug under the CONTROLLED SUBSTANCES ACT.

> Shooting PG is a terrible hassle, you have to burn out the alcohol first, then freeze out the camphor and draw this brown liquid off with a dropper—have to shoot it in the vein or you get an abscess, and usually end up with an abscess no matter where you shoot it. Best deal is to drink it with goof balls [and likely die of an overdose—R.R.L.].
> —William Burroughs, *Naked Lunch* (1959)

Parest. [METHAQUALONE hydrochloride, Parke, Davis & Company] a nonbarbiturate hypnotic–sedative. Manufacturer recommends 200–400 milligrams before retiring. Sold as Parest-200 and Parest-400; the former contains 200 milligrams of methaqualone and has a light turquoise blue opaque cap and light green opaque body, and the latter contains 400 milligrams and has a blue cap and light green opaque body. The capsules are printed P/D 572 and P/D 574, respectively. Among illicit methaqualone users there is some mystique attached to Parest—perhaps to the 400-milligram capsules since they obviously contain more of the drug. They are called, erroneously, "super Sopors" and "super Quaalude."

parica. [Yekwana Indian] hallucinogenic snuff prepared by Venezuelan Indians from bark of trees belonging to the genus VIROLA, a member of the same family as the NUTMEG. Compare YAKEE.

partying. enjoying HEROIN sociably; sharing it with others.

pass. a transfer of drugs, as in "I paid him, and we arranged a place to make the *pass*."

PCP. PHENCYCLIDINE.

PDR. [*Physicians' Desk Reference*] the BOOK.

peace pill. PHENCYCLIDINE.

peaches. [from the color] BENZEDRINE tablets.

peaking. attaining the highest stage of intensity of the LSD TRIP.

pearls. AMYL NITRITE.

pellets. LSD capsules.

pentazocine. [1,2,3,4,5,6-hexahydro-cis-6, 11-dimethyl-3-(3-methyl-2-butenyl)-2, 6-methano-3-benzazocin-8-ol] a synthetic-opiate ANALGESIC. Pentazocine was first synthesized at the Sterling-Winthrop Research Institute in 1961; it is a member of the benzomorphan chemical family. It was then marketed by Sterling-Winthrop Laboratories under the name TALWIN. The drug was introduced to much press fanfare and touted as a nonaddicting painkiller, as effective as MORPHINE and not producing TOLERANCE.

Administered intravenously, a 40-milligram dose of pentazocine has the analgesic effects of 10 milligrams of morphine; a 120-milligram dose taken orally has approximately the same effect. Talwin has been marketed ever since as an analgesic of similar potency to CODEINE not subject to federal narcotics controls.

Nonetheless, pentazocine is an addicting drug. The user feels euphoria and tolerance does develop, especially to its euphoria-producing effects. A small number of users have developed PSYCHIC and PHYSICAL DEPENDENCE on the drug, with WITHDRAWAL SYMPTOMS less severe than morphine or HEROIN. Withdrawal symptoms include nausea without vomiting, loss of appetite, sleeplessness, constant sweating, and intermittent periods of tenseness, nervousness, depression, and anxiety. The withdrawal symptoms cause sufficient discomfort to motivate the user to seek out more pentazocine to alleviate them. Many cases of pentazocine abuse are related to medical use and supplies come from overprescription, excessive fillings of prescriptions by pharmacists, and diversion of supplies from hospitals. The users are often of the mistaken belief that pentazocine is not addictive. There is also evidence of "street" use of pentazocine, although it is regarded warily by addicts because it can cause hallucinations. Pentazocine is also a mild narcotics antagonist of about one-fiftieth the strength of NALLINE; thus its use by a person physically dependent upon heroin would precipitate mild withdrawal symptoms. Abusers either inject or take the drug orally. Injection of the drug (accompanied, in the reported cases, by an asthma drug) caused five deaths. The coroner theorized that the deaths were due to the talcum powder used to "bind" the pentazocine tablets. The drug is not subject to the CONTROLLED SUBSTANCES ACT.

Pentothal Sodium. [thiopental sodium, Abbott Laboratories] a very short-acting BARBITURATE hypnotic and sedative. When administered intravenously, Pentothal induces unconsciousness rapidly and suddenly; hence, it is used, alone or in combination with other drugs, as an anesthetic for minor and brief surgery; it is also administered before a general anesthetic to place the patient in a receptive state.

Along with other barbiturates, Pentothal is used as an adjunct to psychotherapy (narcoanalysis or narcotherapy). In amounts too small to induce anesthesia, the drug lowers the patient's inhibitions, makes him communicate more freely repressed emotional conflicts, and increases his responsiveness to suggestion by the therapist. Like AMYTAL, the drug is used in an analogous way as a so-called truth serum by the law-enforcement agencies, especially as an aid to total recall of an event or conversation which the subject cannot remember in a normal, conscious state. Naturally the suggestibility induced by the drug makes the "truth" elicited heavily dependent upon the interrogator's skill in avoiding planting any suggestions in subjects which would cause them to alter their memories in a way they think would please the interrogator.

Overdosage of Pentothal Sodium can cause fatal respiratory depression and paralysis. It is sold only in solution and ampuls for injection intravenously and should be administered only by a trained anesthetist with emergency equipment such as oxygen, in case respiratory depression does occur. A Schedule III drug under the CONTROLLED SUBSTANCES ACT. Compare NITROUS OXIDE.

people, the. high-level HEROIN distributors. Also called KILO CONNECTION.

pep pills. AMPHETAMINE pills.

per. a prescription.

Percobarb. [OXYCODONE hydrochloride and hexobarbital, with other ingredients, Endo Laboratories Inc.] a semisynthetic derivative of MORPHINE combined with a BARBITURATE and used as a hypnotic, sedative, and analgesic. Manufacturer recommends in cases of mild-to-moderate pain causing sleeplessness, e.g., headache, bursitis, neuralgia. Prolonged, excessive use can result in PHYSICAL DEPENDENCE upon both the oxycodone and the hexobarbital. When physical dependence develops, the WITHDRAWAL SYMPTOMS are close to those of morphine dependence in severity. Percobarb is sold in blue and yellow capsules, each containing 4.5 milligrams of oxycodone hydrochloride and 100 milligrams of hexobarbital, and as blue and white capsules, each containing one-half as much oxycodone and hexobarbital. Recommended dosage: one tablet every six hours. A Schedule II drug under the CONTROLLED SUBSTANCES ACT.

Percodan. [OXYCODONE hydrochloride and other analgesic ingredients, Endo Laboratories Inc.] similar to PERCOBARB except that it contains no BARBITURATE. Sold as yellow scored tablets, each containing 4.50 milligrams of oxycodone, and pink scored tablets containing one-half as much oxycodone. Percodan has reportedly found popularity among addicts in California. Compare EUCODAL. A Schedule II drug under the CONTROLLED SUBSTANCES ACT.

peter. CHLORAL HYDRATE, a sedative.

pethidine. [international generic name] MEPERIDINE.

peyote. [from Nahuatl *peyotl,* silk cocoon or caterpillar's cocoon; from the white, woolly tufts growing out of the surface part of the cactus] a small gray-brown cactus, *Lophophora williamsii,* with small spineless heads, or buttons, barely protruding from the earth (resembling mushrooms) and a long carrot-shaped root. The hallucinogenic properties of peyote were known to the Aztecs, who considered it divine. In remote areas Mexican Indians descended from the Aztecs continue to use it as a divine cure, in religious worship, and as a vehicle for communicating directly with divine spirits.

In the latter part of the nineteenth century, Indians in the United States learned of peyote's properties during forays into Mexico and brought it back to their homelands. They used it in religious rites and to heal the sick, and gradually a cult grew up around the cactus. This cult, which incorporated elements of Christianity, was formally organized as the First-born Church of Christ, later the Native American Church. The church and the peyote rite spread among North American Indians regardless of tribal barriers, so that today the Native American Church claims 200,000 members from all tribes in the United States and Canada.

At first the Bureau of Indian Affairs attempted to discourage the use of peyote by the Indians, with the tacit cooperation of several state governments which considered peyote in the class with alcohol for Indians (actually, use of the drug may cut down alcoholism), but it gradually became recognized that peyotism as practiced by the Indians was a sincere religion, and the courts have upheld it as such under the Bill of Rights. Peyotism does not interest all Indians, most of whom prefer either the white man's Christianity or a revival of their own native religions. Those who practice it have faith in its efficacy as a cure-all and a true belief—indeed a worship of the cactus itself—in the sacred character of the altered states of consciousness, especially visions, induced by the drug.

In the traditional peyote rite, the cactus is prepared by cutting off the tops of the plant, slicing them into disks (the mescal buttons), which are dried in the sun and then either crushed and boiled in water to make a tea or eaten raw, sometimes chewed until softened and swallowed whole. The buttons have a bitter taste, which has been compared to that of dried orange rind, and a nauseating odor. Nausea usually accompanies ingestion.

Characteristic physiological effects include dilation of the pupils, chills, and vomiting. Subjective effects include anxiety, terror, minor intensifying of sensual impressions, heightened auditory acuity, dislocation of visual perspective, depersonalization (the breaking down of distinction between self and other), mental stimulation and heightened clarity of thought, intensification of colors of surrounding objects, and brilliantly colored visions of shifting, nonobjective shapes, often, but not necessarily, perceived with the eyes closed. Peyote contains at least eight active alkaloids, but it is MESCALINE that causes the hallucinations.

Peyote does not induce PHYSICAL DEPENDENCE, and there are no WITHDRAWAL SYMPTOMS upon discontinuance of use. Among the Indians, some cases of apparent PSYCHIC DEPENDENCE or repeated, habitual use have been observed, but by far the majority of the Indians use it infrequently and only during their religious ceremonies, which are held informally upon weekends, usually sponsored by a family as a partly social occasion. Cases of psychosis linked to use of the drug are practically nonexistent among the Indians. The peyote ceremony is rich in Indian symbolism, contributes to the psychic health of the tribe, and use of peyote is effectively supervised. A limited TOLERANCE probably develops to the effects of peyote, since it does to the active alkaloid mescaline; however, this has not been documented, and cases of regular use, over a span of weeks, have been reported. If so, it would follow that there would be a CROSS-TOLERANCE to LSD-25 and PSILOCYBIN.

The visions never resembled familiar objects; they were extremely definite, but yet always novel; they were constantly approaching, and yet constantly eluding, the semblance of the known things. I would see thick, glorious fields of jewels, solitary or clustered, sometimes brilliant and sparkling, sometimes with a dull rich glow. Then they would spring up into flower-like shapes beneath my gaze, and then seem to turn into gorgeous butterfly forms or endless folds of glistening, iridescent, fibrous wings of wonderful insects; while sometimes I seemed to be gazing into a vast hollow revolving vessel, on whose polished concave mother-of-pearl surface the hues were swiftly changing. I was surprised, not only by the enormous profusion of the imagery presented to my gaze, but still more by its variety.
— Havelock Ellis, *The Contemporary Review* (1898)

The technichimekas (the genuine Chichimekas) know herbs and roots, their properties and their effects. They also know of peyotl. Those who eat peyotl take it instead of wine, as well as the poisonous mushroom nanacatl [teonanacatl]. They assemble somewhere in the prairie, dance and sing all day and all night. The next day they meet again and weep to excess. With their tears they wash their eyes and clear their brains (i.e., return to reason, see clearly again). . . . The plant peyotl, a kind of earth nopal, is white, grows in the northern parts, and produces in those who eat or drink it terrible or ludicrous visions. This inebriety lasts two to three days and then disappears. The Chichimekas eat considerable amounts of the plant. It gives them strength, incites them to battle, alleviates fear, and they feel neither hunger nor thirst. It is even said that they are protected from every kind of danger.
— Sahagun, *Historia general de las cosas de Nueva España* (seventeenth century), in Louis Lewin, *Phatastica: Narcotic and Stimulating Drugs* (1964)

The white man goes into his church house and talks *about* Jesus; the Indian goes into his tepee and talks *to* Jesus.
— J. S. Slotkin, *The Peyote Religion,* The Free Press of Glencoe, New York (1956)

Some of them, they say that the great teacher *Peyote* teaching forever, the Peyote. That's the way they find out, the Peyoters, old Peyoters. Even next meeting I go, I'll find something; next one, I'll find something. Keep on going like that; you'll never get to end. There's no end to it; it is forever.
— J. S. Slotkin, *Transactions of the American Philosophical Society* (1952)

peyotl. PEYOTE.

P.G. PAREGORIC.

pharmaceuticals. pills with the manufacturer's name on them; considered more reliable by illicit buyers. Compare CIBA, QUAALUDE, SOPOR.

phenadoxone (CB-11). a SYNTHETIC OPIATE analgesic, equivalent to MORPHINE. An injection of 10 to 20 milligrams produces analgesic effects equal to those produced by 10 milligrams of morphine, lasting one to three hours. PHYSICAL DEPENDENCE results after prolonged use, with WITHDRAWAL SYMPTOMS less severe than those of morphine dependence. A Schedule II drug under the CONTROLLED SUBSTANCES ACT.

phenazocine. a SYNTHETIC OPIATE analgesic somewhat more potent than MORPHINE. A dose of 3 milligrams injected subcutaneously gives analgesia equal to that produced by 10 milligrams of morphine, lasting four to five hours. PHYSICAL DEPENDENCE occurs after prolonged use, with WITHDRAWAL SYMPTOMS between those of METHADONE and morphine dependence in severity. A Schedule II drug under the CONTROLLED SUBSTANCES ACT.

phencyclidine. An analgesic–anesthetic used in veterinary medicine. Injected intravenously it will produce a trancelike state of unconsciousness with analgesia. Toxic effects include hallucinations, agitations, catatonic rigidity, disorientation, incoordination, vomiting, numbness, and skin rash. The drug seems to have found its way into the illicit market as a hallucinogenic drug; dealers tout it as LSD, MESCALINE, or PSILOCYBIN. Mixed with other drugs it is called ANGEL DUST, a mixture that is supposed to contain LSD. Trade name is Sernylan (Parke, Davis). Slang names: hog, elephant, PCP, peace pills, and angel dust. Compare METHYPRYLON, another piperidine derivative.

phenos. phenobarbital, SECONAL, or RED BIRDS.

> We also dealt for red capsules of *phenos,* two of which, with hot water, produce a forgetting high.
> —Piri Thomas, *Down These Mean Streets* (1967)

pholocodine. (also called morpholinylethylmorphine) a semi-synthetic derivative of MORPHINE, which is more effective orally. A dosage of 10 to 15 milligrams taken orally gives analgesia equivalent to 10 milligrams of morphine injected, lasting four to five hours. PHYSICAL DEPENDENCE occurs after prolonged use, but the WITHDRAWAL SYMPTOMS are less severe than those of CODEINE dependence. A Schedule II drug under the CONTROLLED SUB-STANCES ACT.

physical dependence. physical dependence occurs with certain drugs after prolonged administration in sufficient dosages induces an adaptive alteration in the body which erupts in a stereotyped set of WITHDRAWAL SYMPTOMS, peculiar to the drug, when its ingestion is stopped. These withdrawal symptoms may also be set off, in the case of certain drugs, by another drug which antagonizes the action of the original one. The withdrawal symptoms will remain dormant as long as the drug or its analog is administered in sufficient quantities.

Physical dependence unaccompanied by PSYCHIC DEPENDENCE can occur. In the case of certain of both physical– and psychic–dependence-producing drugs, TOLERANCE to some or all of the drug's effects, including the lethal dose, may develop, so that the user has to increase the dosage in order to obtain the effects of previous dosages. If the drug is one which causes physical dependence, the user must also increase the dosage to avoid withdrawal symptoms as tolerance increases.

DRUGS PRODUCING PHYSICAL DEPENDENCE

morphine type (Tolerance develops to all actions, including the lethal dose if the increase in intake is carefully regulated.)

barbiturates, nonbarbiturate hypnotics, and sedatives; minor tranquilizers (Tolerance to the sedative effects, but not the lethal dosage, develops.)

alcohol (Some degree of tolerance develops; withdrawal symptoms, such as delirium tremens, are similar to those of the barbiturates, which are effective in alleviating them, just as alcohol partially relieves barbiturate withdrawal symptoms.)

picked up. smoked MARIJUANA, as in "when you've *picked up* gauge and feel great."

piece. [a share, hence a ration of NARCOTICS, since the 1930s; also, an underworld term for ounces since the 1930s—*EP*. A piece is a measure, but in the HEROIN traffic no measure is undiluted, and it thus is also a symbolic share of a monetary pie, cut up by importers, wholesalers, and PUSHERS] *1*. an amount of heroin, diluted with quinine and MILK SUGAR, and purchased by the pusher or by the wholesaler, who dilutes it more and packages it for sale to addicts. Usually 1/2 kilogram (1.1 pounds) of heroin makes up fifteen pieces. Each piece yields thirty to thirty-six teaspoons of heroin, which in turn are diluted and put into BAGS: twenty-five $5 bags make a BUNDLE and fifteen $3 bags make a half bundle or half load (see CLEAN, CUTTING, DECK UP). Of course, the amount the piece is diluted determines how much pushers can further dilute it and in turn how many packages they can make and sell, and thus their profits. The heroin average pushers buy from a wholesaler with direct access to high-level sources of supply is today diluted much more than it was ten years ago, and so they can convert it to fewer packages. *2.* a gun.

> "A lot of the junk today I could either put in my coffee or on a cake 'cause it's mostly sugar and quinine. The stuff is very weak. It's not like it used to be. Like when I first started, the purest you could get was 97.6 or something close to that, and a *piece* of that stuff, if you could get that, by the time it went through all the channels, being cut all them times, you could still cut it maybe seven to one or eight to one, like make eight pieces out of one piece. And then at that time, for a piece, you'd pay maybe $200. Now today, if you buy your piece, you'd be very lucky if you could get a three-to-one cut, make three pieces out of one for $500 or $600. It's that weak. Today if you were buying an ounce and cutting it and bagging it, a $5 bag would actually cost you, I mean me, maybe $2. So there's a $3 profit on each bag you sell. So if you get a hundred bags, that's $300 profit, plus you still have your money to recop with. And I could sell in a day maybe close to two hundred bags, maybe more, sometime less. On a good night I could sell maybe a piece, a piece and a half."
>
> —pusher in James Mills, *The Panic in Needle Park* (1966)

pilde. South American Indian name for BANISTERIOPSIS CAAPI.

pill. [pellet of OPIUM, also called "yen pox"—*MM,* 1946. The opium is heated to melt it, and the resulting pellet can be placed in a pipe. *Obsolete.* Now popular slang for prepared, proprietary remedies with an invidious connotation] BARBITURATE or AMPHETAMINE tablets or capsules, as in "on *pills.*" Compare PILLHEAD.

pillhead. [from *hophead,* an OPIUM addict; see HEAD] a habitual, heavy user of BARBITURATES or AMPHETAMINES (usually by implication opposed to MARIJUANA, LSD, HEROIN, etc.).

piminodine. a SYNTHETIC OPIATE analgesic, slightly more potent than MORPHINE. A dose of 7.5 to 10 milligrams injected subcutaneously produces analgesic effects equal to those of 10 milligrams of morphine, lasting two to four hours. Repeated, regular use can result in PHYSICAL DEPENDENCE, with WITHDRAWAL SYMPTOMS less severe than those of morphine dependence and similar to those of MEPERIDINE dependence. A Schedule II drug under the CONTROLLED SUBSTANCES ACT.

pin. [usually rolled thinner than an ordinary cigarette] a MARIJUANA cigarette.

pinhead. a thinly rolled MARIJUANA cigarette.

pinks. SECONAL, a BARBITURATE.

pinned. constricted; used of the pupils of the eye. Constriction is characteristic of use of HEROIN, MORPHINE, etc. The opposite effect is produced by HALLUCINOGENS, such as LSD-25, and by MARIJUANA, AMPHETAMINES, and ATROPINE-like drugs. The medical term for constriction of the pupils is *miosis* and for enlarged pupils is *mydriasis*. Pupillary action is controlled by the parasympathetic and sympathetic nervous systems of the autonomic chain.

pipe. a large vein. Compare TRACKS, MAINLINE, PIT.

Piper methysticum. see KAVA.

pipiltzintzintli. [Nahuatl] Aztec name for a mint, SALVIA DIVINORUM, said to have hallucinogenic properties.

Piptadenia. a hallucinogenic snuff is made by South American Indians by pulverizing the seeds of the legumes *Piptadenia peregrina, P. colubrina,* and *P. macrocarpa,* belonging to the mimosa family *(Leguminosae).* Among different tribes it is known variously as yopo, niopo, cohoba, and huilca. These tribes are centered in the Orinoco basin of Colombia and Venezuela and in the Peruvian Andes, where huilca, *P. macrocarpa,* is thought to be used as a hallucinatory snuff, though little is known of it. Piptadenia intoxication produces convulsive movements and uncontrolled dancing, inability to control the movements of the limbs, and stimulation of the senses. These may be followed by periods of madness, or the users sink into a deep, nightmare-filled sleep. The Indians use it in orgies, to heighten their physical courage, for divination of the future, and to give them prowess in battle. Chemical analysis of the snuff has identified its chief alkaloid as BUFOTENINE. Piptadenia may also contain DMT.

pit. the main vein leading to the heart, considered the "original main line" and the best vein to inject for some addicts.

pituri. a shrublike plant, *Duboisia hopwoodii,* belonging to the potato family *(Solanaceae),* whose leaves are chewed by Australian aborigines and which contains the alkaloid SCOPOLAMINE. The leaves must first be mixed with ashes of an acacia, *Acacia salicina,* which acts chemically, when chewed, to release the alkaloid in the pituri. The leaves have a stimulating effect, at first, which the natives prize, because it enables them to travel long distances without food; later it produces stupefaction and narcosis. Not to be confused with Australian tobacco, which the aborigines also chew.

place. the setting or locale, whether favorable or hostile, of an LSD TRIP.

Placidyl. [ETHCHLORVYNOL, Abbott Laboratories] a nonbarbiturate hypnotic-sedative used for insomnia. Manufacturer's recommended dosage: 500 to 1,000 milligrams at bedtime, depending upon the severity of the insomnia. PSYCHIC and PHYSICAL DEPENDENCE upon Placidyl will develop on regular doses as low as 1,000 milligrams per day over a period of time. WITHDRAWAL SYMPTOMS upon abrupt discontinuance of the drug resemble BARBITURATE withdrawal symptoms. Incipient withdrawal symptoms include loss of appetite, nausea, anxiety, tremor, loss of coordination, slurring of speech, perceptual distortions, irritability, agitation, and delirium. Severe symptoms include convulsions, delirium, and possibly death unless the original dose is restored and the patient is gradually weaned off the drug under medical supervision. The drug has been used in suicides and suicide attempts. The lethal dose has ranged from 7,000 to 49,000 milligrams, although patients have recovered, after comas lasting several days, from doses ranging from 7,500 to 60,000 milligrams. Sold in maroon 100- and 200-milligram tablets, maroon 500-milligram capsules stamped "Abbott," and green 750-milligram capsules stamped "Abbott." A Schedule IV drug under the CONTROLLED SUBSTANCES ACT.

plant. *1.* a hiding place or a cache. *2.* to place narcotics or other drugs in premises belonging to a suspected addict or user, then raiding them, a practice sometimes employed by narcotics police.

plastic hippie. a part-time or weekend HIPPIE; one who pretends to be a hippie without being committed completely to the hippie way of life.

point. hypodermic needle.

poison. HEROIN, COCAINE.

poison act. federal narcotics laws.

poison people. poison (HEROIN) addicts.

She had a bent-up spoon that she cooked stuff [heroin] in for the *poison people.*
—Claude Brown, *Manchild in the Promised Land* (1965)

poke. [variant (?) of TOAK] a puff of a MARIJUANA cigarette.

poly-drug use. MULTIHABITUATION.

pop. [from *pop*, to fire a pistol, cause a shot or bang; a *shot* of a drug—*EP* from around 1925] *1.* to shoot HEROIN subcutaneously. *2.* to swallow a PILL. Compare BANG, DROP. *3.* arrest.

popped. to be picked up by the police, as in "I got *popped* last week."

poppers. small vials containing AMYL NITRITE, which are broken in a handkerchief and inhaled.

The law [in California] refuses liquor to anyone under twenty-one, but permits eighteen-year-olds to buy amyl nitrite for cardio-sexual stimulation.
—John Sherlock, "The Hollywood Bachelor Observed," *Cosmopolitan* (August, 1967)

popping. [short for SKIN POPPING since around 1946—*EP*] *1.* injecting drugs subcutaneously. *2.* Swallowing pills.

population. at the U.S. Public Health Service (Narcotics) Hospital, Lexington, Kentucky, the inmates. To be "in population" is to be allowed to mix normally with the other inmates, following withdrawal from the drug and "orientation" (counseling).

positive. a good mental state, an UP. Compare NEGATIVE.

pot. [from Mexican Indian *potaguaya,* marijuana; since the 1950s] MARIJUANA.

potentiate. [from Latin *potentia,* power] to make a drug more effective or more powerful, usually by means of synergistic action with a second drug. Alcohol potentiates the effect of many drugs; depressant drugs generally potentiate one another. (Manufacturers sometimes say that a drug that potentiates another is *additive* to it.)

potlikker. a tea brewed from MARIJUANA waste, i.e., seeds and stems, which users say gives them a satisfactory HIGH (the seeds contain the plant's ACTIVE PRINCIPLE in small quantities).

pound. five dollars.

P. R. PANAMA RED.

Preludin. [phenmetrazine hydrochloride, Geigy Pharmaceuticals] central nervous system stimulant similar to an AMPHETAMINE, used in dieting to depress the appetite. The drug promotes a stimulated state and a feeling of well-being and is sometimes used in excess for these effects. TOLERANCE develops, as well as PSYCHIC DEPENDENCE. Abrupt cessation after long-term use results in severe depression and fatigue. Heavy doses may produce acute paranoid schizophrenia, as do the amphetamines. Overdose may result in coma, convulsions, and death. Manufacturer's recommended dosage is 50 to 75 milligrams per day. Sold in the form of pink, square, scored 25-milligram tablets or Endurets, round, pink delayed-release 75-milligram tablets. Jack Ruby was reportedly using these pills excessively at the time he murdered Oswald, though no connection between this use and the shooting was officially established. Subject to Schedule II of the CONTROLLED SUBSTANCES ACT.

Prinadol. [PHENAZOCINE, Smith Kline & French Laboratories] a SYNTHETIC OPIATE. Manufacturer recommends as a narcotic analgesic, adjunct to anesthesia, for relief of postoperative pain, and in acute and chronic pain. Continued, regular use will lead to PHYSICAL DEPENDENCE. Recommended single dose is 2 milligrams. A Schedule II drug under the CONTROLLED SUBSTANCES ACT.

Prolixin. [flupenazine hydrochloride, E. R. Squibb & Sons] a phenothiazine derivative, classified as a MAJOR TRANQUILIZER and used in severe anxiety and tension states and severe mental disorders, especially schizophrenia. In tension and anxiety states, manufacturer's recommended oral dosage is 1 to 2 milligrams daily; in severe mental disorder, 2.5 to 10 milligrams daily, with 20 milligrams daily the maximum. It is claimed to have longer-lasting action than CHLORPROMAZINE and to have fewer hypotensive (lowering of the blood pressure) and sedative effects than the other phenothiazines, to which it is otherwise similar. Supplied in coated, pink 1-milligram, yellow 2.5-milligram, and green 5-milligram tablets with trademark inscribed, as an orange-flavored elixir, and in solution for injection.

Prunicodeine. [CODEINE, terpin hydrate, and other ingredients, Eli Lilly and Company] cough syrup. Each 30 cubic centimeters (about 6 teaspoonfuls) contains 60 milligrams (1 grain) of codeine sulfate and 175 milligrams of terpin hydrate (120 milligrams of codeine provides analgesic effects equal to those of 10 milligrams of MORPHINE). Prolonged use can result in both PSYCHIC DEPENDENCE and PHYSICAL DEPENDENCE, with WITHDRAWAL SYMPTOMS less severe than morphine. Recommended dosage: 1 teaspoonful every three hours. Sold without prescription in many states, but federal Narcotic Registry number and record of sale required.

psilocybin. hallucinogenic alkaloid in certain mushrooms. Average hallucinogenic dose is 20 to 60 milligrams. Subject to Schedule I of the CONTROLLED SUBSTANCES ACT. See MUSHROOMS, MAGIC.

psychedelic. [Greek, *psyche,* soul, and *delos,* visible, evident] mind-manifesting; consciousness-expanding; introducing new, strange, or dramatically altered perceptions, sensory experiences, illusions, visions, and subconscious material into the conscious mind, thus "expanding" it in ways that are beyond the capacity of ordinary experience. Drugs such as LSD, MESCALINE, PSILOCYBIN, DMT, and CANNABIS are considered to have this effect. See HALLUCINOGEN.

psychic dependence. a craving for the pleasurable mental effects produced by a drug, such as euphoria, elation, stimulation, sedation, hypnosis, hallucinations, sensory acuity, etc., and a strong psychological need or craving for this drug-induced state in preference to the normal state, so that drug users find its repetition necessary to their well-being. Withdrawal of psychic-dependence-producing drugs, especially central nervous system stimulants, while it produces no specific physical symptoms, may result in a mild to serious depression, so unpleasant to users that they may continue increasing their dose to forestall it, eventually triggering a psychosis with severe irruption of symptoms the drug had suppressed.

With mild hallucinogenic drugs, e.g., MARIJUANA, sudden withdrawal generally produces neither mental nor physical symptoms, but heavy use may be followed by vague anxiety upon cessation of the drug. True psychic dependence does not occur with the more potent hallucinogens, though their use might be frequent and users may become strongly preoccupied with the drug, seeking to repeat its mental state in preference to a normal one to such an extent that their personalities change, they drop out of their former lifestyles, and they orient their lives around the drug. Often, though, the novelty of such drugs' effects wears off and users simply stop with little discomfort.

DRUGS PRODUCING PSYCHIC DEPENDENCE
BUT NO PHYSICAL DEPENDENCE

cocaine (No tolerance develops; severe depression and/or psychotic symptoms may accompany withdrawal after prolonged heavy use, motivating the resumption of use).

marijuana (Insignificant tolerance develops.)

hashish (Some degree of tolerance may develop; some degree of physical discomfort upon withdrawal after prolonged use has been observed.)

amphetamines (Tolerance develops to a considerable degree, but it is selective; i.e., insomnia and hyperexcitability caused by the drug continue, while increasing doses are necessary to sustain the drug's euphoriant effects. If use has masked symptoms of fatigue, abrupt withdrawal will often be accompanied by exhaustion and severe depression and a strong temptation to return to the drug.)

khat (Not known.)

LSD (Complete tolerance develops after only three days.)

psilocybin (Tolerance develops rapidly.)

mescaline (Tolerance develops rather more slowly.)

morning glory seeds (Not known.)

psychoactive. altering the subjective state; altering perception and consciousness.

psychotogenic. producing hallucinations and psychotic behavior.

psychotomimetic. *1.* imitating a model psychosis. *2.* descriptive of drugs whose effects were thought to produce model psychosis. Since the drug experience is in some ways different from a psychosis, though in other aspects resembling one, the word is not favored, and HALLUCINOGENIC and PSYCHEDELIC are used to describe those drugs.

There are considerable differences between LSD-induced and schizophrenic symptoms. The characteristic autism and dissociation of schizophrenia are absent with LSD. Perceptual disturbances due to LSD differ from those due to schizophrenia and, as a rule, are not true hallucinations. Finally, disturbances of consciousness following LSD do not resemble those occurring in schizophrenia.
—B. Manzini and Saraval, in *Delysid (LSD-25)*, *Annotated Bibliography Addendum No. 3*, Sandoz Pharmaceuticals (1961)

psychotropic. [Greek *psyche,* soul, and *trope,* a turning] changing the consciousness; opposite of CEPHALOTROPIC.

puff. to smoke OPIUM.

pure. [circa 1940] relatively undiluted HEROIN.

> Old "Weeping" fell dead outside a shooting gallery in Saint Paul. Musta' shot some "pure," cause a lookout on the sidewalk heard him mumble before he croaked, "Well kiss my dead mammy's ass if this ain't the best 'smack' I ever shot."
> —"Iceberg Slim," *Pimp. The Story of My Life* (1967)

purple hearts. [from their color and rounded diamond shape] *1.* LUMINAL tablets. *2.* in Great Britain, Drinamyl (see DEXAMYL), a combination of a BARBITURATE and an AMPHETAMINE.

push. [from PUSHER, since around 1920—*EP*] to peddle drugs.

pusher. [from *pusher,* a passer of counterfeit money; since around 1920—*EP*] a low-level peddler of narcotics who sells directly to the addict in the street. Pushers, often addicts themselves, buy their drugs from wholesalers, who in turn get theirs from the importer via courier. Also, a seller of MARIJUANA, LSD, PILLS, etc., but not HARD NARCOTICS, frequently called a DEALER or the SOURCE.

pushing. *1.* peddling narcotics. *2.* peddling MARIJUANA, LSD, PILLS, etc., but not NARCOTICS. See DEALING.

put his (your) trip. preaching the superiority of one's own LSD experience and, by implication, oneself and one's philosophy, as in "Timothy Leary is out of favor with the HIPPIES because he's trying too hard to *put his trip* on everybody else"; i.e., a rebellion against other people's structuring or defining their own LSD experience by holding it up as a model.

put in writing or paper. to conceal drugs between a split postcard or to saturate a letter with soluble drugs; for smuggling into prison.

put on a crosstown bus. "put someone in a dilemma."—Seymour Fiddle, *Portraits from a Shooting Gallery* (1967)

put somebody on. give him some MARIJUANA to smoke—*MM*, 1946. Compare TURN ON.

pyrahexyl. (also called synhexyl) derivative of the ACTIVE PRINCIPLE of CANNABIS. When it is swallowed in capsule form, the effects are similar to those of cannabis. It has been used experimentally in the treatment of drug withdrawal and depressive states.

Q q

q'at. KHAT.

Quaalude. [METHAQUALONE, William H. Rorer, Inc.] a nonbarbiturate hypnotic–sedative recommended for insomnia and daytime sedation. Manufacturer recommends 150 to 300 milligrams for sleep and 75 milligrams for daytime sedation. PSYCHIC and PHYSICAL DEPENDENCE with WITHDRAWAL SYMPTOMS will occur after prolonged, heavy use. Sold in 150-milligram white scored tablets and 300-milligram white scored tablets, with "Rorer" stamped on them.

quarter. $25. Compare NICKEL, DIME, CENT.

quarter bag. about 1 ounce of MARIJUANA, worth $25.

quill. folded matchbook cover used to sniff a drug. The drug (HEROIN or COCAINE) is placed in the fold and then inhaled through the nose. Compare SCOOP.

R r

ragweed. low-potency MARIJUANA.

rainbow. [from the capsule, blue at one half, red at the other, and dark red where the two overlap] TUINAL capsule.

rainy-day woman. MARIJUANA cigarette.

rap. [from *rap*, to perjure oneself, to swear a false oath, around the seventeenth century; hence, *rap*, to speak, to acknowledge someone, since the 1870s—*EP*. Not from *rapport* (see RAPPING), although its use among drug users of middle-class origins, who know the meaning of rapport, may have given it a subtle shift from its meaning among criminals and narcotic addicts] *1.* to talk, especially to talk the jargon of the addict's life. *2.* to gossip, converse. *3.* talk, used as a noun, as in "while I'm going through my *rap*," i.e., while I'm speaking my piece (under the influence of drugs).

rapping. ["Achieving rapport with random talk"—*Time* (1967); but see RAP] *1.* talking. *2.* random free-form conversation.

rat. an addict who is working as a police informer.

Rauwolfia serpentina. a small climbing shrub of the family *Apocynaceae,* indigenous to India and neighboring countries, known in English as snakeroot. In India, the root is ground into powder and used medicinally for snakebite, hypertension, insomnia, and insanity. Its tranquilizing effects have been known there for 2,500 years. It is now used by Western medicine as a TRANQUILIZER, rarely in its powdered form, usually in the chemical derivative RESERPINE.

reader. [prescription for narcotics since around 1925—*EP*] prescription for narcotics, obtained from a doctor by misrepresentation (BRODY) or bribery. Compare MAKING A CROAKER FOR A READER, SCRIPT, PER.

red. PANAMA RED.

red and blues. [from the two-colored capsule] TUINAL capsules.

red birds. [from the color] SECONAL capsules.

red chicken. Chinese HEROIN.

red devils. [from the color] SECONAL capsules.

red dirt marijuana. MARIJUANA growing wild. Compare WEED MARIJUANA.

red rock. Chinese HEROIN in granular form. Compare BROWN ROCK.

reds. [from the color] SECONAL capsules.

reefer. [since around 1925; usually plural—*EP*. Perhaps from GRIFA, (Mexican) MARIJUANA] marijuana cigarette.

reserpine. one of the alkaloids found in RAUWOLFIA SERPENTINA. It is employed in a variety of preparations as a TRANQUILIZER to alleviate anxiety, combat tension, in agitated psychotic states, hypertension, rapid heartbeat, and tension headache. It should not be used where there is evidence of depression. The drug is said to exercise its calming effect unaccompanied by loss of motor control and disequilibrium. Unlike some tranquilizers, it has no anticonvulsant or antihistaminic effects. The phenothiazine derivatives are generally preferred in psychiatric practice. Usual dosages range from 0.1 to 1.0 milligram. Reserpine appears to have a low abuse potential, and is not seen in the illicit market.

rifle range. the withdrawal ward in a narcotics hospital.

rig. equipment for injecting drugs. Compare OUTFIT, WORKS, KIT, BIZ.

righteous. *1.* good quality, potent (said of a drug). *2.* a person to be trusted, an addict who won't inform.

righteous bush. MARIJUANA.

ripped. intoxicated by drugs; very HIGH.

rippers. AMPHETAMINES.

Ritalin. [methylphenidate hydrochloride, Ciba Pharmaceutical Co.] an amphetaminelike central nervous system stimulant. Manufacturer recommends for mild depression, for hyperkinetic children, drug-induced lethargy produced by depressant drugs, apathetic or withdrawn senile behavior, and narcolepsy (involuntary sleep). Ritalin is very similar to the AMPHETAMINES in its effects and is abused in similar ways (it can be taken in pill form or injected). TOLERANCE develops to the stimulant effects and severe PSYCHIC DEPENDENCE can develop after continued use. Ritalin intoxication can trigger psychotic episodes, especially when it is injected. Abrupt withdrawal after continuing use may result in a severe depression. Overdosage can result in hallucinations, delirium, convulsions, and coma and must be treated by medical personnel. Average dosage is 20 to 30 milligrams daily. Ritalin is sold in 20-milligram peach-colored tablets, 10-milligram green-colored tablets, and 5-milligram pale yellow tablets, all with "Ciba" stamped on them. It is also sold in 10 milliliter vials. A Schedule II drug under the CONTROLLED SUBSTANCES ACT.

Rivea corymbosa. plant of the bindweed family *(Convovulaceae)*, the seeds of which have hallucinogenic properties. See MORNING GLORY SEEDS.

roach. ["In the jargon of the marijuana addict [*sic*] a man who has smoked half a cigarette is called a 'cucaracha' which literally means cockroach"—Pablo Oswaldo Wolff, 1949. Perhaps from the wriggling motion of the cockroach and also the size, shape, and brownish color resembling a cockroach] butt of a MARIJUANA cigarette. In order not to waste any marijuana, the smoker puffs down to as short a butt as possible, holding it with a toothpick or inserting it in one end of a tightly rolled match folder, or a ROACH HOLDER, when it is too hot for the fingers. Some even eat the remaining marijuana to destroy evidence and because they believe the ACTIVE PRINCIPLE is concentrated in the end. When the butt can no longer be smoked, it is torn open, and the remaining marijuana is put back in the smoker's supply for reuse.

> La cucaracha, la cucaracha,
> Ya no puede caminar,
> Porque no tiene, porque *le Palta*
> Marijuana que fumar.   —Mexican folk song

roach clip. ROACH HOLDER.

roach holder. a thin, pronged instrument, often elaborately decorated, upon which the ROACH is skewered for smoking purposes. Compare CRUTCH, STEAMBOAT.

roach pick. ROACH HOLDER.

rock. granules of HEROIN; this form is for smoking. Compare BROWN ROCK, RED ROCK.

roll. *1.* a wrapped quantity of pills. *2.* a HIGH, as in "Carbona's a deprivation *roll.*"

root. [see JOINT] a MARIJUANA cigarette.

rope. [see HEMP] MARIJUANA.

roses. [from the color] BENZEDRINE tablets.

run. *1.* period of addiction, as in "then I got hooked and had a three-year *run.*" *2.* a period of continuous, heavy AMPHETAMINE use, usually by injection, lasting three to five days and ending when the user sinks into protracted, exhausted sleep (CRASH).

rush. the initial onset of warmth, orgasmlike feelings, euphoria, and physical well-being immediately after the drug has been injected; distinguished from the HIGH, the continuing state of relaxation, tranquilization, and well-being while the drug's effects (the

NOD) last. Intravenous injection produces the quickest, most intense rush. The term was originally applied to HEROIN, then extended to injected AMPHETAMINES. Compare FLASH, FLUSH.

> Then you just take off the strap and squeeze it in. Then you feel that *rush* all over your body and you got your high.
> —addict, quoted in Jeremy Larner and Ralph Tefferteller
> *The Addict in the Street* (1964)

S s

sacrament. LSD-25.

sacred mushrooms. MUSHROOMS, SACRED.

salt shot. an injection of a saline solution to an addict who is unconscious from an OVERDOSE. This treatment, an addict's home remedy, is not medically sanctioned.

Salvia divinorum. a plant with hallucinogenic properties belonging to the mint family. It is used primarily by the Mazatec Indians of Mexico, usually when hallucinogenic mushrooms are not available. The leaves are chewed directly or crushed, steeped in water, and drunk. Their effects are said to be similar to those of the hallucinogenic mushrooms, but less sweeping and shorter lasting. The ACTIVE PRINCIPLE of the leaves is not known. Compare MUSHROOMS, SACRED.

Sansert. [methysergide maleate (1-methyllysergic acid butanolamide maleate), Sandoz Pharmaceuticals] a SEROTONIN inhibitor, chemically related to LSD-25. It is used medically as a preventive treatment for chronic migraine headaches. Manufacturer's recommended average daily dosage is two to four tablets or 4 to 8 milligrams. Illicit users have discovered the drug, which they tout as a substitute for LSD because it produces similar effects. One claimed that 16 milligrams of Sansert gave effects equivalent to 100 micrograms of LSD. Sustained use for over six months is not recommended; the drug should not be administered at all except under constant medical supervision—there are numerous side effects. The drug is available only by prescription. Supplied in bright yellow, sugar-coated 2-milligram tablets.

sassfras. [from (?) the physical resemblance to the sassafras tree] MARIJUANA cigarette, made from marijuana grown in the United States and therefore not so potent as the imported kinds—La Guardia Report, 1944. *Obsolete.*

satch. paper saturated with a soluble drug for smuggling.

scag. HEROIN.

scars. traces left by healing needle marks; black or blue spots. See TRACKS.

> Now people would ask you if you knew someone by describing their *scars.* —Claude Brown, *Manchild in the Promised Land* (1965)

scene. social patterns of drug use in a particular area, usually referring to a college or high school.

> The drug *scene* at Harvard is normally played in private. . . . The pusher takes you around campus, to the places where "the scene" happens (i.e., where students turn on).
> —Richard Goldstein, *One in Seven: Drugs on Campus* (1966)

schmack. [corruption of Yiddish SCHMECK, to sniff] *1.* HEROIN or COCAINE. *2.* by extension, all drugs.

schmeck. [Yiddish, to sniff; from the practice of sniffing drugs, especially heroin; since the 1940s] HEROIN.

schmecker. a HEROIN user.

schoolboy. CODEINE.

scoff. [from tramp's term for food; to take narcotics orally (?); since around 1920—EP] *1.* food. *2.* to eat.

scoop. *1.* a folded matchbook cover. *2.* to sniff COCAINE or HEROIN through a rolled or folded matchbook cover. Compare QUILL.

> I taught him how to *scoop* cocaine . . . before I could get the matchbook scoop up to my nostril again.
> —Claude Brown, *Manchild in the Promised Land* (1965)

> I felt something thrust into my hand and saw a cap and a piece of match-book cover folded into a V-shaped *scoop.*
> "Snort, man," Waneko said. "It's H."
> —Piri Thomas, *Down These Mean Streets* (1967)

scopolamine. also called hyoscine. A nonbarbiturate hypnotic, sedative, and involuntary-muscle relaxant. Scopolamine is the active alkaloid of henbane *(Hyoscyamus niger);* it is also found in *Scopola carniolica,* in the Australian shrub, PITURI, and in all of the potato family *(Solanaceae),* whose members include BELLADONNA and DATURA. They contain the alkaloids ATROPINE and HYOSCYAMINE, which have pharmacological effects similar to scopolamine. In toxic doses, scopolamine, like atropine, can cause excitation, hallucinations, delirium, and other bizarre mental effects.

Scopolamine in large doses can be deadly, and it was known for such properties by the ancient Greeks and Romans. In the Middle Ages the henbane and belladonna plants were used in the manufacture of salves and potions for necromancy and witchcraft. Some authorities believe that the illusions accompanying such rites, e.g., having intercourse with the devil, flying, were produced by belladonna or henbane intoxication.

In the twentieth century scopolamine has been employed as a so-called truth serum. Subjects in a state of hypnosis or "twilight sleep" produced by the drug are more pliable to interrogation, as they are under such BARBITURATES as PENTOTHAL SODIUM. Since the drug can also induce amnesia, it is not frequently used today. In modern medicine scopolamine is used occasionally as a TRANQUILIZER with mental patients; as a preanesthetic tranquilizer, with morphine, to allay anxiety and fear and induce anesthesia; and as an antispasmodic in gastrointestinal disorders and peptic ulcers, because of its action in immobilizing the smooth muscles of the intestine (for further discussion see ATROPINE). Scopolamine has approximately twice the depressant effect on the central nervous system that atropine has; hence it is a more effective sedative and is found (as scopolamine hydrobromide) in a variety of nonprescription sedatives on the market such as Sominex, Sleep-eze, and Compoze. The usual effects of the average medical dose of scopolamine (0.5 milligram) are drowsiness, euphoria, amnesia, and dreamless sleep. Occasionally, bizarre reactions to such small doses will occur, especially when the patient is in pain. Scopolamine also acts to inhibit bodily secretions (saliva, tears, sweat, etc.), to dilate the pupils, and to stimulate the central respiratory system.

Scopolamine is thought to be more toxic than atropine, although this is not certain. Toxic reactions progress, with increase of the dosage, from slight slowing of the heartbeat, dryness of the mouth, rapid heartbeat, dry skin, dilated pupils, and restlessness combined with fatigue to loss of coordination, extreme restlessness, loss of memory, excitement, flushed skin, hallucinations, delirium, and coma. Doses of above 10 milligrams will almost certainly produce these major toxic effects. When death occurs, it is due to paralysis, coma, and resultant respiratory failure. The toxic symptoms may continue for a period of days. With scopolamine, a period of depression and hypnosis may follow the psychotic symptoms. TOLERANCE develops if it is used over a period of time. Some patients take doses of 5 milligrams three times a day, and one taking 54 milligrams a day was reported. The fatal dose is sometimes given as roughly 100 milligrams, although a dose of 500 milligrams has been survived.

PHYSICAL DEPENDENCE upon scopolamine with WITHDRAWAL SYMPTOMS does not occur; presumably PSYCHIC DEPENDENCE upon the drug's sedative effects can develop. The hallucinations, excitement, and euphoria that toxic doses of the drug produce might be sought by some users of other hallucinogenic drugs; however, these effects are quite often frightening and unpleasant in the extreme, and so it is doubtful that anyone would wish to repeat them.

Recent reports on the impressions of patients treated with *scopolamine*, the active principle of henbane, supply more information. They experience a feeling of pressure in the head as if a heavy body rested on it. At the same time an invisible force seems to close their eyelids. Sight becomes vague and all objects seem to be stretched lengthwise. All kinds of visual hallucinations are produced while the eyes are open. For instance, a black circle on a silver background or a green circle on a golden background appears. The eyes then close and sleep sets in. The senses of taste and smell are also frequently affected. When sleeping the individual is surrounded by fantastic apparitions.

—Louis Lewin, *Phantastica: Narcotic and Stimulating Drugs* (1964)

score. [from (?) *score dough,* the price of a BUNDLE of narcotics; the proceeds of a theft; money; among American drug addicts *the score* means "sufficient money to purchase narcotics"; since around 1930—*EP*] *1.* to purchase narcotics.

I was living near 145th and Broadway at that time and I was *scoring* up there. I'd get my six bags, 11 o'clock at night go to work, and the same routine all day.

—addict, quoted in Jeremy Larner and Ralph Tefferteller, *The Addict in the Street* (1964)

2. purchase of narcotics. *3.* acquisition of money by an illegal transaction. *4.* to obtain something, to succeed, as in "I *scored* with her." Compare COP, BUY.

scratch (scratching). [description of addict's compulsion to scratch himself] being an addict.

script. [contraction of prescription] a narcotics prescription. Compare READER, PER.

scrubwoman's kick. naphtha, sometimes used as a cleaning preparation, emits intoxicatory fumes, which produce giddiness, loss of coordination, and sometimes euphoria; scrubwomen are supposed to have enjoyed the practice of inhaling the fumes until they were mildly intoxicated.

seccy. SECONAL.

Seconal. [secobarbital, Eli Lilly and Company] a short-acting, fast-onset BARBITURATE hypnotic and sedative. The hypnotic dosage is 100 milligrams. Excessive long-term use will result in PSYCHIC DEPENDENCE and PHYSICAL DEPENDENCE with severe WITHDRAWAL SYMPTOMS if use is abruptly ceased. Overdosage results in central nervous system depression, respiratory depression, slight constriction of the pupils (though in severe poisoning they may dilate), decreased urine formation, lowered body temperature, and coma; death comes from cessation of the respiratory reflex. Supplied in bright red 32-milligram capsules. Slang names: red birds, red devils, reds. A Schedule II drug under the CONTROLLED SUBSTANCES ACT.

seggy. SECONAL.

Sernylan. PHENCYCLIDINE.

serotonin. also called 5-hydroxytryptamine, enteramine, and 5-HT. A neurohormone found in the nervous system, small intestine, and brain. Neurohormones are chemical messengers which transmit nerve impulses across the synapses between the neuron and the muscle cell, thus activating the muscle. Other neurohormones are adrenalin (epinephrine) and acetylcholine.
   Serotonin is known to activate the smooth muscle of the small intestine, raise blood pressure, and constrict small blood vessels. Its function in the brain is only dimly understood but is thought to

be important, even though less than 1 percent of the body's total supply of serotonin resides there.

Because of its chemical similarity to the indole ring in hallucinogenic drugs such as BUFOTENINE, LSD-25, PSILOCYBIN, and MESCALINE, it is thought to be intimately related with their action, although precisely how is not certain. LSD-25, for example, seems to block the action of serotonin. When the two are placed together on a slice of smooth muscle tissue, nothing happens, although serotonin alone (or LSD alone) causes the muscle to contract. This suggests an analogous action in the brain.

According to one theory, LSD in the brain may compete with serotonin for the monoamine oxidase enzymes (see MONOAMINE OXIDASE INHIBITORS), which normally act upon serotonin to produce metabolites. When serotonin does not metabolize normally, as a result of LSD's monopolizing the necessary enzymes, it may throw off abnormal byproducts, one of which could be bufotenine, which has hallucinatory effects when injected. A similar derangement of serotonin caused by chemicals produced within the body rather than the hallucinogenic drugs may possibly be a cause of schizophrenia. This chemical theory of schizophrenia has yet to be demonstrated. (For another theory see ADRENOCHROME.)

Another theory of the relationship between serotonin and the effects of LSD postulates that serotonin acts as a mediator or inhibitor of nerve messages within the brain, serving to channel them in an orderly manner; that LSD replaces serotonin but is a weaker inhibitor and, thus, more messages are transmitted. According to this theory, the brain's regulatory center becomes overloaded, like a telephone switchboard suddenly jammed with incoming calls and lighting up on every circuit, and the illusions, pseudo hallucinations, distortions of normal perception, inflow of subconscious, repressed materials, etc., caused by hallucinogenic drugs are explained as dislocations of the usual orderly patterns of brain function, a figurative storm of suddenly unleashed material beating against the consciousness in sheets and waves.

Another theory holds that by blocking serotonin LSD induces temporary starvation of message transmissions; into this vacuum flow subconscious materials, disoriented perceptions of the surrounding environment, and so on, which take over the individual's consciousness.

It is interesting to note that MORPHINE and the TRANQUILIZER CHLORPROMAZINE, often used to reverse the LSD experience, also inhibit the action of serotonin, while RESERPINE, another tranquilizer, acts to stimulate it. All these explanations still have to be demonstrated by experiment.

set. *1.* [term proposed by Timothy Leary] the mental state of a person about to take a drug, encompassing both his state at the time and his deep psychological tendencies. Some LSD theoreticians hold that the set and the SETTING determine the quality of the psychedelic experience, including any adverse reactions. Anyone harboring a latent psychosis (part of his set) might emerge from the LSD with a chronic long-term psychosis; or a novice, frightened, ill at ease in his surroundings, and distrustful of his companions, might have a temporary, acute panic reaction to the drug. But even experienced LSD users, with over a hundred favorable LSD trips under their belts, can experience adverse results. Still, it seems incontrovertible that the person's intelligence, background, imagination, emotional state, and response to suggestion by others will color and provide the content of the hallucinations and emotions experienced while under the influence of a hallucinogenic drug. By the same token, there are always unpredictables in people's makeup at a given point in time, which makes a certain prediction of their reaction to experimental drugs like LSD impossible. *2.* [from (?) stage *set*] a drug-selling and drug-taking locale; a place where a group of addicts and pushers habitually congregate and are known to each other and where drugs are available. Compare LEAVING-THE-SET WALK, SCENE.

> The *set* is on the fifth floor and the floor is creaking an' groaning under the weight of all the coolies that are swinging. You dig the open door of the roof and smell burning pot.
> —Piri Thomas, *Down These Mean Streets* (1967)

setting. the total environment in which hallucinogenic drug-users undergo their drug experiences. A supportive, friendly environment, in which the user is supervised by a trusted person and is surrounded by pleasing objects, colors, and music, rich in associational content and interacting with a favorable SET, is considered most conducive to a favorable experience. In a favorable setting in a therapeutic atmosphere, a patient counseled by a psychiatrist may achieve a positive, therapeutic experience. A supportive setting, however, is no absolute guarantee against an adverse reaction.

set up. *1.* to entrap narcotics users by having informants sell them drugs in the presence of narcotics officers. *2.* to conceal drugs in drug users' residences and then raid them, as in "the cops *set* them *up* for a bust." Compare PLANT.

seventeen-fifty-one. [from the number of the New York State statute] felonious possession of drugs, i.e., in amounts above a statutory minimum which establishes a legal presumption that drugs are being held for purposes of sale.

seventeen-forty-seven B. possession of BARBITURATES, a misdemeanor under New York State law.

shit. [from (?) a deprecation of the quality of diluted heroin on the market, in comparison with that available in the 1920s; see JUNK; or using a socially proscribed word, see CRAP] HEROIN. Nonnarcotics users have taken over the term to some extent and use it to refer to HASHISH, PAREGORIC, LSD, and other drugs.

> Lysergic *shit*
> —R. Fariña, *Been Down So Long It Looks Like Up to Me* (1966)

Shiva. SIVA.

shlook. a puff of a MARIJUANA cigarette. Compare POKE, TOAK.

shooting gallery. *1.* a place where addicts regularly go to inject themselves with their purchases. Some addicts rent out their apartments for this purpose. *2.* the place in a hospital where addicts in withdrawal (or on maintenance therapy) are given their shots or oral doses. Compare RIFLE RANGE.

shooting gravy. injecting "cooked" blood. Sometimes the addicts' blood, drawn back up in the needles while they are injecting, coagulates and clogs the needle. They pour the mixture of blood and NARCOTICS back into their COOKERS, heat it until the blood dissolves, and reinject. Compare BOOTING, GRAVY.

shoot up. inject HEROIN.

> I began mainlining about 3 years ago—maybe 4—after I lost my job, and then I began *shooting up* pretty regular.
> —addict, quoted in Dr. Donald B. Louria, *Nightmare Drugs* (1966)

short. [since around 1930—*EP*] a car. Compare CRACKING SHORTS.

short con. a petty confidence game. Compare LONG CON.

short count. a short weight of a drug given by a supplier to a PUSHER for resale to the addict, the object being to cheat the pusher.

short go. *1.* a shortage. *2.* short weight from the PUSHER's supplier. Compare PANIC, SHORT COUNT.

> Everything was going as good as could be expected, till the panic hit. There was a *short go* on heroin on account of some big wheeler-dealer with millions of dollars worth of the stuff had gotten himself busted and this caused a bad shortage.
> —Piri Thomas, *Down These Mean Streets* (1967)

short piece. an amount of narcotics for sale that has been highly diluted. Compare PIECE, SHORT COUNT.

shove. [variant of PUSH] to sell drugs at the street level.

shying. the technique of cooking OPIUM pellets—*MM*, 1946. *Obsolete?*

sick. suffering from incipient WITHDRAWAL SYMPTOMS.

Siva. the mahadevi, or great god, of the Hindu trinity, who brought CANNABIS to mankind. Taking BHANG or CHARAS often accompanies ceremonies of worship to Siva.

sixteenth. one-sixteenth ounce of diluted HEROIN, a measure for purposes of sale to the addict. Compare PIECE.

sizzle. NARCOTICS carried on the person. Compare CARRYING, HOLDING.

skid bag. [from *skid row,* a gathering place of derelicts; the bottom of the heap] a BAG containing highly diluted HEROIN.

skid row. the convalescent ward at the Lexington, Kentucky, U.S. Narcotics Hospital.

skin. cigarette paper for rolling MARIJUANA cigarettes.

skinning. SKIN POPPING.

skin popping. [perhaps from *pop,* to burst or break; or from *pop,* to fire a pistol; leading to shoot, and to shoot, i.e., inject, drugs; compare BANG; since the 1920s—*EP*] injecting a narcotic subcutaneously or intramuscularly. The onset of the drug's effects is not so immediate as it is with MAINLINING (injecting intravenously). Neophytes often pass through three modes of taking the drug on their way to addiction: SNIFFING or snorting, skin popping, and mainlining. The practice of skin popping is also resorted to by old addicts whose veins are "used up." Skin popping often results in sores and boils on the body, through which tetanus bacillus enters. In New York City 75 percent of all tetanus cases are addicts; 50 percent of these cases are fatal. Compare INFECTION.

skin shot. a subcutaneous injection of a drug. Compare SKIN POPPING.

sleepers. BARBITURATES or other hypnotic–sedatives.

sleepwalker. HEROIN addict.

smack. [corruption of SCHMECK] HEROIN.

smashed. intoxicated on drugs. Compare RIPPED, ZONKED, WIPED OUT, SPACED, WASTED, STONED.

smeck. SCHMECK.

smoke. MARIJUANA, as in "He was dealing *smoke.*"

snakeroot. RAUWOLFIA SERPENTINA.

snappers. [the glass vials are *snapped* open so that the contents can be inhaled] AMYL NITRITE vials.

sniffing. inhaling HEROIN or COCAINE in powdered form through the nostrils. Compare SCHMECK, SNORT.

> Looking dead at Alfredo, I inhaled, first through one nostril, then through the other. Then turning quickly, away I went into the cold, cold street. Almost immediately I felt a burning sensation in my nose, like a sneeze coming. I pulled out my handkerchief and had barely enough time to put it to my nose when the blood came pouring out. *Man,* I thought, *this cap has blown out the insides of my nose.* But in a few seconds the bleeding stopped just as it started.
>
> Now the night lights seemed to get duller, my awareness of things delayed. But the music was clearer and I felt no pain, nothing at all. I seemed sort of detached. I felt a little sick in my belly, but the good-o feeling was better. I saw Trina coming to meet me and I crossed the street and walked toward her, walking real light, real dreamy and slow, so she would have to meet me more than halfway. Sometimes I'd make her walk all the way to me, but tonight I felt good.
>
> —Piri Thomas, *Down These Mean Streets* (1967)

snop. MARIJUANA or a marijuana cigarette.

snort. *1.* to inhale HEROIN or COCAINE through the nose. *2.* an inhalation of heroin or cocaine. *3.* COCAINE.

> When you *snort* heroin, you know, it got a bad, bitter taste, like a taste

that would turn your stomach inside out. It got some way-out taste. I couldn't snort because I couldn't take that taste; so I started shooting up.   —addict, quoted in Jeremy Larner and Ralph Tefferteller
The Addict in the Street (1964)

snow. [from the white, flaky appearance; since around 1900] COCAINE crystals.

soaper. [from SOPOR] METHAQUALONE.

sodium succinate. MESCALINE antagonist; it reverses the hallucinogenic effects of the drug.

soft drugs. nonnarcotic drugs, such as MARIJUANA, AMPHETAMINES, HALLUCINOGENS, BARBITURATES. "Soft" drugs may, of course, be addictive.

soma. an intoxicating beverage made from the juices exuded from stems of an unknown plant (possibly *Asclepias acida* or CANNABIS) and used ceremonially by priests and nobles in ancient India. Legend says that after drinking soma the god Indra was inspired to create the universe. Because restrictions were placed upon the drug's use in ancient times and it was replaced by yoga as a religious technique, its certain identity has been lost.

Sominex. See SCOPOLAMINE.

Somnafac. [METHAQUALONE hydrochloride, Smith Miller & Patch, Inc.] a nonbarbiturate hypnotic–sedative. Manufacturer recommends for the elderly, for those who cannot take BARBITURATES or other hypnotics, and for those for whom other hypnotics are not effective. Methaqualone usage can result in PSYCHIC and PHYSICAL DEPENDENCE, with WITHDRAWAL SYMPTOMS upon abrupt cessation of the dosage. Recommended dose is 200 to 400 milligrams; it is not recommended that Somnafac be taken for a period longer than four weeks. Sold in two-tone, blue 200-milligram capsules and dark blue 400-milligram capsules (Somnafac Forte).

Sopor. [METHAQUALONE, Arnar-Stone Laboratories] a nonbarbiturate hypnotic–sedative. Manufacturer recommends for sedation, insomnia, patients who cannot take other hypnotics, and brain-damaged elderly people. Recommended dose ranges from 75 milligrams for daytime sedation on up to 300 milligrams for sleep. Sold in pale green 75-milligram tablets, white 150-milligram tablets, and pink 300-milligram tablets, all with the initials "AS" stamped on them.

source, the. *1.* a supplier of drugs. *2.* a high-level supplier of narcotics to PUSHERS. Compare BIG MAN, PEOPLE, KILO CONNECTION.

spaced. [perhaps from a sensation of floating in space, the dislocation of the time sense caused by hallucinogenic drugs, or the floating HIGH from BARBITURATES or AMPHETAMINES] *1.* in a state of altered consciousness induced by a drug, originally a HALLUCINOGEN, such as MARIJUANA, HASHISH, or LSD, but now any drug. *2.* out of communication; in a state of pent-up inarticulateness as one undergoes the mental effects of a hallucinogenic drug; high.

spaced out. SPACED.

sparkle plenties. [after Sparkle Plenty, a character in "Dick Tracy"] AMPHETAMINES.

speed. [from SPEEDBALL; or from the stimulant effects of the drug] *1.* AMPHETAMINES, usually METHEDRINE. *2.* speedball.

speedball. [term—and practice—originated among GIs during the Korean conflict] HEROIN and COCAINE or AMPHETAMINE (DESOXYN is most common) injected as a mixture. The cocaine or amphetamine enhances the RUSH, while the heroin tempers the unpleasant extremes of the cocaine exhilaration and perhaps prolongs the KICK. Compare BOMBITA, FLASH.

> The reason for a *speed* is you get this tremendous girl [cocaine] kick that lasts only about one-half hour, and after it sort of starts dying off you have this almost buzzing sensation in all of your body and everything. But it becomes definitely sensuous, you know, all of a sudden and then after that it is just beginning to wear off, then wham, it's just like you made the boy [heroin] *then.* It comes on with this flash and everything. It's as though it holds off, you know, until the girl can operate.
> —Helen Macgill Hughes (ed.), *The Fantastic Lodge* (1961)

speed freak. a heavy intravenous user of methamphetamines (METHEDRINE and DESOXYN).

spike. hypodermic needle.

splash. AMPHETAMINES.

split. [SYNANON term] to run away, leave, break off treatment.

splits. probably a TRANQUILIZER, identity unknown.

Splits were common [in prison]. They're round white pills with a groove across the middle, some sort of tranquilizer. If you swallow one with a glass of hot water, you get a gone high that's almost like heroin. . . .

"That damn fool, he got some splits and it's bad enough to swallow them like he does, three or four at a gulp, but he went and crushed them and copped some works, an eye dropper and a needle, and shot himself up. His heart stopped."

—Piri Thomas, *Down These Mean Streets* (1967)

spoon. *1.* [from the tiny spoons used to ladle out the HEROIN] *2.* a measure of pure heroin, about 1/16 ounce, i.e., the unit by which the wholesaler often sells it to the PUSHER, who then cuts it and puts it in bags. There are, very roughly, seven bags to a spoon. *3.* an ordinary teaspoon (usually with handle bent) used for dissolving heroin over heat prior to injecting it. *4.* a measure of COCAINE, about a quarter of a teaspoon. Compare BAG, CUTTING, PIECE, SIXTEENTH.

spring. to treat another to a MARIJUANA cigarette.

square. *1.* anyone who does not use drugs. Compare STRAIGHT, LAME. *2.* a conventional cigarette.

S.S. a suspended sentence.

Remember I said in the Automat that when a junkie gets busted he rats on a couple of connections to get an *SS*—a suspended sentence?

—narcotics detective in James Mills,
The Panic in Needle Park (1966)

star dust. COCAINE.

stash. a hiding place for drugs and drug-taking equipment. Taping to the inside of a toilet tank is a common stash. See HOLD, HOLDING.

There are essentially two schools of thought. The first is the extreme one-up method of *stashing in the most obvious place.* On the coffee table labeled in plain sight. This is the preferred style in your upper socio-economic circles. The opposite point of view is the place *where it cannot be.* Inside the ice cubes or within brick walls, for example. Both obviously unsuitable due to the preparations involved. A third viewpoint does exist: this is the reactionary non-holder, his thesis being *never hold* [keep drugs on the premises]. A fourth view, not worthy of prime attention, is the *off-pad* scheme. On the roof stash, or the clothesline stash. The object here is to avoid direct holding. If you smoke you must hold sometime. Stash in your own home. Avoid unnecessary losses that can result from accidental stash uncovery. A cause for great paranoia.

—The Marijuana Newsletter No. 2 (March 15, 1965)

steamboat. [from the resemblance to a steamboat smokestack] to inhale the butt of a MARIJUANA cigarette stuck in a hole in a toilet roll, the hand enclosing one end, the mouth on the other end. Since the butt is too short and hot to hold in the fingers, it is inserted in the roll, which traps the smoke to be inhaled. Thus none of the smoke escapes, and it is cooled. Marijuana users believe that the concentration inhaled mixed with air, or "hyperventilated," is greater in potency.

stick. *1.* [from *stick of tea,* a thinly rolled cigarette—*MM,* 1946] a MARIJUANA cigarette purchased already rolled. *2.* [from Yiddish *schtick,* a technique, especially a characteristic bit of theatrical business] a favored criminal technique or mode of con; a style of life or criminal's modus operandi.

> Way down he was tickled that I wanted to imitate his *stick* of being.
> —Piri Thomas, *Down These Mean Streets* (1967)

sting. [from *sting,* to rob or defraud; verb since the 1800s; noun since around 1920—*EP*] a robbery, theft, illegal obtaining of money from a victim.

> I could uh . . . use uh my particular accent and have them believin' one thing . . . and the others was—would be takin' the *sting* off, you know?
> —addict in Seymour Fiddle,
> *Portraits from a Shooting Gallery* (1967)

stone. [from STONED, high on a drug; also, a stone is smooth, hard, solid, final] completely, finally, ultimately (good).

> . . . so cold it [a Coca-Cola] hurt my throat clear round to the back of my neck. But it was *stone* good.
> She was really a good-looking blip, stone-smooth.
> —Piri Thomas, *Down These Mean Streets* (1967)

stone addict. [see STONE; one becomes completely, fully stoned quickly; also (?) the idea of finality, of being ultimately stoned, completely achieving the goal of drug use] an addict who has rapidly acquired a strong habit.

stoned. in a state of drug-induced intoxication, elation, or euphoria, in a pleasant stupor. Compare HIGH.

stool. [from *stool pigeon,* police informer] *1.* to give information to police on illicit narcotics activities. *2.* to cooperate with police in trapping narcotics users.

STP. [DOM (4-methyl-2,5-dimethoxy-a-methylphenethylamine), Dow Chemical Company; probably from the brand name of a motor oil additive, "scientifically treated petroleum," which promises added power] a synthetic hallucinogenic drug chemically related to AMPHETAMINE and MESCALINE, STP achieved notoriety in the summer of 1967, when hospitals began receiving cases marked by psychotic reactions to the drug. Ten such cases were admitted in eleven days in San Francisco; one chronic psychosis and a possible death were also reported. It was believed that several thousand capsules containing the drug had been distributed free at a San Francisco be-in in April or May. The capsules were described by police as white with blue spots (later a New York biweekly described them as orange).

Use of the initials was variously attributed to members of the Hells Angels motorcycle gang (the motor-oil additive) and to Timothy Leary ("serenity, tranquillity, and peace"). At any rate, the drug was undoubtedly real, and its effects were said to be both more dramatic and longer lasting than those of LSD, three to four days as opposed to eight to twelve hours, although it was less potent on a weight-for-weight basis.

The tranquilizing drug CHLORPROMAZINE, frequently administered to calm an LSD taker who has had a panic psychotic reaction, was found to intensify and worsen adverse reactions to STP, leading some doctors to believe that STP, like chlorpromazine, resembled ATROPINE and hence one POTENTIATED the other. Another report called the drug BZ, a top-secret "nerve gas" being experimented on by the Army. When at last the Food and Drug Administration obtained samples and analyzed them, they announced it was a mescaline derivative.

A BDAC chemist then noticed the similarity of the drug's formula to that of an experimental drug, DOM, upon which Dow Chemical had applied for a patent. A check with the company revealed that the formulas were in fact identical. Whether STP represented the theft of Dow's formula, a leak of supplies of the actual drug (it had been sent to some scientific investigators and was being proposed for use in mental illness), or the independent discovery of some underground chemist could not be determined. Although some experienced users of HALLUCINOGENS praise it, others say that it carries more risk of a psychotic reaction than any other drugs; one writer said the odds were sixty to forty against a good TRIP.

Another writer, close to the drug underground, reported that the "manufacturer" was distributing the drug free of charge.

All veterans concur on the overwhelming power of *STP*. They speak of a maelstrom of relentless energy. "A feeling," said [Richard]

Alpert, "that it's going to do it to you whether you like it or not." The energy seems to manifest itself physically. "You feel like your body is a conductor for tens of thousands of volts," said a user. "I was desperate for a ground." People tripping on STP physically tremble with the energy sensation. It is a stretching, quivering, shaking experience. Many have emerged from STP with a sudden concern for physical health. "We have need to be strong," said one. "We need protein. The macrobiotic diet is bad news."

The relentless rush of energy is often a frightening experience. "Acid is like being let out of a cage," explained one user. "STP is like being shot out of a gun. There's no slowing down or backing up. You feel like your brakes have given out. . . ."

A key to survival in the STP experience seems to be an ability to surrender to the energy flow of the drug. Resisting the rush or holding back can lead, many report, to an incredibly frustrating uptight experience.

STP seems to lack the disorientation of acid. Although the audio and visual hallucinations are vivid, a girl explained, "Everything looks like it does when you're straight. It's like being on the other side of a glass wall." There also seems to be less identity confusion than under LSD. "You know who you are," she said. Many have found that they could easily function—make telephone calls, find cabs,—shortly after the peak of the STP experience. These things can be difficult to do after an intense LSD experience.

Another recurring report about STP is a sensation of timelessness. Alpert calls it "a totally NOW orientation." Past and future seem to dissolve in an electric present. As time was lost, Alpert recalled, "I felt that I had lost something human. I felt that I had lost my humanity."

But the most enticing, and clearly the most disturbing aspect of STP is that, unlike LSD, it seems to have a cumulative effect. It is a long trip to begin with. The direct effects last about 14 hours, and a stoned aftermath may continue until asleep.

The next morning, many STP initiates have discovered that they still felt high, or at least "different." It is a mild feeling, but a persistent one. Generally rated a "good" feeling, it seems to last indefinitely. . . .

Some people claim to have discovered intense telepathic powers in STP. Another curious aspect of STP, a user explained, is that at the peak of the experience you tend to think that everyone else has taken the drug. He described his experience:

"I got out of the cab on St. Mark's Place. It was three in the morning and the street was full of people, standing around. The sky was glowing, like it was flaming. I thought it was the Second Coming or something. I was absolutely convinced that It had just happened or would happen in seconds. And I thought everyone else knew it. How do you react when you're convinced? I was completely stoned."

—Don McNeill, *The Village Voice* (April 13, 1967)

straight. [from *getting straight,* getting one's affairs straightened out; also, perhaps, from *straight,* in the sense of being sexually normal] *1.* in a state of narcotics-induced normality with concomitant forestalling of WITHDRAWAL SYMPTOMS, as in "I need a shot to get *straight."* 2. not using drugs. *3.* not possessing drugs on the person. *4.* SQUARE, middle-class. *5.* a nonmarijuana cigarette. *6.* detoxified, sober.

straighten out. *1.* to prevent WITHDRAWAL SYMPTOMS. *2.* to restore the HEROIN addict to a normal, anxiety-free state of mind. Compare STRAIGHT.

> Like I might find old Joe Schmo today and buy three bags from him and find that one bag *straightens* me *out.* Now, okay, so I'll time my shots and get away with fifteen dollars today. Tomorrow I can't find Joe Schmo so I go find Larry the Jerk, and I buy three off him and one won't straighten me out, and maybe three won't straighten me out.
> —addict, quoted by James Mills, in *The Drug Takers* (1965)

stramonium. an alkaloid (occurring in jimson weed, DATURA STRAMONIUM, a plant of the same family as BELLADONNA and henbane), which is actually the alkaloids ATROPINE and HYOSCYAMINE. Stramonium can cause mental confusion and sluggish thinking or make the user preternaturally excited with accompanying hallucinations. In large doses, it produces narcosis, coma, stupefaction, convulsions, and death. It is sometimes used in asthma remedies. Compare DATURA, ASTHMADOR.

street, on the. the addict's milieu; by extension, to be using drugs.

street, the. [from the addict's necessity of constantly searching (HUSTLING) for drugs, purchasing on street corners, committing petty thefts to get money for drugs, etc.; similar to *pounding the pavements*] where addicts spend much of their time; hence, addicts' lives, in which they devote their time to finding drugs and are incapable of working at a regular job.

> It seems that addicts in general find it difficult to tolerate prolonged interpersonal contacts when there is no means of running away from them. . . . It is no accident that our patients refer to the world outside [of the U.S. Public Health Service Hospital, Lexington, Kentucky] as *"the street";* they cherish their mobility, the opportunity to escape difficult relationships very highly.
> —psychiatrist in James Mills, *The Panic in Needle Park* (1966)

strung. STRUNG OUT.

strung out. [from (?) *stringy,* reflective of the addict's emaciated appearance, or from (?) the sense of stringing something along, drawing it out, stringing along with something; since the 1950s] *1.* badly addicted to a drug. *2.* thin and sick looking because of long-term addiction. Compare EMBALAO. *3.* unable to obtain sufficient drugs to keep comfortable.

stuff. narcotics, or any drugs.

stumblers. [from the loss of motor control induced by drug intoxication] hypnotic–sedative drugs, especially BARBITURATES.

sugar weed. MARIJUANA soaked in a solution of sugar and water, which makes it weigh more, but also adheres it in block form; users sometimes refer to it as "curing." Said to decrease potency.

sweet lucy. MARIJUANA.

swingman. PUSHER, peddler, CONNECTION.

Synalgos-DC. [Drocode (dyhydrocodeine) bitartrate and other ingredients, Ives Laboratories] a CODEINE derivative used to relieve mild to moderate pain. Supplied in blue and gray capsules containing 16 milligrams of dyhydrocodeine. Manufacturer's recommended dosage is two capsules initially, then one or two capsules, two or three times daily. A Schedule III drug under the CONTROLLED SUBSTANCES ACT.

Synanon. [from an addict's mispronunciation of *seminar*] a communal-living program for the rehabilitation of drug addicts, in which the addicts help cure each other, through group therapy, mutual reinforcement, companionship, and social pressure. The members of each Synanon house are all addicts or former addicts; they stay as long as they like but are discouraged from leaving until they are judged capable of remaining off drugs—it is hoped permanently—though no "cures" are claimed. The stages of therapy are as follows:

1. Withdrawal from drugs; confinement to the house. No outside contacts.
2. When withdrawn from drugs and apparently off them, the member continues to live in the house but can work at an outside job.
3. Working and living outside the house; "cured."

"Cures" are estimated at 10 percent; apparently very few have progressed to phase 3, except those who have stayed in the movement and set up new branches of Synanon or work at Daytop Lodge, a similar program located in Staten Island, New York, and numerous other encounter-group therapeutical programs such as Phoenix House, Narcotics Anonymous, and Odyssey House. Like members of Alcoholics Anonymous, Synanon addicts are "cured" by replacing their drug addiction with an addiction to the "movement."

> We haven't been at this long enough to know for sure about cures. I won't pronounce anybody cured for at least five or six years. Not until some of our graduates go out there and come up against the things an adult must face—like losing a house, or a job or a child—without using drugs.   —Chuck Diederich, founder of *Synanon,*
> in Richard B. Stolley, *The Drug Takers* (1965)

synhexyl. PYRAHEXYL.

synthetic opiates. the class of synthetic MORPHINE substitutes (opioids) which resemble morphine in many of their actions and sometimes their chemical structures yet also differ in their actions, depending upon the synthetic. All induce some degree of PHYSICAL DEPENDENCE, though with many the WITHDRAWAL SYMPTOMS are less severe than those of morphine addiction. By the same token, many are of greater analgesic potency than morphine. The principal chemical types of synthetics are:

1. meperidine (pethidine) and such related drugs as alphaprodine, anileridine, and piminodine.
2. substituted morphinans, of which levorphanol is the most potent and important.
3. diphenylheptane derivatives such as methadone.

system, the. addicts' TOLERANCE, as in "They took too much heroin for *the system* and O.D.-ed."

T t

tabs. capsules containing LSD-25. Compare PELLETS.

taken off. to be robbed of money or drugs, as in "I was standing in the hall about to shoot up, but I got *taken off* by three men from the neighborhood."

take off. *1.* to get HIGH. *2.* to inject narcotics. Compare FLY, WINGS. *3.* to rob. Compare RIPPED.

take-off artists. addicts who support their habits by robbing other addicts or pushers.

taking care of business. what addicts do on the STREET; implies that they have things under control, that they are obtaining money for their fixes. Compare HUSTLING.

taking off. robbing.

taking on a number. smoking MARIJUANA.

tall. [from the idea of height, i.e., HIGH] in a drug-induced state of euphoria.

Talwin. [PENTAZOCINE hydrochloride, Winthrop Laboratories] a synthetic opiate analgesic. Manufacturer recommends in moderate to severe pain. Thirty milligrams of Talwin is the equivalent of 10 milligrams of MORPHINE or 75 to 100 milligrams of MEPERIDINE. TOLERANCE, PSYCHIC and PSYCHOLOGICAL DEPENDENCE on Talwin develop after prolonged use. WITHDRAWAL SYMPTOMS are of less severity than those associated with HEROIN dependence. The recommended injection is 30 milligrams; the recommended oral dose is 50 milligrams. Talwin is sold in ampuls for injection and 50-milligram, peach-colored tablets with "Winthrop" stamped around the circumference on the front.

tapita. [from diminutive of Spanish *tapa*, cork, plug, cap, meaning little cap] a bottle cap used for cooking HEROIN.

tapping the bags. the practice by PUSHERS of taking a small amount of HEROIN from their BAGS before selling them to the addict.

Taractan. [chlorprothixene, Roche Laboratories] a MAJOR TRANQUILIZER structurally similar to the phenothiazines. Used in severe mental and emotional disorders arising out of schizophrenic states. TOLERANCE and PHYSICAL DEPENDENCE do not occur, although gastritis, nausea, vomiting, tremulousness, and dizziness may follow abrupt cessation after long-term use. Manufacturer's recommended dosages range upwards from 25 to 50 milligrams three or four times a day, as needed; high dosages sometimes cause drowsiness. Supplied in red coated tablets with "ROCHE" inscribed on them, and in ampuls and liquid for injection.

taste. *1*. small amount of HEROIN or other drug proffered as a gift. *2*. a shot or sniff of heroin or another drug.

tar. gum OPIUM suitable for smoking.

tea. [from the physical resemblance to marijuana leaves chopped up for smoking; since the 1930s—*EP*] MARIJUANA.

> Watch your gums on that stick of *tea*
> and get high with me.
> It sends me gate and I can't wait
> I'm viper mad.   —marijuana song, around the 1940s

tea bag. smoking MARIJUANA, as in "in the *tea bag.*"

tea head. [see HEAD] a frequent, often heavy, habitual MARIJUANA smoker.

tea pad. rooms in apartments or pup tents on the roof in Harlem where MARIJUANA was sold and users gathered and smoked communally in the 1930s and 1940s.

tecata. HEROIN.

Tedral. [theophylline, ephedrine hydrochloride, and phenobarbital, Warner-Chilcott Laboratories] a bronchodilator with sedative for the relief of bronchial asthma, asthmatic bronchitis, and broncho-spastic disorder. Ephedrine is a stimulant and the phenobarbital is added to counteract it. There are reports of abuse of this drug which, because of the ephedrine and phenobarbital, would give a high of a sort. Sold in white, uncoated, scored tablets containing 130 milligrams of theophylline, 24 milligrams of ephedrine hydrochloride, and 8 milligrams of phenobarbital (Tedral-25—half pink, half pink-spotted white tablets—contains 25 milligrams of butabarbital).

telepathine. HARMINE.

ten-cent pistol. a HEROIN bag that actually contains poison. Compare HOT SHOT.

tens. 10-milligram AMPHETAMINE tablets.

teonanactl. [Nahuatl, God's flesh] Aztec name for hallucinogenic mushrooms. See MUSHROOMS, SACRED.

terpin hydrate. a nonnarcotic cough suppressant (a turpentine derivative in a high percentage of alcohol) sometimes taken for a sedative effect. See BLUE VELVET.

tetrahydrocannabinol. the euphorically ACTIVE PRINCIPLE in CANNABIS. When cannabis is smoked, it is believed that tetrahydrocannabinol is changed less than any of the other resinous materials found in the hemp leaves and thus is more highly concentrated in the smoke. In experiments, however, natural HASHISH given to animals had more potency than the sublimate remaining after smoking. Nearly eighty derivatives of natural tetrahydrocannabinol have been compounded, but it was not reproduced synthetically until 1966. Compare PYRAHEXYL.

Texas tea. MARIJUANA.

THC. TETRAHYDROCANNABINOL.

Theo-Nar. [contains NOSCAPINE, Key Pharmaceuticals, Inc.] a cough-reflex depressant containing an alkaloid of OPIUM. Each delayed-release tablet contains 30 milligrams of noscapine, a nonaddicting alkaloid of opium. Recommended for symptoms of bronchial asthma and emphysema.

third eye. in the psychedelic drug cult, the inward-looking eye, the new vision into self that drugs provide.

thirty-three-oh-five. [from the number of the statute] under New York State law, possession of narcotics, a misdemeanor when the amount held is below the minimum required for presumption of holding for purpose of sale, a felony.

Thorazine. [CHLORPROMAZINE hydrochloride, Smith Kline & French Laboratories] a MAJOR TRANQUILIZER, a phenothiazine derivative. PHYSICAL DEPENDENCE does not occur but abrupt withdrawal after long-term use will produce gastritis, nausea and vomiting, dizziness and tremulousness. Recommended in moderate-to-severe tension, apprehension, and anxiety; mild alcohol withdrawal; and schizophrenic and manic-depressive states. The drug has been used in panic reactions induced by hallucinogenic drugs such as LSD-25, but there are a number of possible side effects and simply talking patients out of their fears is often as effective. Recommended doses range from 10 to 25 milligrams. Sold in tablets, vials, ampuls, suppositories, and concentrate. In overdoses symptoms range from drowsiness to lowered blood pressure to cyanosis (blue skin), perspiration, rapid pulse, and respiratory depression.

throwing rocks. committing violent crimes.

thrupence bag. [from *pound,* five dollars, or *nickel,* five dollars] a bag of MARIJUANA costing $2.50.

At Columbia, marijuana is sometimes given as a Christmas present (one pusher revealed that he specially packages $2.50 doses of

marijuana—which he calls a *"thrupence bag"*—for purchases by Columbia students around Christmas time).
     —Richard Goldstein, *One in Seven: Drugs on Campus* (1966)

thrusters. AMPHETAMINE pills.

thumb. a fat MARIJUANA cigarette.

ticket, the. LSD-25.

tie. a belt or tourniquet used to distend the vein for an injection.

tie off. TIE UP.

tie up. to tighten a tourniquet around the arm in order to distend
the vein for injection.

tighten somebody's wig. to give him some MARIJUANA to
smoke—*MM,* 1946. *Obsolete.*

tighten up. to give someone some drugs.

tin. *1.* a can of smoking OPIUM. *2.* a tobacco can of MARIJUANA.
Compare CAN, LID.

tingle. a RUSH, or onset, of HEROIN's effects felt immediately in the
abdomen or across the chest.

TJ. Tijuana, Mexico; popular rendezvous for American tourists
purchasing MARIJUANA.

tlitliltzen. [Nahuatl, black] Aztec word for the black, hallucinogenic MORNING GLORY SEEDS.

TMA. [3,4,5-trimethoxyphenyl-*B*-aminopropane] a synthetic
HALLUCINOGEN of greater potency than MESCALINE but less than
LSD-25.

toak. also toke. *1.* a puff of a MARIJUANA cigarette. *2.* smoking the
entire cigarette, as in "a few *toaks* and he was high." Compare POKE.

toast. addicts' song.

     A ballad about "the life," the underworld and gray world through
     which the addicted pass for a period of time; generally handed down
     in prisons and hospitals.
          —Seymour Fiddle, *Portraits from a Shooting Gallery* (1967)

toke. TOAK.

toke pipes. tiny, short-stemmed pipes in which MARIJUANA is
smoked.

toke up. [from *toke*] to light up a MARIJUANA cigarette.

tolerance. the cumulative resistance to the pharmacological effects of a drug, gradually increased as use continues and the system adapts to it, sometimes selective as to the effects tolerated. Tolerance has set in when repeated administration of a given dose produces a decreasing effect, or increasingly larger doses must be administered in order to obtain the effects of the original dose. Compare ADDICTION, BARBITURATES, HEROIN, PHYSICAL DEPENDENCE, PSYCHIC DEPENDENCE.

tooies. TUINAL capsules.

tools. equipment for injecting drugs, mainly HEROIN. Compare GIMMICKS, WORKS, BIZ, KIT.

Top. a brand of wheat-straw cigarette paper, impregnated with different flavors, in which loose MARIJUANA is rolled for smoking.

topi. PEYOTE.

torn up. intoxicated by a drug.

torpedo. drink containing CHLORAL HYDRATE. Compare MICKEY FINN.

torture chamber. a jail where an addict can't obtain drugs.

tossed. searched for drugs.

> I don't get *tossed* too often. One time I got tossed three days in a row. . . . But they never find anything on me. Not because I'm clean. I'm never clean. I've almost always got works or pills or something. But they can't look where I carry the things. And when they're tossing me I start crying and screaming and making a scene and they get nervous. —addict in James Mills, *The Panic in Needle Park* (1966)

toss out. to feign WITHDRAWAL SYMPTOMS in order to obtain narcotics from a doctor. Compare WINGDING, BRODY.

toy. *1.* a small box of OPIUM. *2.* a hypodermic needle.

tracked up. [from TRACKS, needle scars caused by repeated injections] covered with blue healed and semihealed scars from a hypodermic needle.

> I shot up every day and I was pleased in a funny way that my arm wasn't *tracked up* like a trolley car run.
> —Piri Thomas, *Down These Mean Streets* (1967)

tracks. [from (?) the appearance, and in the sense of *traces*] *1.* veins collapsed from too frequent narcotics injections. *2*. needle scars from frequent injections in the form of blue or black spots with a tatooed appearance. Compare LINES, PIT.

> *Tracks* are marks, like a long black streak coming down your arm directly over your vein; that comes from hitting in the same place so much. Now when you skin-pop you hit all over your body; you can't keep up with the tracks. You lose them. They just keep falling off.
> —addict, quoted in Jeremy Larner and Ralph Tefferteller,
> *The Addict in the Street* (1964)

train arrived. a shipment of drugs has been successfully smuggled into prison.

tranquilizers. term for a number of drugs which have a depressant effect on the central nervous system, relieve anxiety and tension, and sometimes relax the skeletal muscles. Unlike hypnotic–sedative drugs, such as BARBITURATES, tranquilizers generally do not cause hypnosis, drowsiness, or loss of alertness (except in amounts larger than necessary for therapy). However, there are many exceptions to this rule, and frequently the tranquilizers offer little to recommend them over barbiturate sedatives in calming anxiety and tension (and are usually higher priced). Tranquilizers are usually classified both pharmacologically and chemically as MAJOR TRANQUILIZERS and MINOR TRANQUILIZERS, terms which reflect their therapeutic use.

trap. a hiding place for drugs. Compare STASH.

travel agent. [suggested by the LSD TRIP; since the 1950s] *1*. LSD-25. *2*. an LSD PUSHER.

trey. a $3 BAG of HEROIN. Compare DECK, THRUPENCE BAG, NICKEL BAG.

trick. *1*. an act of sexual intercourse by a prostitute. *2*. an illegal technique for making money.

trip. *1*. to take a hallucinogenic drug. *2*. the hallucinogenic drug experience.

trips. LSD.

tripsville. San Francisco.

tryptamine. nonhallucinogenic chemical from which the hallucinogenic drugs DMT, LSD, BUFOTENINE, and PSILOCYBIN can be derived.

Tuazole. European brand of METHAQUALONE.

Tuinal. [amobarbital sodium and secobarbital sodium, Eli Lilly and Company] a short- to intermediate-acting BARBITURATE hypnotic and sedative, combining in equal amounts AMYTAL and SECONAL. Recommended dosages: for sedation 3/4 grain (50 milligrams); for hypnosis 1 1/2 to 3 grains (100 to 200 milligrams). The lethal dose is approximately twelve times the hypnotic dose. Tuinal is sold in 3/4-grain (50 milligrams), 1/2 grain (100 milligrams), and 3-grain (200 milligrams) capsules with blue body and orange cap. Slang names: tooies, rainbows, red and blues. A Schedule II drug under the CONTROLLED SUBSTANCES ACT.

turned out. introduced to the fast life, or drugs.

turn on. [from (?) the mechanical sense of turn on a light, machine, etc.; since the 1950s] *1.* to introduce someone else to drugs, as in "I *turned* him *on*." *2.* to take drugs oneself, as in "We copped some pot and *turned on.*" *3.* to become intoxicated from drugs, as in "he was *turned on.*" *4.* by extension, any positive, satisfying, exhilarating experience.

turp. TERPIN HYDRATE cough syrup.

Tussanil-DH. [dihydrocodeine bitartrate and other ingredients, Misemer Pharmaceuticals] a cough syrup containing a CODEINE derivative. Each 5 cubic centimeters (1 teaspoonful) of the syrup contains 1.66 milligrams of dihydrocodeine bitartrate. In sufficiently large dosages it can produce PSYCHIC DEPENDENCE and PHYSICAL DEPENDENCE. A Schedule V drug under the CONTROLLED SUBSTANCES ACT.

twenty-five. LSD-25.

twist. MARIJUANA.

twisted. *1.* suffering WITHDRAWAL SYMPTOMS. *2.* under the influence of drugs. Compare BENT.

tying up. wrapping a cord, necktie, belt, etc., around the upper arm so as to distend the vein, preparatory to an intravenous shot of HEROIN. Compare DO UP.

U u

U.C. undercover agent.

uncle. [from Uncle Sam] a federal narcotics agent.

up. *1.* in a state of intoxication, HIGH, from some drug, especially a stimulant of the AMPHETAMINE type. *2.* a stimulant drug.

up and down the lines. [from *lines,* veins] collapsed or thromboid veins all over the arm. Compare TRACKS.

upper. an AMPHETAMINE pill.

uppie. an AMPHETAMINE pill.

ups. AMPHETAMINE pills.

uptight. [in the sense of being hemmed in, back against the wall] *1.* objectively in a tight situation with the law: the evidence is against you. *2.* tense, worried, feeling hemmed in. *3.* touchy, defensive, flaring up with hostility. Compare PARANOIA.

using. taking drugs.

V v

Valium. [diazepam, Roche Laboratories] a MINOR TRANQUILIZER and skeletal-muscle relaxant. Used in alleviating neurotic tension and anxiety states and in controlling muscle spasms (as in cerebral palsy). Manufacturer's recommended dosages: 2 to 5 milligrams, two or three times daily, in mild to moderate neuroses; up to 5 to 10 milligrams three or four times daily in severe neurotic reactions. Prolonged, heavy dosage can result in PHYSICAL DEPENDENCE with severe WITHDRAWAL SYMPTOMS similar to BARBITURATE withdrawal (convulsions, tremor, abdominal and muscle cramps, and sweating) if drug is abruptly ceased. Overdose results in intoxication similar to alcoholic or barbiturate intoxication; Valium has been used successfully in suicides, and depressant drugs POTENTIATE its effects if taken along with it. Supplied in white 2-milligram and yellow 5-milligram tablets inscribed with "ROCHE."

Valmid. [ETHINAMATE, Eli Lilly and Company] a nonbarbiturate hypnotic. According to the manufacturer, the hypnotic dose is 500 milligrams at bedtime, which can be repeated as late as three to four hours before arising, in the event the patient wakes up, without residual sedation ("drug hangover"). Massive doses of Valmid can cause death through depression of the respiratory center. The drug has a euphoric effect on some persons, especially former alcoholics or disturbed persons, who may develop a PSYCHIC DEPENDENCE upon it. Prolonged, heavy use produces PHYSICAL DEPENDENCE and severe WITHDRAWAL SYMPTOMS upon abrupt cessation of the drug. Supplied in 0.5-gram (7 1/2-grain) peach-colored tablets with "DISCKETS" inscribed upon them. A Schedule IV drug under the CONTROLLED SUBSTANCES ACT.

vendedor. [Spanish, seller, salesman] a PUSHER, narcotics peddler.

Veronal. See BARBITURATES.

vinho de jurumena. a narcotic beverage prepared from the seeds of *Mimosa hostilis* by the Pancaru Indians of Brazil. A closely related genus is PIPTADENIA. It is a HALLUCINOGEN and is used by the Indians in religious ceremonies and magical rites. Contains an alkaloid first named nigerine but latter identified as DMT, a hallucinogen and the ACTIVE PRINCIPLE of the plant.

violated. arrested for a parole violation, as in "I stopped seeing my P.O. [parole officer] and started back on drugs and then I got *violated* again and went in for three months."

vipe. [from viper] to smoke MARIJUANA. *Obsolete.*

viper. [from the sense that marijuana renders one as dangerous and unpredictable as a viper; since the 1930s—*EP*] a MARIJUANA smoker. *Obsolete.*

> When your pipes get dry
> Then you know you're high
> Everything is dandy

You truck on down to the candy store.
But you don't get no peppermint candy
Then you know your body's sent
You don't care if you don't pay rent.
Light a tea and let it be
If you're a viper.   —'If You're a Viper" (around 1940)

Virola. a genus of tree belonging to the NUTMEG family *(Myristicaceae)* whose resin is used by Indians of the Colombian Amazon to make an intoxicating snuff, which they call *yakee* or *parica.* Species include *Virola colophylla, V. calophylloidea,* and perhaps *V. elongata.* The ACTIVE PRINCIPLE is believed to be MYRISTICIN (ELEMICIN), which is also found in nutmeg and is responsible for its hallucinogenic effect. The resin is collected by stripping the bark before the sun is up, scraping it off, and boiling it to a thick paste which is dried, pulverized, sifted, and mixed with ashes of wild coca stems. Compare MDA, MMDA.

> I took about one-third of a teaspoonful [of the snuff] in two inhalations using the characteristic V-shaped bird-bone snuffing tube. This represents about one-quarter the dose that a diagnosing medicine man will take to bring on an eventful state of unconsciousness. . . . Within fifteen minutes, a drawing sensation was felt over the eyes followed very shortly by a strong tingling in fingers and toes. The drawing sensation in the forehead gave way to a strong and constant headache. Within a half hour, the feet and hands were numb and sensitivity of the fingertips had disappeared. . . . Shortly after eight, I lay down in my hammock, overcome with a drowsiness, which, however, seemed to be accompanied by a muscular excitation except in the hands and feet. About nine-thirty, I fell into a fitful sleep which continued, with frequent awakenings, until morning. . . . The witchdoctors see visions in color, but I was able to experience neither visual hallucinations, nor color sensations. The large dose used by the witch-doctor is enough to put him into a deep but disturbed sleep, during which he sees visions and has dreams which, through the wild shouts emitted in his delirium, are interpreted by an assistant. That it is a dangerous practice is acknowledged by the witch-doctors themselves. They report the death, about 15 years ago, of one of their number . . . during a yakee intoxication.
> —Richard E. Schultes, *Psychedelic Review* (1964)

vol. VOLUNTEER.

volunteer. at the U.S. Public Health Service (Narcotics) Hospital, Lexington, Kentucky, one who commits himself for treatment of narcotics or BARBITURATE addiction and is free to leave any time.

voyager. person under the influence of LSD-25.

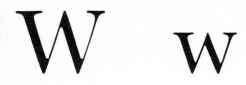

wake-up. the addict's first morning injection. Compare EYE OPENER, MORNING SHOT.

wallbangers. [British; from the user's loss of muscular coordination while intoxicated] Mandrax (METHAQUALONE).

waste. to use up, destroy, pulverize, obliterate, kill.

> Indio pushed another stick [marijuana cigarette] in my hand. I *wasted* it down to nothing.
> —Piri Thomas, *Down These Mean Streets* (1967)

wasted. *1.* passed out from acute drug intoxication. *2.* see WASTE.

water. [methamphetamine users believe the drug is chemically close to water] AMPHETAMINE, especially methamphetamine (METHEDRINE and DESOXYN).

watering out. undergoing narcotics WITHDRAWAL SYMPTOMS without the aid of drugs. Compare COLD TURKEY, A LA CANONA.

wedges. flat LSD-25 tablets.

weeding out. [from *weed*, MARIJUANA] smoking marijuana.

weed marijuana. low-potency MARIJUANA growing wild in the United States.

weekend habit. using narcotics irregularly, on weekends. Compare CHIPPYING, ICE CREAM HABIT.

weekend warrior. an irregular drug user.

weight. a supply of, measure of drugs for sale. Compare PIECE.

> Give her her *weight* for the week. . . . He said that these were the people into all the cocaine weight and that he was going to cut me into them.   —Claude Brown, *Manchild in the Promised Land* (1965)

whacked. diluted, adulterated, CUT; usually said of HEROIN.

wheat. [probably from the wheat-straw paper used in rolling the cigarette] MARIJUANA.

wheel. a car. Compare CRACKING SHORTS.

whistling (I came in). [from the idea of the wind whistling through an old house; the addict's clothes are threadbare, and the wind is whistling through him in this manner—Seymour Fiddle, *The Language of Addiction*] entering a hospital very sick, run down, and impoverished.

white lady, the. HEROIN or COCAINE. Compare WHITE STUFF, SNOW.

white light. a hallucination of a blinding white light, accompanied by a feeling of omniscience, said to be produced by STP.

> Within forty minutes I was peaking, experiencing what I can only describe as *white light,* whatever that might be.
> —editorial, *Innerspace* (1967)

whites. BENZEDRINE pills.

white stuff. [since the 1920s] COCAINE, MORPHINE, or (usually) HEROIN.

wig. [from *hair, head* extended to mean the mind, and *wig out,* lose one's wig, i.e., mind; *"wig,* head or hair; wig-trig, idea"—*MM,* 1946] *1.* the mind. *2.* to be upset, excited, panicky. *3.* to WIG OUT, to be crazy.

> So I says, "What's with you? You *wig* already?"
> —William Burroughs, *Naked Lunch* (1959)

wig out. abrupt, usually euphoric, dramatic alteration of subjective mood under the influence of a drug. Compare BLOW YOUR MIND, FREAK OUT, FLIP OUT.

wild Geronimo. [around the 1940s] a drink consisting of BARBITURATES dissolved in an alcoholic beverage.

winder. a VOLUNTEER for treatment at the U.S. Public Health Service (Narcotics) Hospital, Lexington, Kentucky; one who can leave at any time, and thus who *winds* in and out.

wingding (throw a). feigned WITHDRAWAL SYMPTOMS to get a doctor to give one narcotics. Compare TOSS OUT.

wings. *1.* the first MAINLINE shot. *2.* learning how to take narcotics in this way.

> He gave me my *wings*—my first mainline shot.
> —James Mills, in *The Drug Takers* (1965)

wiped out. acutely intoxicated from a drug.

wired. *1.* addicted to HEROIN. Compare STRUNG OUT. *2.* HIGH on AMPHETAMINES.

withdrawal symptoms or syndrome. a cluster of characteristic reactions, and behavior, of varying intensity, depending on the amounts of the drug taken and the length of time used, sometimes fatally severe, which ensue upon abrupt cessation of a drug upon which the body has PHYSICAL DEPENDENCE. The withdrawal syndrome varies with the drug. An antagonist drug, which acts to reverse the effect of the addictive drug, will precipitate withdrawal symptoms when it is administered; however, not all drugs to which physical dependence develops have antagonist drugs. These symptoms often can be controlled only by carefully spaced, decreasing dosages of the drug upon which there is dependence or a related drug.

CHARACTERISTIC WITHDRAWAL SYNDROMES

drug dependence of the morphine, opiate type: appears within a few hours of last dose. Reaches peak intensity in twenty-four to forty-eight hours. Subsides spontaneously. Symptoms: anxiety, restlessness, generalized body aches, insomnia, yawning, tears, running nose, perspiration, contraction of the pupils, gooseflesh, hot flushes, nausea, release of the bowels, diarrhea, rise in body temperature, rise in respiratory rate, rise in systolic blood pressure, abdominal cramps, seminal ejaculations, muscle cramps, dehydration, and loss of body weight. Nalline and levallorphan will precipitate these symptoms.

drug dependence of the barbiturate type: appears within sixteen to twenty-four hours of cessation of drug-taking. Reaches peak intensity in two or three days. Subsides slowly. There is no antagonist which will precipitate the withdrawal syndrome. Symptoms: anxiety, involuntary twitching of muscles, tremor of hands and fingers, progressive weakness, dizziness, distortion in visual perception, nausea, vomiting, insomnia, weight loss, sudden drop in blood pressure when addict stands, epileptic type of seizure and severe convulsions (possible death from exhaustion or heart failure), delirium tremens, and, later, a major psychotic episode accompanied by paranoid reactions, schizophrenic reactions with delusions and hallucinations, withdrawn semistuporous state, and/or disorganized panic, depending upon the individual. Alcohol will at least partially suppress the withdrawal syndrome.

drug dependence of the alcoholic type: appears with the following symptoms: tremors, sweating, nausea, rapid heartbeat, rise in temperature, jerky reflexes, and, in severe cases (where the consumption has been in large amounts over a long period), convulsions, and delirium tremens (confusion, disorientation, delusions, and vivid auditory and visual hallucinations). The withdrawal syndrome can be suppressed by barbiturates. Compare COCAINE, ALCOHOL, OPIUM, TRANQUILIZERS.

working. obtaining money for drugs. Compare HUSTLING, TAKING CARE OF BUSINESS.

works. equipment for injecting HEROIN, consisting of needle; bottle cap or spoon (COOKER) for dissolving heroin over heat; eyedropper bulb or baby's pacifier; eyedropper; paper collar packed around the junction of the dropper and the needle; belt, string, or cord (for wrapping tightly around the arm to distend the vein—TYING UP); small bottle of distilled water in which to dissolve the heroin and cook it. Compare FIX, GIMMICKS, ARTILLERY, BIZ, KIT, COLLAR, COTTON.

wrap. innocuous-looking covering of a package of marijuana or other bulky drug in which it is transported or shipped in the mail. Compare STASH.

> Beware of a smelly stash. This might be scented by trained POTHEAD HOUNDS which are occasionally toured through bus depots and similar baggage scenes, sniffing out stashes poorly packaged. *A bad wrap can burn you. . . .* Important things to remember about packaging are: Use no identifying or implicating containers, wrap in both foil and plastic film. Another layer of brown paper might help, especially if you plan to stash under the kitty-litter, a very good spot where a good wrap really makes a difference.
>
> —*The Marijuana Newsletter No. 2* (March 15, 1965)

Y y

yage. AYAHUASCA.

yaje. AYAHUASCA.

yakee. hallucinatory snuff prepared by Yekwana Indians from the VIROLA plant.

yellow jackets. [from the color] NEMBUTAL capsules.

yellows. NEMBUTAL capsules.

yen. [from Chinese *yen-yen* or *inyunfun*, OPIUM habit; one suffering with *inyun;* hence a strong need; since the 1880s—*EP*] now, any craving. Compare COP SICKNESS, YENNING.

> I felt my throat blend in and out with the *yen.* The taste that takes place even before you get the junk in your system. All of a sudden, I felt like nothing mattered, like if all the promises in the world didn't mean a damn, like all that mattered was that the stuff is there, the needle is there, the yen is there and your veins have always been there.　　　　—Piri Thomas, *Down These Mean Streets* (1967)

yen hok. [since the 1880s—*EP*] needle used to cook OPIUM pellets. *Obsolete?*

yenning. [from YEN] experiencing incipient WITHDRAWAL SYMPTOMS. See COP SICKNESS (quotation).

yen pok. [since the 1880s—*EP*] pellet of OPIUM prepared for smoking. *Obsolete?*

yerba. [from Spanish, *hierba,* grass, weed, herb, and *mala hierba,* weed, bad character, marijuana] MARIJUANA. Compare GRASS, HERB, WEED.

yopo. hallucinogenic snuff made by Otomac Indians of the Orinoco Valley from PIPTADENIA.

Z z

zap. [from the noise made by the ray gun in "Buck Rogers," a science-fiction comic strip and radio series] *1*. to (symbolically) defeat someone, as in "I *zapped* him with love." *2*. to (literally) kill, hurt, or overpower someone with violence or a weapon.

zigzag. a brand of wheat-straw cigarette paper, impregnated with different flavors, in which loose MARIJUANA is rolled for smoking.

ZNA. mixture of dill weed and monosodium glutamate, smoked for an alleged hallucinogenic effect.

zonked. HIGH, highly intoxicated from a drug; overdosed.

Appendix I

Nonsynthetic derivatives of opium, morphine, and cocaine.
Source: Federal Bureau of Narcotics.

Opium, powdered, granulated, or deodorized, or tinctures or extracts of opium.
Mixed alkaloids of opium and their salts.
Morphine and its salts.
Codeine and its salts.
Thebaine and its salts.
Noscapine and its salts.
Papaverine and its salts.
Cotarnine and its salts.
Narceine and its salts.
Ethylmorphine and its salts.
Apomorphine and its salts.
Nalorphine (N-allylnormorphine) and its salts.
Hydromorphone (dihydromorphinone) and its salts.
Metopon (methyldihydromorphinone) and its salts.
Dihydrocodeine and its salts.
Hydrocodone (dihydrocodeinone) and its salts.
Oxycodone (dihydrohydroxycodeinone) and its salts.
Cocaine and its salts.
Ecgonine and its salts.
Levorphan and racemorphan (3-hydroxy-N-methylmorphinan) and their salts.
Levomethorphan and racemethorphan (3-methoxy-N-methylmorphinan) and their salts.
Dihydromorphine (3,6-dihydroxy-N-methyl-4,5-epoxymorphinan) and its salts.
Oxymorphone (14-hydroxy-dihydromorphinone) and its salts.
Pholcodine (morpholinylethylmorphine) and its salts.

Appendix II

Generic names of synthetic opiates. *Source: Federal Bureau of Narcotics.*

ACETYLMETHADOL
ALLYLPRODINE
ALPHACETYLMETHADOL
ALPHAMEPRODINE or NU-1932

ALPHAMETHADOL
ALPHAPRODINE or NU-1196
ANILERIDINE
BENZETHIDINE
BETACETYLMETHADOL
BETHAMEPRODINE or NU-1932
BETAMETHADOL
BETAPRODINE or NU-1779
CLONITAZENE
DEXTROMORAMIDE
DIAMPROMIDE
DIETHYLTHIAMBUTENE
DIMENOXADOL
DIMEPHEPTANOL
DIMETHYLTHIAMBUTENE
DIOXAPHETYL BUTYRATE
DIPHENOXYLATE
DIPIPANONE
ETHYLMETHYLTHIAMBUTENE
ETONITAZENE
ETOXERIDINE
FENTANYL
FURETHIDINE
HYDROXYPETHIDINE
ISOMETHADONE
KETOBEMIDONE
LEVOMETHORPHAN, RACEMETHORPHAN (its racemic and levorotatory forms and their
    salts, but excepting its dextrorotatory form and its salts)
LEVOMORAMIDE
LEVOPHENACYLMORPHAN
LEVORPHANOL, DEXTRORPHAN, RACEMORPHAN, NU-2206
METAZOCINE
METHADONE
METHADONE-INTERMEDIATE
MORAMIDE-INTERMEDIATE
MORPHERIDINE
NORACYMETHADOL
NORLEVORPHANOL
NORMETHADONE
NORPIPANONE
PETHIDINE
PETHIDINE-INTERMEDIATE-A
PETHIDINE-INTERMEDIATE-B
PETHIDINE-INTERMEDIATE-C
PHENADOXONE or CB-11
PHENAMPROMIDE
PHENAZOCINE
PHENOMORPHAN (its racemic and levorotatory forms, but excepting its dextrorotatory
    form and its salts)

PHENOPERIDINE
PIMINODINE
PIRITRAMIDE
PROHEPTAZINE
PROPERIDINE
RACEMORAMIDE
TRIMEPERIDINE

Appendix III

Schedule I drugs under the Controlled Substances Act of 1970.
Source: Bureau of Narcotics and Dangerous Drugs.

Hallucinogens including LSD-25, mescaline, peyote, DMT, psilocybin, psilocin, marijuana, tetrahydrocannabinols
Heroin
Ketobemidone
Levomoramide
Racemoramide
Benzylmorphine
Dihydromorphine
Morphine Methylsulfonate
Micocodeine
Nicomorphine

Appendix IV

Schedule II drugs under the Controlled Substances Act of 1970, as revised in 1973. (Note: amobarbital (Amytal), secobarbital (Tuinal), pentobarbital (Nembutal) and secobarbital (Seconal) were added to the list subsequently.) *Source: Bureau of Narcotics and Dangerous Drugs.*

Adanon Hydrochloride
Ad-Nil (Medics)
Ad-Nil No. 2 (Medics)
Adipo (Sig)

Adjudets Troches (Ives)
Alodan (Gerot)
Alphaprodine
Alphaprodine Hydrochloride

Alphetamine 10 Capsules (Alpha)
Alphetamine 15 Capsules (Alpha)
Alvodine Ethanesulfonate (Winthrop) Ampules 1 ml.
Alvodine Ethanesulfonate (Winthrop) Tablets 50 mg.
Am Plus (Roerig)
Amagesic (Caldwell and Bloor)
Amba-Dex (Moffet)
Amba-Dex-TD (Moffet)
Ambar Extentabs (Robins)
  No. 1
  No. 2
Ambardex Tablets (Phila. Caps. Co.)
Ambar Tablets (Robins)
Ambi-Dex (Buffalo)
Ambodex (Testagar)
Amcodex Dakaps (Amco)
Am-Dex (Superior)
Amdram 7 1/2 Tablets (Dram)
Amedrine (Methamphetamine)
Amerital (Merit)
  Capsules 7.5 mg.
  Capsules 15 mg.
Amfadiol (Philips Roxane)
Amfodex (Phila. Caps. Co.)
Amidone Hydrochloride
Amitrene (Normand)
Amo-Dextro (Rocky Mountain)
  Tablets
  Capsules No. 1
  Capsules No. 2
Amo-Dextrosule Jr. (Storck)
Amo-Dextrosule Sr. (Storck)
Amo-Dextrosule Sr. Timesule (Arnar-Stone)
Amo-Dexules (Recsei)
  Capsules No. 1
  Capsules No. 2
Amobese (Cole)
Amodex (various)
  Capsules
  Tablets
Amodex Junior (Testagar)
Amondex Timed Capsules (Testagar)
Amordex (Palmedico)
Amorex Injection (Mallard)
Ampha-Cel Plus (Paramount)
Amphamed (Amphetamine Sulfate)
Amphamine Tablets (Naman)
Ampha-Mix Tablets (Sonnenberg)
Amphaplex (Palmedico)
  Injection
  Tablets 10 mg.
  Tablets 20 mg.

Ampharb (Harvey)
Amphate (various)
Amphcaps (Manne)
  Capsules 10 mg.
  Capsules 20 mg.
Amphe-Gum (Prof. Drug Service)
Amphebarb Tablets (Jabert)
Amphecaps-R Capsul (direct)
Amphecell (Allan)
Amphedex (various)
  Capsules 10 mg.
  Capsules 15 mg.
  Tablets
Amphedrine (Van Pelt Brown)
Amphedrine-M (Van Pelt Brown)
Amphedroxyn (Lilly)
Amphehist Capsules (Consol. Midland)
Amphemine Tablets (Prof. Drug Service)
Amphepyrilate Capsules (Consol. Midland)
Ampherex (Royce)
Am-Phet (Paul Maney)
Am Phet Capsules (M. J. Labs)
Amphet-A-Barb (Archer-Taylor)
Amphet-A-Barb Forte (Archer-Taylor)
Amphet-O-Phen (various)
  Capsules
  Tablets No. 1
  Tablets No. 2
  Tablets No. 3
Amphetamine
Amphetamine and Methylcellulose (Bariatric)
Amphetamine Dextro and Amobarbital (Vitarine)
Amphetamine HCL-1 (various)
  DL, Powder
  Vials
Amphetamine Phosphate, Dextro
Amphetamine Reducing Capsules (Davis-Edwards)
  No. 1
  No. 2
  No. 3
Amphetamine Sulfate Dextro (various)
Amphetamine w/ Amobarbital (West-Ward)
Amphetamine-10 (Alpha)
Amphetamine-20 (Alpha)
Amphetaminum (Amphetamine Sulfate)
Amphetavite Tablets (Len-Tag)
Amphetidisin (Allan)
Amphetidisin-10 (Allan)
Amphetoplex (Vitamix)
Amphetoplex Injectable (various)
Amphetose Tablets (Jabert)
Amphex (Algro)

Amphobarb No. 1 (Kay)
Amphobarb No. 2 (Kay)
Amphobese (various)
  Capsules
  Tablets No. 1
  Tablets No. 2
Amphocell Tablets (Wolins)
Amphoids-S (Gold Leaf)
Amphone (various)
Amphorbarb (CMC)
Amphovite (Tri-State)
Amphovite Improved Capsules (Tri-State)
Amsustain (Key)
Amvicel (Stuart)
Amvicel-X10 (Stuart)
Amvicel-X15 (Stuart)
Amvidex Timecaps (Caldwell and Bloor)
An-Du-Hist (Philips Roxane)
Anadrex (Anahist)
Analstat (Bush)
Anileridine
Anorex (Tenn. Pharm.)
Ante-Mens (Haberle)
Antussal (Vale)
Apadex (various)
Apamine (Stillco)
A.P.C. with Demerol (Winthrop) Tablets 30 mg.
A.P.C. with Meperidine HCl (Wyeth) Tablets 30 mg.
Apetain Granutabs (Tutag)
Apetain w/Amobarbital (Tutag)
Apodol (Squibb Injection) 25 mg./cc.
Apodol (Squibb) Tablets 25 mg.
Apomorphine
Apomorphine Hydrochloride
Apomorphine HCl (Lilly) Tablets Hypodermic 1/10 gr.
Apomorphine Methylbromide
Apomorphine-10-Methyl Ether
Apomorphine Hydrochloride (Merck) Powder 5 gr.
Appetrol Tablets (Wallace)
Appetrol-Sr Capsules (Wallace)
Apyrilene-Deoxie (Foy)
Arcodex (Arcum)
  Capsules
  Capsules No. 2
Arda Timed Capsules (Testagar)
Ardex 10 (Arden)
Ardex 15 (Arden)
Armadex 1 (Arden)
Armadex 2 (Arden)
Armodex (Arden)
AT-1053 Hysobel No. 3 (Zemmer)

B & O Supprettes (Webster) Suppositories No. 15-A
B & O Supprettes (Webster) Suppositories No. 16-A
Bamadex (Lederle)
  Sequels
  Tablets
Bamite (First Texas)
Barbadex (Kirkman)
Bardex (various)
  Capsules
  Tablets No. 1
  Tablets No. 2
  Tablets No. 3
Bar-Dex (Mercury)
Barbidex (Davis and Sly)
Barbidex TDC (Canfield)
Bariatric Formula (Bariatric)
  No. SS2
  No. SS3
  No. SS5
  No. 75A
  No. 75B
  No. 75D
  No. 75F
Bariatric Formula (Table Rock)
  No. 37
  No. 38
Barmine Tablets (Tutag)
Bartime Capsules (various)
Benzamphetamine (Amphetamine Sulfate)
Benzebar (S.K. & F.)
Benzedrine (S.K. & F.)
  Capsules 15 mg.
  Tablets 5 mg.
  Tablets 10 mg.
Benzoylecgonine
Benzoylpseudotropeine
Benzoyl-Psi-Tropeine
Betafen (Amphetamine Sulfate)
Bezitramide
Bifran Tablets (Strasenburgh)
Biphetamine 7 1/2 (Strasenburgh)
Biphetamine 12 1/2 (Strasenburgh)
Biphetamine 20 (Strasenburgh)
Biphetamine-T 12 1/2 Capsules (Strasenburgh)
Biphetamine-T 20 Capsules (Strasenburgh)
Bluzedrin (Amphetamine Sulfate)
Boldine
Bontril (Carnrick)
  Tablets No. 1
  Tablets No. 2
Bufeta Compound (Burrough Bros.)
Buta-Dexsules (Normal)

Capsules 10 mg.
Capsules 15 mg.
Butalgin

C and B Tonic (Caldwell and Bloor)
C.T. Blue No. 1-CVK (Durst)
C.T. Gray No. 1-DCQ (Harvey)
C.T. Green No. 1-CSE (Harvey)
C.T. Green No. 1-CYK (Durst)
C.T. Mottled Pink No. 1-CDO (Arrow)
C.T. Natural No. 1-14966 (Caldwell and Bloor)
C.T. Natural No. 2-AGG (Hiss)
C.T. Pink No. 1-CTJ (Caldwell and Bloor)
C.T. Pink No. 1-CVL (Durst)
C.T. Pink No. 1-CVW (Harvey)
C.T. Purple No. 1-CVN (Durst)
C.T. White No. 1-CAS (Lafayette)
C.T. White No. 1-CBU (Arrow)
C.T. Yellow No. 1-BMP (Caldwell and Bloor)
C.T. Yellow No. 1-CTF (Harvey)
C.T. Yellow No. 1-CVM (Durst)
Cafaryl (Elder)
Calaformula w/ Amphetamine Sulfate (Eric Kirk)
Calate (Marsin)
Carcell (various)
Carcell-Ten (Garde)
Carrtime-10 (various)
Carrtime-15 (various)
Cel Obese (Paramount)
Cel-Am-Vite Capsules (Nysco)
Celdex (Rocky Mountain)
Cell O-B (Ruckstuhl)
Cell-O-Dex Tablets (Fellows Testagar)
Cell-O-Rex No. 2 (Ruckstuhl)
Cello-Bese (Halsom)
Cellodex Tablet (various)
Cellomine (Kenyon)
Celludex Tablets (various)
Celludex-Plus (North American)
Cellukraft Special (Kraft)
Cellulet Tablets (various)
Cellutabs (Kraft)
Cendex Cenule (various)
Cendexal (various)
Chlor-Anodyne (Parke-Davis)
Chlorprophenpyridamine w/ D-Amphet. Sulfate (Coral)
Coca
Coca Leaves
Cocaine
Cocaine (various) Crystals

Cocaine (Penick) Flakes
Cocaine (Penick) Granules
Cocaine (various) Powder
Cocaine Hydrochloride
Cocaine Hydrochloride (Lilly) Solvets
Cocaine Hydrochloride (Merck) Granules
Cocaine Hydrochloride (Merck) Powder
Cocaine Hydrochloride (various) Crystals
Cocaine Sulfate
Cocaine Sulfate (various)
Codeine
Codeine (Merck) Crystals
Codeine (various) Powder
Codeine Hydrochloride (various)
Codeine Phosphate (Horton and Converse) Ampules 1 gr./cc.
Codeine Phosphate (Intra Products) Inject. 30 mg./cc.
Codeine Phosphate (Intra Products) Inject. 60 mg./cc.
Codeine Phosphate (Kirkman) Tablets 1/2 gr.
Codeine Phosphate (Kirkman) Tablets 1 gr.
Codeine Phosphate (Kirkman) Tablets Triturate 1/2 gr.
Codeine Phosphate (Lilly) Tablets Hypodermic 1/4 gr.
Codeine Phosphate (Lilly) Tablets Hypodermic 1/2 gr.
Codeine Phosphate (various)
Codeine Phosphate (various) Ampules 1/2 gr./cc.
Codeine Phosphate (various) Tablets Hypodermic 1 gr.
Codeine Phosphate (Wyeth) Tubex 30 mg./cc.
Codeine Phosphate (Wyeth) Tubex 60 mg./cc.
Codeine Phosphate with Ipecac Compound (Lilly) Syrup
Codeine Sulfate
Codeine Sulfate (Lilly) Ampules 30 mg./cc.
Codeine Sulfate (Lilly) Tablets 1/4 gr.
Codeine Sulfate (Lilly) Tablets 1/2 gr.
Codeine Sulfate (Lilly) Tablets 1 gr.
Codeine Sulfate (Lilly) Tablets Hypodermic 60 mg.
Codeine Sulfate (Penick) Crystal
Codeine Sulfate (various) Powder
Codeine Sulfate Tablets Hypodermic 7.5 mg.
Codeine Sulfate (various) Tablets Hypodermic 15 mg.
Codeine Sulfate (various) Tablets Triturate 60 mg.

Codeine Sulfate (various) Tablets Triturate
30 mg.
Codeine Sulfate (various) Tablets
Hypodermic 30 mg.
Codeine Sulfate (various) Tablets Triturate
15 mg.
Corparid (Sutliff and Case)
Cradex (Craig)
Cradex B No. 1 (Craig)
Cradex B No. 2 (Craig)
Crystodex (Crystal)
Curban Capsules (Pasadena)
No. 1/2
No. 1 1/2
No. 3
Curban-P (Pasadena)
Curbetite-La (Amfre-Grant)
Cycotin (Reed and Carnrick)
Cydril (Tutag)

D.A.S. (various)
Capsules 10 mg.
Capsules 15 mg.
Tablets 5 mg.
Tablets 10 mg.
Tablets 15 mg.
D-A-S (La Crosse)
Capsules
Tablets
D-A-Cap (Kenyon)
Capsules No. 1
Capsules No. 2
Capsules No. 3
D-Amphetamine Sulfate
D-Amfetasul (Pitman-Moore)
D-Amphetamine Hydrochloride
D-Amphetamine Methylcellulose & Dical-
cium Phos (Interstate)
D-Ampel-Kaps (Grail)
No. 1
No. 2
D-Amphetamine Carboxymethylcellulose
D-Amphetamine Methylcellulose/Dicalcium
Phosphate (Interst.)
D-Ampho-Caps 10 (Kare)
D-Ampho-Caps 15 (Kare)
D-Ampho-Sed 10 (Kare)
D-Ampho-Sed 15 (Kare)
D-Cap (Kenyon)
D-Citramine (Preston)
D-Desoxyephedrine HC1
D-Desoxyepedrine Hydrochloride
D-Dextro Tablets (Firks)

D-8-Desamine (Starr)
DA-10 Timcaps (Vanol)
Dapco-S (Schlicksup)
Daprisal (S.K. & F.)
DAS w/ Methocell (Plymouth)
DAS-Amobarb Timcap II (Coral)
Daycap (various)
Daycap-AM (various)
Daycap-B (Ethical)
Delatropin (Eastern Research)
Delfetamine (Eastern Research)
Tablets 30 mg.
Tablets 10 mg.
Delfeta-Sed Tablets (Eastern Research)
Delfeta-Sed Plus T (Eastern Research)
Delsox No. 4 (Queen City)
Deltolate (Mallard)
Demerol APAP (Breon) Tablets
Demerol Compound (Breon) Tablets
Demerol Hydrochloride (various) Tablets 50
mg.
Demerol Hydrochloride (various) Vials 50
mg./cc.
Demerol Hydrochloride (various) Vials 100
mg./cc.
Demerol Hydrochloride (Winthrop) Am-
pules 25 mg.
Demerol Hydrochloride (Winthrop) Am-
pules 50 mg.
Demerol Hydrochloride (Winthrop) Am-
pules 75 mg.
Demerol Hydrochloride (Winthrop) Am-
pules 100 mg.
Demerol HCl (Winthrop) Disp. Syr. 50 mg.
(1 cc.)
Demerol HCl (Winthrop) Disp. Syr. 50 mg.
(2 cc.)
Demerol HCl (Winthrop) Disp. Syr. 75 mg.
(1 cc.)
Demerol HCl (Winthrop) Disp. Syr. 75 mg.
(2 cc.)
Demerol HCl (Winthrop)
Disp. Syr. 100 mg. (1 cc.)
Disp. Syr. 100 mg. (2 cc.)
Demerol Hydrochloride (Winthrop) Powder
Vials
Demerol Hydrochloride Elixir (Winthrop)
50 mg./5 cc.
Demerol Hydrochloride (Winthrop) Tablets
100 mg.
Demerol Hydrochloride with Scopolamine
(Winthrop) Vials
Demerol Lotusate (Winthrop) Tablets
Deofed (Drug Products)

Des-O-Bese 10 Capsules (various)
Des-O-E Tablets (Wendt-Bristol)
Des-Oxa-D (Walker)
Desamine (Starr)
 Capsules 10 mg.
 Capsules 15 mg.
 Tablets 5 mg.
 Tablets 10 mg.
Desarex (Desert)
 Capsules No. 1
 Capsules No. 2
Desarex-A (Desert)
 Capsules No. 1
 Capsules No. 2
Desbutal Capsules (Abbott)
Desbutal 10 (Abbott)
Desbutal 15 (Abbott)
Desoxamin (High)
Desoxedrine (Testagar)
Desoxyn (Abbott)
 Tablets 2.5 mg.
Desoxy-Plex (Bush)
Desoxyephedrine (Upjohn)
Desoxyn (Abbott)
 Ampules
 Gradumets 5 mg.
 Gradumets 10 mg.
 Gradumets 15 mg.
 Tablets 2.5 mg.
 Tablets 5 mg.
Desyphed (Winthrop)
Detrex (Mallard)
Dex-A-Barb 10 (Bell)
Dex-A-Barb 15 (Bell)
Dex-A-Mine 15 (Bell)
Dex-Am-Bar Capsules (Naman)
Dex-Am-Caps (Naman)
Dex-Am-Fet Tablets (Moffet)
Dex-Am-Vite Capsules (various)
Dex-Amo (Kenyon)
Dex-Amo 10 Tablets (Rasman)
Dex-Amo 15 Tablets (Rasman)
Dex-B-Plex (United Research)
Dex-Cel (Schlicksup)
Dex-O-Cel (Airhart)
Dex-Ob (Tully)
 Tablets 10 mg.
 Tablets 15 mg.
Dex-Sed (Carrtone)
Dex-Sed-10 (various)
Dex-Sed-15 (various)
Dex-Sules (Normal)
 Capsules 10 mg.
 Capsules 15 mg.

Dexa-Key Slocaps (Key)
Dexa-Pyramine Injection (various)
Dexabar No. 1 (Medco)
Dexabar No. 2 (Medco)
Dexabar Tablets (Myers-Carter)
Dexabar-15 Capsules (Paramed)
Dexabarb (various)
 Capsules No. 1
 Capsules No. 2
 Capsules No. 3
 Tablets
Dexabese (Donley-Evans)
Dexabute Plus Tablets (Southwell)
Dexacap (various)
Dexacaps w/ Amobarbital (United)
Dexacel Special Form No. 1229 (Wester-
 field)
Dexacell Tablets (Phila. Caps. Co.)
Dexadan Capsules (Daniels)
Dexadur (Wynn)
Dexafet Tablets (Betan)
Dexagesic Tablets (Coast)
Dexahist (Tyler)
Dexalme (Meyer)
Dexalme-S (Meyer)
Dexalone (Wynn)
Dexam 10 Capsules (Robinson)
Dexam 15 Capsules (Robinson)
Dexamine (Kay)
 Tablets 5 mg.
 Tablets 10 mg.
 Vials
Dexamine (various)
 Liquid
 Tablets 5 mg.
 Tablets 10 mg.
 Vials
Dexamine-B (Kip)
Dexamine-B Tablets (Kip)
Dexamine No. 2 (Kay)
Dexamo (various)
 Capsules No. 1
 Capsules No. 2
 Tablets No. 10.
 Tablets No. 15
Dexamo T.D. Tablet (various)
 Tablets 5/30
 Tablets 10/60
 Tablets 15/90
Dexamo-Tidisin (Allan)
Dexamobarb (various)
 Capsules 10/60
 Capsules 15/60
 Capsules 15/100

Capsules T.D. 10/60
Capsules T.D. 15/60
Tablets 15/60
Tablets 5/32
Dexamobard No. 1 (Consol-Midland)
Dexamobard No. 2 (Consol-Midland)
Dexamobard No. 3 (Consol-Midland)
Dexamocaps (United)
Dexamosed (Mayrand)
Dexamosed-TD (Mayrand)
Dexamyl (S.K. & F.)
    Capsules No. 1
    Capsules No. 2
    Elixir
    Tablets
Dexaphet (Domed)
Dexaplex 15 Capsules (Coast)
Dexaplus 5-30 Tablets (Gateway)
Dexaplus-TD 10-60 Capsules (Gateway)
Dexaplus-TD 15-60 Capsules (Gateway)
Dexaplus-TD 15-90 Capsules (Gateway)
Dexased Tablets (Midwest and Vitec)
Dexasequals (Lederle)
    Capsules 10 mg.
Dexasequals (Lederle)
    Capsules 15 mg.
Dexaslim (Domed)
Dexaspan (USV)
Dexaspan-B (USV)
Dexatal Tablets (various)
Dexatal-TDC No. 1 (Hartford)
Dexatal-TDC No. 2 (Hartford)
Dexbutal S R No. 1 Capsules (Churchill)
Dexbutal Tablets (Churchill)
Dexcel Tablets (Naman)
Dexedrine (S.K. & F.)
    Capsules 5 mg.
    Capsules 10 mg.
    Capsules 15 mg.
    Elixir
    Tablets
Dexibar (Barre)
Dexibar-B (Barre)
Dexigan Capsules (Arlo)
Dexime Timecaps (United)
Dexime w/Amobarbital (United)
Dexital (Cenci)
Dexital Capsules (Bruner-Tillman)
Dexivite Spaned-Cap (Indianapolis)
Dexobarb (Jabert)
Dexobarb No. 1 (Jabert)
Dexobarb Fortis (Jabert)
Dexobarb Fortis No. 2 (Jabert)
Dexobarbital (Rondex)

Dexobarbital-TR No. 1 (Rondex)
Dexobarbital-TR No. 2 (Rondex)
Dexobard (Robinson)
Dexobee Capsules (Laser)
    No. 1
    No. 2
Dexocaps (Jabert)
Dexocel Capsules (United)
Dexol (Century)
Dexophate (Jabert)
Dexostan (Stanlabs)
    Capsules 10 mg.
    Capsules 15 mg.
Dexostan w/ Amobarbital (Stanlabs)
    Capsules No. 1
    Capsules No. 2
    Capsules No. 3
    Capsules TD No. 1
    Capsules TD No. 2
    Tablets
Dexstim (Central) Vials
Dextro-Amphetamine (H. Sonnenberg)
Dextro-Amphetamine Hydrochloride
    Capsules
    Powder
    Tablets 5 mg.
    Tablets 10 mg.
Dextro-Amphetamine Phosphate Powder
    (Arenol)
Dextro-Amphetamine Sulfate (various)
    T.D. Capsules 10 mg.
    T.D. Capsules 15 mg.
    Powder
    Tablets 5 mg.
    Tablets 10 mg.
Dextro-Barb-TD (Prof. Drug Service)
Dextro-Cel (Superior)
Dextro-Cel-Vite Capsules (Interstate)
Dextro-Cell (various)
Dextro-Profetamine (Clark and Clark)
Dexotime (Hamilton)
Dexoval (Vale)
Dexpro Elixir (Robinson)
Dexpro 10 (Robinson)
Dexpro 15 (Robinson)
Dexrex Capsules (Jonco)
Dexseco Capsules (Robinson)
Dexserprine 5 Tablets (Nysco)
Dexspan Capsules (Kip)
Dexspan-S Capsules (Kip)
Dexstim (Central)
    Tablets 5 mg.
    Tablets 10 mg.
Dextramose (Rupp and Bowman)

Dextrisal (Plymouth)
Dextro Capsules (various)
Dextro Amphetamine w/ Amobarbital E
  (A.P.P.)
  Capsules No. 1
  Capsules No. 2
  Tablets
Dextro Carboxy Tablets (Richlyn)
Dextro No. 2 Timed Cap. (Blaine)
Dextro Teen-Tabs No. 3 15 mg. (Rugby)
Dextro Unicelles (Hiss)
Dextro-Am-Bital (Columbia)
  Capsules No. 1
  Capsules No. 2
  Tablets
Dextro-Amo No. 1 Capsules (Tracy)
Dextro-Amo No. 2 Capsules (Tracy)
Dextro-Amo No. 3 Capsules (Tracy)
Dextro-Amobarb (various)
Dextro-Fetamine Elixir (Vita-Fore)
Dextro-Obicaps w/ Amobarbital (Gotham)
Dextro-Obitabs 15 mg. (Gotham)
Dextro-Obitabs 30 mg. (Gotham)
Dextro-Frolongsules (Wolins)
Dextro-Timecaps 60 (Jabert)
Dextro-Timecaps 90 (Jabert)
Dextrobar (various)
Dextrobarb (various)
  Liquid
  Tablets
Dextrobarbital (Barry-Martin)
Dextrocaps (Len Tag)
Dextrocel (Lannett)
Dextrocell Tablets (Jones and Vaughan)
Dextrolen (Len Tag)
Dextrofate-TD Capsules (various)
Dextrolett Tablets (Studebaker)
Dextrolett-B Tablets (Studebaker)
Dextromine Capsules (Rocky Mt. Pharmacal)
Dextroneed-T Capsules (Hanlon)
Dextroplex Tablets (Naman)
Dextropyrin Tablets (Studebaker)
Dextrosule (various)
  Capsules 15 mg.
  Capsules 7.5 mg.
Dextrulose (Evron)
Dextromine Injection (Rocky Mt. Pharmacal)
Dexules Capsules (various)
  No. 1
  No. 2
Diapep Tablets (K.L.R.)
Dicodid Bitartrate (Knoll) Powder

Dicodid Bitartrate (Knoll) Tablets Soluble 5
  mg.
Dicodrine
Dietamine Injection (Key)
Diocurb (Tutag)
Dihydrocodeine
Dihydrocodeine Bitartrate
Dihydrocodeinone
Dihydrocodeinone Hydrochloride
Dihydrocodeinone Resin Complex
Dihydrocodeinone Terephthalate
Dihydrohydroxycodeinone
Dihydrohydroxymorphinone
Dihydromorphinone
Dihydromorphinone Hydrochloride
Dilaudid Cough Syrup (Knoll)
Dilaudid Hydrochloride (Knoll) Ampules 1
  mg.
Dilaudid Hydrochloride (Knoll) Ampules 2
  mg.
Dilaudid Hydrochloride (Knoll) Ampules 3
  mg.
Dilaudid Hydrochloride (Knoll) Ampules 4
  mg.
Dilaudid Hydrochloride (Knoll) Powder
Dilaudid Hydrochloride (Knoll) Suppositories 3 mg.
Dilaudid Hydrochloride (Knoll) Tablets
  Compounding 30 mg.
Dilaudid Hydrochloride (Knoll) Tablets
  Soluble 1 mg.
Dilaudid Hydrochloride (Knoll) Tablets
  Soluble 2 mg.
Dilaudid Hydrochloride (Knoll) Tablets
  Soluble 3 mg.
Dilaudid Hydrochloride (Knoll) Tablets
  Soluble 4 mg.
Dilaudid Sulfate (Knoll) Vials 2 mg./cc.
Dilocol (Table Rock) Liquid
Dinarkon
Dionin (Merck)
Diphenoxylate
Diphetamine (Tutag)
Diphylets (Tutag)
Diphylets w/Amobarbital (Tutag)
Direcel (Direct)
Diurobese (Biber)
DL-Amphetamine Hydrochloride
DL-Amphetamine Phospate
DL-Desoxyephedrine Hydrochloride
DL-Desoxyephedrine w/ Thyroid (Davis and
  Sly)
DL-Methamphetamine
DL-Methamphetamine Hydrochloride

DLsoxoid (Queen City)
Dobo-TD Capsules (Klug)
Dobo-Sed-TD (Klug)
D.O.E. (Tilden-Yates)
D.O.E. Tablets (various)
Dolophine Hydrochloride (Lilly) Ampules
10 mg./cc.
Dolophine Hydrochloride (Lilly) Syrup
Dolophine Hydrochloride (Lilly) Tablets 5
mg.
Dolophine Hydrochloride (various)
Tablets 7.5 mg.
Dolophine Hydrochloride (Lilly) Tablets 10
mg.
Domafate (Haag)
Capsules 10 mg.
Capsules 15 mg.
Tablets
Domapen (Haag)
Capsules
Tablets
Donnagesic Extentabs No. 2 (Robins)
(Codeine 1 1/2 gr.)
Dopbese (Philadelphia)
Dovers Powder
Dovers Powder Syrup
Doxephin (Methamphetamine)
Doxyfed (Raymer) Tablets
Doxyfed w/ Phenobarbital (Raymer)
Dramamine-D (Searle) Tablets
Dramphetamine Computabs (Dram)
Drinalfa (Squibb) Injection 20 mg./cc.
Drinalfa (Squibb) Tablet 5 mg.
Drocode Bitartrate (Atlas) Mult. Dose Vials
30 mg./cc.
Dromoran
Ducevim-T (Bernhoft)
Ducevim-T Forte (Bernhoft)
Ducodol
Duo-Amphet Duracap (Phila. Caps. Co.)
Duoampho (Kenyon)
Duo-Gesic (Frederick Trout)
Du-Oria Tablets (Ascher)
Dura-Dex (Bonar)
Duratabs (Wynn)
Durophet (Amphetamine Sulfate)
DVB-10 (Norwood)
DVB-15 (Mayrand)
Dysonil (Circle)

Ecgonine
Ecgoninebenzoyl Ester
Ecgoninebenzoyl Ethyl Ester
Ecgonine Cinnamoylmethyl Ester
Ecgonine Phenylacetylmethylester

Ecgonine Hydrochloride
Edrisal with Codeine 1/4 gr. (S.K. & F.)
Edrisal with Codeine 1/2 gr. (S.K. & F.)
Efroxine (Strasenburgh) Tablets
Eldertonic Elixir (Mayrand)
EN-1530
Erythroxylon Coca
Escodex 1 and 2 (Esco)
Escodex-A1 (Esco)
Escodex-A2 (Esco)
Eskatrol Spansules (S.K. & F.)
Ethyl Benzoyl Ecgonine
Ethyl Morphine
Ethyl Morphine Hydrochloride (Mallinc-
krodt)
Ethylmorphine Hydrochloride (Penick)
Powder
Eucodal
Evrodex Tempules (Evron)
Expectomint (Research)

Fedra-Thy (Cole)
Fentanyl
Fentanyl Citrate
Ferndex No. 1 Kronocaps
Ferndex No. 2 Kronocaps
Fetamin (Mission)
Fiosal (Medco)
Fordex Injection (Fellows-Testagar)
Forfetamine No. 3 (Cabot)
Formacaps (Plymouth)
Formula No. 2 SF 1368 (Bariatric)
Formula No. 2 SF 1369 (Bariatric)
Formula No. 3 SF 1362 (Bariatric)
Formula No. 3 SF 1363 (Bariatric)
Formula No. 5 SF 1365 (Bariatric)
Formula No. 37 (Bariatric)
Formula No. 38 (Bariatric)
Formula No. 39 (Bariatric)
Formula No. 277 (Hiss)
Formula No. 1720 (Jan)
Formula No. 1800 (Jan)
Formula No. 12 (Spencer-Mead)
Four Amphetamine Compound No. 751
(Darby)

Genetak Capsules (General)
Geralix (Ruckstuhl)
Gerisitone (Pharmacole)
Gerobit (Methamphetamine)
Gerone (Pitman-Moore)
Gerovit (Methamphetamine)
Gevrestin (Lederle)
G.I. Tran (Westerfield)
Gobewin Tablets (Winston)

Green Reducing Formula (Kraft)
Green Reducing Formula Mild (Kraft)
Gum Opium

Hetamine (Dumas-Wilson)
Heterocodeine
Histamic-SR (Metro)
Histamic-SR SF.670 (Net-Med)
Hist-Cxa-Mine (Walker)
H-M-C No. 1 (Abbott) Tablets Hypodermic
H-M-C No. 2 (Abbott) Tablets Hypodermic
Hourdex No. 1 Capsules (Delta)
Hourdex No. 2 Capsules (Delta)
H.S. Capsules Green No. 2-AKL (Hiss)
H.S. Capsules No. 3 Green No. 2-AFV (Hiss)
H.S. Capsules Red No. 2-AMD (Eric Kirk
    and Gray)
Hycodan (Endo) Powder
Hy-Dex-Barb Capsules (High)
Hydex (Moore Kirk)
Hydrocodin
Hydrocodone
Hydrocodone Bitartrate
Hydromorphinol
Hydromorphone
Hymorphan
Hysobel (Zemmer)
    Tablet
    Tablet No. 2
    Tablet Forte

Ibiozedrine (Amphetamine Sulfate)
Innovar (McNeil) Injection Ampules
Ipecac and Opium Powder (Penick)
Ipecac and Opium Powder Purified (Mal-
    linckrodt)
Isoadanon
Isoamidone
Isococaine
Isomethadone
Isomethadone Hydrobromide
Isomethadone Hydrochloride
Isonipecaine

Kirkobee No. 3 (Kirk)
Knidex-TD (Knight)
Knidex-Ten Capsules (Knight)
Kraftoplex (Kraft)
Kraftquad No. 3 (Kraft)
Krodin (Kraft)

Laevomate-PM (Jabert)
    Capsules 5 mg.
    Capsules 10 mg.

Tablets 5 mg.
Tablets 10 mg.
Lamodex (Tri-State)
    No. 1
    No. 2
Lanazine (Lannet)
    Tablets 5 mg.
    Tablets 10 mg.
Lasodex-10 (Tri-State) Capsules
    Lasodex-15 Caps
Laudicon
Leptamine Tablets (Bowman)
    Lipsett 10 mg.
    Tablets 5 mg.
    Tablets 10 mg.
Leritine (M.S. & D.) Ampules
Leritine (M.S. & D.) Tablets 25 mg.
Leritine (M.S. & D.) Vials
Levetamine (Abbott)
Levo-Dromoran (Roche) Ampules 2 mg.
Levo-Dromoran (Roche) Tablets Oral 2 mg.
Levo-Dromoran (Roche) Vials 2 mg./cc.
Levomethorphan
Levomethorphan Hydrobromide
Levonor (Cooper-Tinsley)
Levorphan
Levorphanol
Levorphanol Tartrate
Lifo-Dex Injection (New Mexico)
Linampheta (Lincoln)
Lowedex CTR (Lowe)
Lurline (Fielding)
Lynnprodex Injection (Lynn)

M-Dex No. 1 and 2 (Misemer)
M-Dex No. 10 (Echos)
M-Dex No. 15 (Echos)
M-Dex No. 2 (Echos)
M-Dex 10 (Misemer)
M-Dex 15 (Misemer)
Magalin Tablets (Westerfield)
Maigret (Ferndale)
Mardex 15-S (Mardale)
Meda-Plex (Medco)
Medex (Medco)
Medexin (Haberle)
Mepergan (Wyeth) Capsules
Mepergan (Wyeth) Tubex 50 mg.
Mepergan (Wyeth) Vials 25 mg./cc.
Mepergan Fortis (Wyeth) Capsules
Meperidine Hydrochloride
Meperidine Hydrochloride (various) Am-
    pules 25 mg./cc.

Meperidine Hydrochloride (various) Ampules 50 mg./cc.
Meperidine Hydrochloride (various) Ampules 75 mg./cc.
Meperidine Hydrochloride (various) Ampules 100 mg./cc.
Meperidine Hydrochloride (various) Tablets 50 mg.
Meperidine Hydrochloride (various) Vials 50 mg./cc.
Meperidine Hydrochloride (various) Vials 100 mg./cc.
Mephenon
Mepho-D (Walker)
Mercodinone (Merrell) Tablets 5 mg.
Meridil
Metalose (Tutag)
Metazocine
Metazocine Hydrochloride
Metha-Dex (Sonnenberg)
Methadex (Nysco)
Methadone
Methadone Hydrochloride
Methadone Hydrochloride (Horton and Conv.) Tabs. 10 mg.
Methadone Hydrochloride (various) Vials 10 mg./cc.
Methamphetamine Hydrochloride Vials 20 mg. (various)
Methamphetamine Hydrochloride (various)
Powder
Tablets 5 mg.
Oral Liquid
Methamphetamine Sulfate (various)
Methamphetamine with B-Complex (Franklin)
Methamphin (Rorer)
Methajade (M.S. & D.) Syrup
Methedrine Hydrochloride (B.W. & Co.) Ampules 20 mg./cc.
Methedrine Hydrochloride (Burroughs-Wellcome)
Methedrine Tablets 5 mg. (Burroughs-Wellcome)
Methobenzmorphan
Methorphan
Methorphinan
Methoxyn (Kenny Pharm)
Methyl Dihydromorphinone
Methyl Dihydromorphinone Hydrochloride
Methyl Morphine
Methylphenidate
Methylphenidate Hydrochloride
Metopon
Metopon Hydrochloride Capsules 3 mg.

Milidex (various)
Miller-Drine (Miller)
Minadit
Monetamine (Northwest Labs)
Monophos (Harvey)
Monophos Tablets (Tilden-Yates)
Morphine
Morphine (Parke-Davis) Vials 1/4 gr./cc.
Morphine (Penick) Crystal
Morphine (Penick) Powder
Morphine Acetate
Morphine Acetate (Merck) Anhydrous
Morphine Acetate (Penick) Powder
Morphine Bimeonate (Penick) Solution
Morphine Hydrochloride (Lilly) Elixir
Morphine Hydrochloride (various) Powder
Morphine Sulfate
Morphine Sulfate (Lilly) Ampules
Morphine Sulfate (Lilly) Tablets Hypodermic 1/8 gr.
Morphine Sulfate Tablets Hypodermic 1/2 gr.
Morphine Sulfate (Lilly) Tablets Hypodermic 1/2 gr.
Morphine Sulfate (Merck) Crystals
Morphine Sulfate (various) Ampules 8 mg./ml.
Morphine Sulfate (various) Ampules 10 mg./cc.
Morphine Sulfate (various) Ampules 15 mg./cc.
Morphine Sulfate (various) Cubes
Morphine Sulfate (various) Powder
Morphine Sulfate (various) Tablets Hypodermic 1/6 gr.
Morphine Sulfate (various) Tablets Hypodermic 1/4 gr.
Morphine Sulfate (various) Vials 1/4 gr./cc.
Morphine Sulfate (1/4 gr./cc.) and Atropine (Horton-Conv.) Vial
Morphine/Atropine (Merrell) Ampules 10 mg. w/ 0.4 mg.
Morphine/Atropine (Merrell) Tablets 15 mg. w/ 0.4 mg.
Morphine Sulfate and Atropine Sulfate (Massengill) Vials
Morphine Sulfate and Atropine Sulfate (Moore Kirk) Ampins
Morphine with Atropine (Lilly) Ampules
Morphine with Atropine (Lilly) Tablets Hypodermic
Morphine with Atropine Ampules (Merrell) 10 mg. w/ 0.4 mg.
Morphothebaine
Myalate (Grail)

Nalertan (Neisler)
Nectadon (Merck) Powder
Neo-Artycal No. 2 (Queen City)
Neoprobestine (Jabert)
Nexorin Capsules (Dorsey)
Nicogesic Plus (Lemmon)
Niripase (Northrup)
Nisalco-Plus (Queen City)
Nisentil (Roche) Ampules 40 mg.
Nisentil (Roche) Ampules 60 mg.
Nisentil Hydrochloride
Nisentil (Roche) Vials 60 mg./cc.
Nobese Tablets (Edwards)
Nodalin (Table Rock) Tablets
Normadrine (Van Pelt-Brown)
Normadrine Solution (Van Pelt-Brown)
Normeperidine
Normin (De Leon)
Norodin (Endo)
Norpethidine
Novadex (Perry)
Nucleon and Amphetamine (Park)
Nucodan (Endo) Tablets
Numorphan Hydrochloride (Endo) Ampules 1 mg./cc.
Numorphan Hydrochloride (Endo) Ampules 1.5 mg./cc.
Numorphan Hydrochloride (Endo) Suppositories 2 mg.
Numorphan Hydrochloride (Endo) Suppositories 5 mg.
Numorphan Hydrochloride (Endo) Tablets 10 mg.
Numorphan Hydrochloride (Endo) Vials 1 mg./cc.
Numorphan Hydrochloride (Endo) Vials 1.5 mg./cc.
Nutrix Vitamin-Mineral Syrup (Wabash)

O-B-C-T (various)
Obamide (Fisher)
Obecarb (Bush)
Obedex Lozenges (United Research)
O-Bedex Lozenges (Lustgarten)
Obedrill (B.L.B.)
Obedrin (Massengill)
   Capsules
   Tablets
Obedrin-LA (Massengill)
Obesan (Dunhall)
Obesilin (Lincoln)
Obesonil (Lincoln)
Obestrol (Crestmed)
Obetamine (Davis and Sly)
Obetrim (Sylvania)

Obetrol (various)
   Tablets 10 mg.
Obeval (Vale) Tablets 20 mg.
Obi-Tri-Phet Injection (Gotham)
Obocell (Neisler)
Obocell Complex (Neisler)
Obocell-TF (Neisler)
Obolip (Lakeside)
Omnopon
Opidice (Boyle)
Opium
Opium Extract
Opium Extract (various)
Opium Fluidextract
Opium Granulated
Opium Granule (various)
Opium Poppy
Opium Powder (various)
Opium Powdered
Opium Tincture
Opium Tincture Deodorized (Lilly)
Opium with Belladonna (Horton and Converse) Suppos. 1 gr.
Opium with Belladonna (Wyeth) Suppositories 1 gr. w/ 1/4 gr.
Oxycodone
Oxycodone Hydrochloride
Oxydess (Chimedic)
Oxydrin (Grant)
Oxyfed (Cole)
Oxymorphone
Oxymorphone Hydrochloride

Palobese (Palmedico)
Pancodine
Panrexin-TP (Pan American)
Pantopon (Roche) Ampules 1/3 gr.
Pantopon (Roche) Tablets Hypodermic 1/3 gr.
Papaveretum
Papine (Battle) Liquid
Papine Hydrochloride
Paradex-10 Capsules (Paramed)
Paradex-15 Capsules (Paramed)
Paradexsets No. 3 (Paramount)
Paramorphine
Parkoplex (Park)
Pelladex-10 (Coast)
Pelladex-15 (Coast)
Pellcaps (Kirkman)
   Tablets 10 mg.
   Tablets 15 mg.
Pen-Phetamine (Clark and Clark)
Percobarb (Endo) Capsules
Percobarb-Demi (Endo) Capsules

Percodan (Endo) Tablets 5 mg.
Percodan-Demi (Endo) Tablets
Perke-One (Ascher) Capsules
Perke-Two (Ascher) Capsules
Permadex 10 Capsules (Croyden-Browne)
Permadex 15 Capsules (Croyden-Browne)
Permadexal Capsules (Croyden-Browne)
Pethidine
Pethidine Hydrochloride
P.F. No. 7777 (Moffet)
P.F. No. 1466 (Table Rock)
Phantos-10 (Cooper-Tinsley)
Phantosine-DLA Capsules (Cooper-Tinsley)
Phedoxe-4B (Elder) Tablets
Phedrisox (Ascher)
Phedrisox Vials
Phenazocine
Phenethylazocine
Phenmetrazine
Phenmetrazine HCl
Pheta 5 Delacaps (Sig)
Pheta 10 Delacaps (Sig)
Pheta 15 Delacaps (Sig)
Phetabar (Moore Kirk)
Phetobese (Cole)
Piminodine
Piminodine Dihydrochloride
Piminodine Ethanesulfonate
Plimasin (Ciba) Tablets
Preludin (Geigy)
Preludin Endurets (Geigy)
Prelu-Vite (Geigy)
Premodrin (Premo)
  Capsules 25 mg.
  Capsules 50 mg.
  Elixir
Pretension (Quaker City)
Prevamodex 15 (Rand)
Prevamodex 60 (Rand)
Previdex 10 (Rand)
Previdex 15 (Rand)
Prinadol (S.K. & F.) Ampules 2 mg./cc.
Prinadol (S.K. & F.) Vials 2 mg./cc.
Private Formula No. 1-DGN
Private Formula No. 4651 (Halsom)
Probese-P
Probestine (Jabert)
  Capsules
  T.D.
Profetamine Hydrochloride (Archer-Taylor)
Profetamine Phosphate (Clark and Clark)
Prolaire (Stuart)

Prolaire-B (Stuart)
Pro-Meperdan
Providex Tablets (Reid-Provident)
Pseudococaine
Pymadex Timed Capsules (Fellows-Testagar)
Pyrdex Injection (Savage)
Pyriladex (various)
Pyrilamine Maleate w/ Dextro-Amphetamine (United Res.)

Quadamine (Tutag)
Quatra-Mak 20 TD (Jabert)

R/Amphetamine (Prof. Drug Service)
R.A.S. (Stayner)
  Tablets 5 mg.
  Tablets 10 mg.
Rabudex (Lynn)
Rabudex-GR (Lynn)
Racemethorphan
Racemic Dromoran
Racemorphan
Racemorphan Hydrobromide
Racephen (Ives-Cameron)
Raphetamine Phosphate (Strasenburgh) Vial
Red Expectorant (Wendt-Bristol)
Redex Jr. (Tri-State) Capsules
Redexcel (Central)
Reducell (Bush) Tablets
Reducing Capsules 10 mg-No. 2 SF. 1234 (Davis-Edwards)
Reducing Capsules 10 mg-No. 3 SF. 1235 (Davis-Edwards)
Reducing-Tabs 10 mg-No. 1 Grey (Davis-Edwards)
Reducing-Tabs 10 mg-No. 2 White (Davis-Edwards)
Reducing-Tabs 10 mg-No. 3 Pink (Davis-Edwards)
Reducing-Tabs 15 mg-No. 3 Blue (Davis-Edwards)
Reducing-Tabs 15 mg-No. 3 Pink (Davis-Edwards)
Reducto (Arcum) Tablets
Revamodex 15 (Rand)
Revamodex 60 (Rand)
Revicaps (Lederle) Capsules
Revidex (Rand)
Ritalin Hydrochloride (Ciba)
  Tablets 5 mg.
  Tablets 10 mg.

Tablets 20 mg.
Vials 10 ml.
Ritonic (Ciba) Capsules
Robese Inj. (Rocky Mt. Pharmacal)
Rogesic (Rocky Mountain)
Rohist-Plus (Rocky Mountain)
Rotase (Northrup) Capsules
Rotase-Mitte (Northrup) Tablets
RU-Ludin (Rudy Klein)
RX No. 644 (Kirkman)
RX 4016 Papine (Blue Line)
RX No. 4087 (Zemmer)
RX No. 4100 (Zemmer)
RX No. 4109 (Zemmer)
RX No. 4135 (Zemmer)

Salcetol with Morphine Sulfate (Tilden-Yates) Tablets
S.C. Lavender No. 3-AXQ (Harvey)
S.C. Yellow No. 3-AVG (Scheumann)
Seco-Synatan (Neisler) Tabules
Secodex (Hart) Capsules
Secodex Capsules (Cumberland)
Sedadex (Novocol)
Semoxydrine (Massengill) 5 mg. Tablets 7.5 mg.
Senigesic (Caldwell and Bloor)
Sertrim Tablets (Arnell)
Sertrim-RA (Arnell) Tablets
Slodex Tablets (Mid-Atlantic)
Slo-Jaydex (Mid-Atlantic)
Span-RD (Metro-Med) Capsules
Span-RD 12 (Metro-Med) Capsules
Spandex-B (Bock) Capsules
Spasmalgin
Special Amphetamine Formula No. 751
Special Amphetamine Formula Capsules No. 351 (Rugby)
Special Amphetamine Formula (United)
Special Dextro-Amphetamine Formula No. 182 (United)
Special Formula Capsules No. 1 (Halsey)
Special Formula Capsules No. 3 (Halsey)
Special Formula Capsules No. 6 (Halsey)
Special Formula Capsules No. 7 (Halsey)
Special Formula No. 00 Capsules SF 1290 (Pharmex)
Special Formula No. 51 (Penn State)
Special Formula SF No. 1291 (Bariatric)
Special Formula SF No. 1292 (Bariatric)
Special Formula T-208 (Schlicksup)
Special Formula T-209 (Schlicksup)
Special Formula T-210 (Schlicksup)

Special Formula RX T-214 (Schlicksup)
Special Formula Tablets (Davis-Edwards)
Special Formula Time Release SF No. 1293 (Bariatric)
Special Formula Triangular Pink (Bariatric)
Standex (Standex) Capsules
Stedytabs-Delfeta-Sed (Eastern Research)
Stedytabs-Delfetamine 30 mg. (Eastern Research)
Stimalose (Irwin-Neisler)
Stimdex (Ulmer) Tablets
Stimdex Injection (New Mexico)
Sublimaze (McNeil) Ampules 0.05 mg./cc.
Sulphet-AB Ovules No. 2 (Vita Elixir)
Synatan (Neisler) Tablets
Synatan Forte (Neisler) Tablet
Syndrox (McNeil) Elixir Tablets
Syntil (McNeil) Tablets

T-125 (Bell)
T-131 (Bell)
T-135 (Bell)
T-145 (Bell)
T-146 (Bell)
T-147 (Bell)
T-148 (Bell)
Tablet No. 1-ALK (Physicians Supply)
Tablet No. 1-BLN (Davis and Sly)
T-Tonic (Tennessee)
TD-10-60 (St. Louis)
Teen-Tabs No. 3 15 mg. (Rugby)
Teenette (Foy)
Tega-Dex-10 (Ortega)
Tega-Dex-15 (Ortega)
Teon No. 1 Timecaps (Winters)
Teon No. 2 Timecaps (Winters)
Thebaine
Theptine Elixir (S.K. & F.)
Three in One (Rocky Mountain)
Tidex (Don Hall)
Tidex Depacaps (Hall)
    Capsules 10 mg.
    Capsules 15 mg.
Tidex Tablets (Allison)
Timed Tobie Capsules (Testagar)
Timed Tridex (Testagar)
Timed Tridex Jr. (Testagar)
Toni Ampho-Cellulose (TMCO)
Toni Dextrobarb (TMCO)
Tragesin (Vale)
Trand (Buffingtons)
Transed (various)
Tre-Dextro Tablets (Phila. Caps. Co.)

Tri-Zine G Tablets (Virtal)
Tri-Zine Tablets (Virtal)
Triangle Reducing Tablets No. 1 (Davis-Edwards)
Triangle Reducing Tablets No. 2 (Davis-Edwards)
Tridex (Testagar)
Tridex Jr. Timed (Testagar)
Tridex Timed (Testagar)
Triodex w/ Amobarbital (Ruckstuhl)
Triphex (Tennessee)
Tropacocaine
Truxillo Coca
Two-Bar-Dex (Arden)
Tydex Capsules (Tyler)
   10 mg.
   15 mg.
Tydex-Plus (Tyler)
Tymafast No. 1 Capsules (Mason)

Uni-Chlor-Dex TDC (United Research)
Unitryl Tablets (Myers-Carter)
Unitryl-S.A. Capsules (Myers-Carter)

Videxemin (S.K. & F.)
Vio-Dex Capsules (Rowell)
Vio-Dex Timelets (Rowell)
   Tablets 10 mg.
   Tablets 15 mg.
Vitec Complex w/ Desoxyphedrine (Vitec)
Vitobese (Detroit)

Zamitam (Marion)
   No. 1
   No. 2
Zamitol (Marion)
   No. 1
   No. 2
Zil-A-Gen (Walker)

Appendix V

Schedules III, IV, and V drugs under the Controlled Substances Act of 1970, as revised in 1973. *Source: Bureau of Narcotics and Dangerous Drugs.*

A-Bas (Darby)
A-Bes (Cumberland)
ACA and Codeine (Rowell)
   Capsules 16 mg.
   32 mg.
   Tablets 16 mg.
   32 mg.
A.C.A.P. (Halsom)
A.C.A. with Dovers (Private Formula)
ACD Caps (Philips Roxane)
ACD S.C. Blue Tabs (Philips Roxane)
ACD S.C. Red Tabs (Philips Roxane)
ACD Tabs Pink Children's (Philips Roxane)
A-D-A Capsules (LaCrosse)
A-N Rectorettes (Oak Ridge)
   Regular
   Infant
A.P.C. and Butabarbital (Park)

A.P.C.I. (Bates)
APC with Dovers (Cord)
A-Sec Suppositories (Webster)
   No. 1
   No. 3
   No. 5
A-66
A. V. M. (Luke)
   Capsules
Abactal (Massengill)
Abadex (ABA)
   No. 1
   No. 2
   No. 3
Abate (Cambridge)
Acaneel and Codeine (Sherman)
Acedoval Tab (Vale)
Acetidine Tablets (M.S. & D.)

Acetidine/Codeine (M.S. & D.)
  Tablets 15 mg.
    30 mg.
Acetofate (Day-Baldwin)
Acetyl Caf-Phen Caps (various)
Acetyl-Dex (Moore Kirk)
Acetylphen Cap. (Haug)
  Capsules
  Tablets
Acoda Zem (Zemmer)
Acogesic (Strasenburgh)
Acotal (Prof. Drug Service)
Actifed-C (B.W. & Co.)
Acutuss with Codeine (Philips Roxane)
Adetate (M.S. & D.)
Adipex (Lemmon)
Adistat (C. O. Truxton)
Adrizine
Agma Cough Syrup (Strong Cobb Arner)
Agrypnal (Phenobarbital)
Aidant with Codeine (P. J. Noyes)
Aidant with Dovers Powder (P. J. Noyes)
Aidco Tablets (Pharmak)
Airo-Sed (Airhart)
Aironol (Airhart)
Airotal (Airhart)
Aladrine (various)
  Tablets
  Suppositories
  Suspension
Alafed (Crest)
  Liquid
  Tablets
Alamine Expectorant (Elder)
Alamine-C (Elder)
Albutal (Medical Arts)
Aldex =3 (Allied Surgical)
Alepsal (Fougera)
Alercap (Truett Labs)
Alerticon Capsules (Consol. Midland)
Aliasis No. 2 (Superior)
Alka-Nux (Maceslin)
Allonal Tablets (Roche)
Almetussin-C (Meyer)
Al-Nal (Cumberland)
  Capsules
  Tablets
Alobese =1 (Allied Surgical)
Alobese =2 (Allied Surgical)
Alobese =3 (Allied Surgical)
Alphenate
Alprine (Ulmer)
Al-Spa (Allied Surgical)
Altinal

Alubarb Elixir (various)
Alurate Elixir (Roche)
Alurate Sodium Tablets (Roche)
Alurate Verdum Elixir (Roche)
Aluro (Foy)
Alutricol (Tutag)
Amabese (Caldwell and Bloor)
Amagesic (Caldwell and Bloor)
Amal
Amaphen Tablets (Trimen)
Amasal-DH Capsules (Defco)
Ambarb Capsules (Manne)
Ambenyl Expectorant (Parke-Davis)
Ambidex Timecaps (Caldwell and Bloor)
Ambrol (Smith Miller and Patch)
Ambusal Tablets (Amine)
Amcobarb Dakaps (Amco)
Amelicrans (Phila. Caps. Co.)
Amethoid (C. S. Ruckstuhl)
Amethoid-Forte (C.S. Ruckstuhl)
Amex Tablets (Pasadena)
Amfebarbs (Gold Leaf)
Amfet-Oxy-20 (Studebaker)
Amgesic Tablets (various)
Amgesic No. 2 Tablets (various)
Ammonium-Chloride Compound Capsules
  (Elder)
Amodril Spancap w/Thyroid (North Ameri-
  can)
Amo-Dureide (Goodrich-Wright)
Amo-Pellcaps (Kirkman)
  No. 1
  No. 2
Amostat (North American)
Am-O-Tabs 1 (North American)
Am-O-Tabs 2 (North American)
Am-O-Tabs 3 (North American)
Amobarbital
Amobarbital Sodium (various)
  Ampules 250 mg.
  Ampules 500 mg.
  Bulk
  Capsules 65 mg.
  Capsules 200 mg.
  Vials 250 mg.
  Vials 500 mg.
  Vials 1.0 mg.
Amocaps P.A. 10 (Vita Fore)
Amocaps P.A. 15 (Vita Fore)
Amodril (North American)
Amosec Capsules No. 2 (Penhurst)
Amosene (Ferndale)
Amosette Kronocap (Ferndale)
Amospan (B.S. & L. Pharm)

Amo-Tran (Superior)
Amotrax Capsules (Jamieson-McKames)
Amozar (North American)
Ampelose Tablets (Blue-Line)
Amperoid (Franklin)
Amperone (Kremers-Urban)
Ampha-Lysin 10 mg. No. 1 (Davis-Edwards)
Ampha-Lysin 10 mg. No. 2 (Davis-Edwards)
Ampha-Lysin 10 mg. No. 3 (Davis-Edwards)
Amphecaps (Direct)
Amphedase (Parke-Davis)
Amphesal (Darby)
Amphestat (Toledo)
Amphetamin-Tabs 10 mg-No. 3 (Davis-Edwards)
Amphetamine Combination No. 1 (Robinson)
Amphetamine Combination No. 2 (Robinson)
Amphetamine Combination No. 3 (Robinson)
Amphetamine and Thyroid (SF 252) (Davis-Edwards)
Amphetamine Compound (Cord)
Amphetamine Compound (Classic)
Amphetamine Compound 15-1 1/2 (Shaw)
Amphetamine Compound 15-3 (Shaw)
Amphetamine Compound 30-3 (Shaw)
Amphetamine Compound No. 1 (Kraft)
Amphetamine Compound No. 2 (Kraft)
Amphetamine Compound No. 3 (Kraft)
Amphetamine Compound Grey =1 (Shaw)
Amphetamine Compound Neutral =2 (Shaw)
Amphetamine Compound Pink =3 (Shaw)
Amphetamine O.B. Compound (Kenyon)
Amphetamine O.B. Compound (Lustgarten)
Amphetamine Reducing Capsules-Half Strength (Davis-Edwards)
Amphetamine Reducing Capsules-15 mg. (Henlein)
Amphetamine Sulfate Combination 5 mg., No. 3 (Lustgarten)
Amphetamine Sulfate Combination 10 mg., No. 3 (Lustgarten)
Amphetamine Sulfate Combination 10 mg., No. 1 (Gray)
Amphetamine Sulfate Combination 10 mg., No. 2 (Lustgarten)
Amphetamine Sulfate Combination 5 mg., C/T (Lustgarten)
Amphetamine Sulfate Combination 5 mg., No. 2 (Lustgarten)

Amphetamine Sulfate Compound No. 1 (Bates)
Amphetamine Sulfate Compound No. 2 (Bates)
Amphetamine Sulfate Compound No. 3 (Bates)
Amphetamine Sulfate Sets 15 mg. (Rugby)
Amphetamine Sulfate Sets 15 mg.-No. 1 (Rugby)
Amphetamine Sulfate w/ Thyroid Aloin and Atropine No. 1 (Evron)
Amphetamine Sulfate w/ Thyroid and Atropine No. 2 (Evron)
Amphetamine Sulfate w/ Thyroid and Phenobarb No. 3 (Evron)
Amphetamine Sulfate w/ Thyroid, Aloin and Atropine (Double Strength) No. 1 (Evron)
Amphetamine Sulfate w/ Thyroid and Phenobarb (Double Strength) No. 3 (Evron)
Amphetaset No. 1 (Rupp and Bowman)
Amphetaset No. 2 (Rupp and Bowman)
Amphetaset No. 3 (Rupp and Bowman)
Amphetaset (Rupp and Bowman)
Amphetasin (Haberle)
Amphetcaps 1-2-3 (Bel-Air)
Amphethyn No. 1 (Park)
Amphethyn No. 2 (Park)
Amphethyn No. 3 (Park)
Amphetosal (Rupp and Bowman)
Amphezine Tablets (Royce)
Amphobese Regular Formula (Starr)
Amphobese Regular Formula Special Formula (Starr)
Amphocaps (Lakehurst)
Amphocaps (Nysco)
Amphocaps, Half Strength (Nysco)
Amphocaps (Jabert)
Amphoid (North American)
Amphoid (Person and Covey)
Ampholoid-1 (Starr)
Ampholoid-2 (Starr)
Ampholoid-3 (Starr)
Ampholoid-A (Starr)
Ampholoid-B (Starr)
Ampholoid-C (Starr)
Amphotabs =1 (Interstate Drug Exchange)
Amphotabs =2 (Interstate Drug Exchange)
Amphotabs =3 (Interstate Drug Exchange)
Amphotabs =1 D.S. (Interstate Drug Exchange)
Amphotabs =2 D.S. (Interstate Drug Exchange)

Amphotabs =3 D.S. (Interstate Drug Exchange)
Amplex (Remson)
Ampsu Capsules (Manne)
Amron (S. J. Tutag)
Amsalin (Neisler)
Amsebarb
Am-Sul Barb Capsules (M. J. Labs)
Am-Sul Jr. Capsules (M. J. Labs)
AMT-10-60-OC (Mills)
AMT-15-60-BY (Mills) Tablets
AMT-15-60-GC (Mills)
Am-Vite (Drug Industries)
Amyaldex (Hiss)
Amylofene (First Texas)
Amylofene Sodium (First Texas)
Amytal (Lilly)
  Elixir 130 mg./30 ml.
  Elixir 259 mg./30 ml.
  Tablets 15 mg.
  Tablets 30 mg.
  Tablets 50 mg.
  Tablets 100 mg.
Amytal and Aspirin (Lilly)
Amytal Sodium (Lilly)
  Ampules 65 mg.
  Ampules 125 mg.
  Ampules 250 mg.
  Ampules 500 mg.
  Pulvules 65 mg.
  Pulvules 200 mg.
  Suppositories
Anadol Tablets
Analgesic No. 2 (Philips Roxane)
Analgesic Ovals (Lampert)
Analgesic Tablets No. 5776 (Savoy)
Analgestine Capsules (Mallard)
Analgestine Forte Capsules (Mallard)
Analpac (Lyons Physician Supply)
Anamine (Detroit First Aid)
Anastress
Analval (Vale)
Analzem No. 2 Tablets (Zemmer)
Andaxin
Aneural
Anexsia-D Tablets (Massengill)
Anexsia with Codeine (Massengill)
Angesic Tablets (Edwards)
Anodynos-DHC (Tilden-Yates)
Anorex-15 (Cabell)
Anorexin Tablets (various)
Anox Capsules (Winston)
Ans (Kenwood Labs)
Anti-Bese (American Tablet and Capsule)

Anti-Bese (Direct)
Anti-Bese T (Direct)
Anti-Bese T (American Tablet and Capsule)
Anti-Bese T-15 (American Tablet and Capsule)
Anti-Nausea Supprettes (Webster)
  Children
  No. 1
  No. 2
Antibesity Tablets (various)
Apalon Tablets (Kessel)
Apap with Dihydrocodeinone (Private Formula)
Apascil
APC/Codeine (various)
  Capsules No. 3
  Tablets No. 2
  Tablets No. 3
  Tablets No. 4
A.P.C. w/ Isobutylallylbarbituric Acid (Davis-Edwards)
A. P. Forte (Walker Corporation)
Appe-Stat (Cooperative)
Apeco (various)
  Capsules
  Tablets
Appetabs (Saron)
Aprobarbital
Aprobarbital Sodium
Aprotal Elixir (Grail)
Aquachloral (Webster)
  Suppositories 5 gr.
  Suppositories 10 gr.
  Suppositories 15 gr.
Ar-Sed Tablets (Arden)
Arbatal (Kay)
Arco Syrup No. 1 (Pharmak)
Arco Syrup No. 2 (Pharmak)
Arcoban (Arcum)
Armide No. 2 (Warren)
Arnetrim Tablets (Arnell)
Artolon
Arvynol (Pfizer)
ASA/Codeine
  Pulvules No. 2
  Pulvules No. 3
  Pulvules No. 4
  Tablets No. 2
  Tablets No. 3
ASC Tablets (Modern Drugs)
Ascaphen (various)
  Capsules
  Tablets
Asco (Charcoal) (E. W. Huen)

Asco (Mottled) (E. W. Huen)
Asco Compound (Sutliff and Case)
    Capsules
Ascodeen-30 (B. W. Co.)
Ascriptin/Codeine (Rorer)
Asper-Sed (Beach)
Asperdeine/Codeine
Asphac G with Codeine (Central Pharmacal)
    Tablets 15 mg.
    Tablets 30 mg.
Asphac-G Tablets (Central)
Asphamal-D Tablets (Central)
Asphenhy (Lynn)
Aspidyne/Codeine
Aspir-Code (various)
Aspir-Phen Tablets (various)
Aspirotabs/Codeine
Aspodyne with Codeine (Blue Line)
    Tablets 15 mg.
    Tablets 30 mg.
Asthnedrin Liquid (Roadex Labs)
Astrobute Tablets (GP Labs)
ASA, Acetophenetidin and DL-
    Amphetamine S04 (Cleveland)
Aspirin/Codeine (various)
Aspirin w/Phenobarbital (various)
A. T. A. (H. R. Cenci)
A. T. A. Amphetamine (Vitamix)
A. T. A. Amphetamine Combination =1,
    Green (Vitamix)
A. T. A. Amphetamine Combination =1,
    Yellow (Vitamix)
A. T. A. Amphetamine Combination =2,
    Pink (Vitamix)
A. T. A. Amphetamine Combination =2,
    Yellow (Vitamix)
A. T. A. Amphetamine Combination =3,
    Pink (Vitamix)
A. T. A. Tablets =1, Green (Vitamix)
A. T. A. Tablets =1, Yellow (Vitamix)
A. T. A. Tablets =2, Pink (Vitamix)
A. T. A. Tablets = 2, Yellow (Vitamix)
A. T. A. Tablets =3, Gray (Vitamix)
A. T. A. Tablets =3, Pink (Vitamix)
Atblaku Formula No. 276 (Hiss)
Atblake Formula No. 252 Capsules (Hiss)
Atblake Formula 276 (Hiss)
Atraxin
Auraplex w/ Amphetamine (Bernhoft)
Auraplex w/ Phenobarb (Bernhoft)
AV-Capsules No. 1 (Paramount Surgical
    Supply)
AV-Capsules No. 2 (Paramount Surgical
    Supply)

AV-Capsules No. 3 (Paramount Surgical
    Supply)
AV-Tabs No. 1 (Paramount Surgical Supply)
AV-Tabs No. 2 (Paramount Surgical Supply)
AV-Tabs No. 3 (Paramount Surgical Supply)
AVA No. 5 Liquid (Modern Drugs)
Axon Syrup (McKesson)
Ayeramate

B-Barb (Foy)
B-Phen Elixir (Wolins)
B-Pheno Tablets (Superior)
    Full-Strength
    Half-Strength
Baby Cough No. 1 (Wynn)
Bakersed Green (W. F. Baker)
Balantrol (Pritchard)
Bamo-400 (Misemer)
Bancaps-C (Westerfield)
Bandyne (Blaine Parker)
Bar-It (Lanpar)
Bar-Jam (Superior)
Bar-Pax Tablets (Bowman)
Banobese-T (Blaine Parker)
Barahist E.C. Liquid (National Pharm)
Barb-Sul Capsules (M.J.)
Barba-Key Slocaps (Key)
Barbamil
Barbamyl
Barba-Niacin (Cole)
Barba-Niacin Forte (Cole)
Barbatose No. 2 Tablets (Vale)
Barbeldonna (Lima)
Barbelixir (Maceslin)
Barbicaine (Cutter)
Barbiclin (Taylor)
Barbico (Jenkins)
Barbicoid (Moore Kirk)
Barbidon Elixir (Supreme)
Barbikote Tablets (Maceslin)
Barbinal (Phillips)
Barbinal Capsules with Codeine (various)
    No. 3
    No. 4
Barbine Tablets (Davis and Sly)
Barbinux (Physicians Supply)
Barbinux w/ Rhubarb (Physicians Supply)
Barbipil Tablets (North American)
Barbipill (Chicago Pharm)
Barbisec Capsules (Kay)
Barbita (Chicago Pharm)
Barbitab Plus (Barre)
Barbitab Tablets (Vista)
Barbital (various)

Powder
Tablets 300 mg.
Barbital Compound (Boyer)
Barbital Hyoscyamus Passiflora Compound
(Zemmer)
Barbital Sodium
   Capsules
   Powder
Barbital-Sodium Solution Veterinary (Syracuse)
Barbitidisin (Allan)
Barbiton Sodium
Barbivis (Chicago)
Barbosec (Rowell)
Barbulen (Len-Tag)
Barcole (Haag)
Barcon-3 Tablets (Tutag)
Barfeine (Bill Moss)
Bariatric Formula 75C (Bariatric)
Bariatric Formula 75E (Bariatric)
Bariatric Formula 80A (Bariatric)
Bariatric Formula 81A (Bariatric)
Bariatric Formula 106 (Bariatric)
Bariatric Special Formula 108 1/2 (Bariatric)
Bariatric Formula G1 (Bariatric)
Bariatric Formula G2 (Bariatric)
Bariatric Formula G3 (Bariatric)
Bariatric Stock No. 81 (Bariatric)
Baritab Plus (Barre)
Barital Elixir (Barry-Martin)
Barkers Cold Capsules (Supreme)
Bar-O-Bex '15' (Barrows Chemical)
Bar-O-Bex '30' (Barrows Chemical)
Bar-O-Bex Super '45' (Barrows Chemical)
Bar-Tabs No. 1 (Barrows Chemical)
Bar-Tabs No. 1A (Barrows Chemical)
Bar-Tabs No. 2 (Barrows Chemical)
Bar-Tabs No. 2A (Barrows Chemical)
Bar-Tabs No. 3 (Barrows Chemical)
Bar-Tabs No. 3A (Barrows Chemical)
   Rplex (Massengill)
Barprin (Cenci)
Barsec Capsules (Maceslin)
Barturate (Davis and Sly)
Bartus Liquid (National Pharm)
   No. 1
   No. 2
Bartuss Jr. Liquid (National Pharm)
Bartwo (Ulmer)
Barval No. 1 Tablets (Durst)
Barval No. 2 Tablets (Durst)
Bateman Drops (R. G. Dunwody)
BBS (various)
   Elixir

Tablets 16 mg.
Tablets 32 mg.
Tablets 49 mg.
Bebital w/ Phenobarbital Tablets (Wilfred)
Bedadol (Ives-Cameron)
Beedex Capsules (Greens Pharm)
Bel-Phen Tablets (Stanlabs)
   No. 1
   No. 2
Beladryl Injectable (Bellevue)
Belap No. 2 Tablets (Haack)
Belatol No. 2 (Cenci)
Bellachar (various)
Belladonna Leaves Extract
Beminal w/ Phenobarbital (Ayerst)
Benecycles Capsules (Bernhoft)
Benesed Liquid (Pharmak)
Beplete (Wyeth)
   Elixir
   Tablets
Berla-Dexatal (Berkeley)
Berla-Sed (Berkeley)
Besertal Tablets (Central)
Bese-Caps (Nysco)
Beta-6 Liquid (Comboceuticals)
Beta-Chlor (Mead Johnson)
Betarb Tablets (Evron)
Bevital (Key)
Bexaphed Capsules (Bexar)
Biatal Tablets (Kendall)
Biatussin AC (Bates Labs)
Biggers HB Cordial (R. G. Dunwody)
Biggers Huckleberry Cordial (Dunwody)
Biobamat
Biogesic (Caldwell and Bloor)
Biotussin GG Syrup (Pharmak)
Bioxyphen Injection (Invenex)
Bipectol Wafers (Vale)
Bipinal Sodium
Biphetacel (Strasenburgh)
Bis, Pec, Opium Tablets (High)
Bised (Bryant)
Bisedalan (Allan)
Bismar Tablets (Delavau)
Bismaster w/ Paregoric (Drug Master)
   Liquid
   Tablet
Bismuth and Salol w/ Paregoric (various)
Bisosed (Buck)
Bistol-Pectin and Paregoric (Penneh Prod.)
Blairserp (Blair)
Blue-Phen (Lemmon)
Bonatuss (various)
Bowtab =1 (Bowman)

Bowtab =2 (Bowman)
Bowtab =3 (Bowman)
B.P. and Paregoric Tablets (High)
B.P. Opium Tab (High)
Bredative-DHC
Brevital Sodium (Lilly)
  Ampules 500 mg.
  Ampules 2.5 gm.
  Ampules 5 gm.
Briadess Tab. (Briar Pharm.)
Briarbit Tab. (Briar Pharm.)
Brietal
Bri-Stan (various)
Bro-Sed (Superior)
Bromi-Chlor Solution (Bowman)
Bromides and Chloral Compound (various)
Bromides w/ Sodium Phenobarbital Elixir
  (Vale)
Bromides-Phenobarbital Special Formula
  4140 (Drug Products)
Bromionyl w/ Barbital (Upjohn)
Bromiphen (McNeil)
Bromital (Moffet)
Bromobarb (Hart)
Broncho-Tussin (First Texas)
Broncchist (Sutliff and Case)
Bronicof Liquid (Jenkins Labs)
Bronsyl Syrup (McNeil)
Brothane Solution (Cole)
Brown Mixture (various)
  Liquid
  Tablets
Bubartal Sodium Injection (various)
Bubartal TT (various)
Bucol AC Liquid (National Pharm)
Bucol Jr. Liquid (National Pharm)
Buethanasia Veterinary Injection (Burns)
Buffered A.P.C. with Codeine (W. T.
  Thompson)
Buladol Capsules No. 2
  Capsules No. 2
  Capsules No. 3
  Capsules No. 4
Burbartal (Columbus)
Burrizem No. 2 (Zemmer)
Busotran Tablets (Klug)
Buta-Reserpine Tablet (Reyman)
Buta-Trol (Pacer)
Butabarb (Hiss)
Butabarb (various)
  Capsules
  Elixir
  Tablets
Butabarbital

Butabarbital Sodium
  Elixir
  Powder
  Tablets 16 mg.
  Tablets 32 mg.
Butabarpal Injection (Philadelphia)
Butacalm No. 1 (Wesley)
Butacalm No. 2 (Wesley)
Butacyl (Queen City)
Butador Capsules (Physicians Prod.)
Butador/Codeine Capsules (Physicians
  Prod.)
  No. 2
  No. 3
  No. 4
Butak (Haack)
Butalbital
Butalix (Vale)
Butalynn (Lynn)
Butalynn-GR (Lynn)
Butamed Elixir (Medics)
Butamid Elixir (Midway Medical)
Butamin Tablets (Mallard)
Butapal (Philadelphia)
Butaparbal (Philadelphia)
Butaphed Tablets (Wendt-Bristol)
Butaphen Elixir (Veltex)
Butaphen Sodium (Veltex)
  Tablets 16 mg.
  Tablets 32 mg.
  Tablets 97 mg.
Butapin No. 1 (Wendt-Bristol)
Butapin No. 2 (Wendt-Bristol)
Butapro (various)
Butarb (Arden)
Butasaron (Saron)
  Tablets 16 mg.
  Tablets 32 mg.
Butasec (Hiss)
Butased 15 (Schlicksup)
Butased-30 (Schlicksup)
Butaserp (Queen City)
Butatab (Palmedico)
Butatal Elixir (Grail)
Butatin Tablets (Winston)
Butatrax (Sutliff)
Butazem (Zemmer)
  Elixir
  Tablets 15 mg.
  Tablets 30 mg.
  Tablets 60 mg.
  Tablets 100 mg.
Butenil
Butes (C.B.S.)

Butesco (Bowman)
Butesco S.X.T. (Bowman)
Butethal
Butex (various)
  Tablets 16 mg.
  Tablets 32 mg.
Butibarbital Elixir (Vita Fore)
Buticaps (McNeil)
  Capsules 15 mg.
  Capsules 30 mg.
  Capsules 50 mg.
  Capsules 100 mg.
Butisec (Hiss)
Butiserpazide-25 Tablets (McNeil)
Butiserpazide-50 Tablets (McNeil)
Butiserpine (McNeil)
  Elixir
  Tablets
Butiserpine-RA Tablets (McNeil)
Butisol-Hyoscyamus Compound Tablets
  (McNeil)
Butisol Sodium (McNeil)
  Elixir
  Tablets 15 mg.
  Tablets 30 mg.
  Tablets 50 mg.
  Tablets 100 mg.
Butisol-RA (McNeil)
  Tablets 30 mg.
  Tablets 60 mg.
Butizide-25 Tablets (McNeil)
Butizide-50 Tablets (McNeil)
Butobarbital
Butrate (Kay)
  Tablets 16 mg.
  Tablets 32 mg.
  Tablets 97 mg.
Butseco S.C.T. (Bowman)

C.C.G. No. 2 Capsules (P. J. Noyes)
C.T. Aspirin w/ Dovers (Elder)
C.T. Blue No. L CTD (Harvey)
C.T. Blue No. 1-CUF (Caldwell and Bloor)
C.T. Brown No. 1-CYC (Caldwell and Bloor)
C.T. Caparin w/ Dovers (Elder)
C.T. Cream No. 1 CXS (Fox)
C.T. Doveram Tablets (Elder)
C.T. Doverlen (Elder)
C.T. Gray No. 1 CUG (Fox)
C.T. Gray (S. F. Durst)
C.T. Gray (Lyons Physician Supply)
C.T. Gray (Heyl Physicians Supply)
C.T. Gray (Caldwell and Bloor)

C.T. Gray (Lyons Physicians Supply)
C.T. Green (Blaine)
C.T. Green No. 1-BDH (Wendt-Bristol)
C.T. Green No. 1-BIV (Caldwell and Bloor)
C.T. Green No. 1-CMR (Carr)
C.T. Green No. 1-CTE (Durst)
C.T. Green No. 1-DAV (Schuemann)
C.T. Green No. 1-DDU (Durst)
C.T. Green No. 1-14422 (Caldwell and
  Bloor)
C.T. Green No. 1-14807 (Caldwell and
  Bloor)
C.T. Green No. 1-15058 (Caldwell and
  Bloor)
C.T. Lavender (Harvey)
C.T. Natural No. 1-ATM (Caldwell and
  Bloor)
C.T. Natural No. 1-BAV (Lyons)
C.T. Natural No. 1-CNV (Lynwood)
C.T. Natural No. 1 CTN (Benet's)
C.T. Natural No. 1-CWP (Raymer)
C.T. Natural No. 1 CXB (Schuemann-
  Jones)
C.T. Natural No. 1-CYL (Durst)
C.T. Natural No. 1-DBK (Durst)
C.T. Natural No. 1-DBL (Caldwell and
  Bloor)
C.T. Natural No. 1-14966 (Caldwell and
  Bloor)
C.T. Orange No. 1 ADU (Schuemann)
C.T. Orange No. LCYB (Caldwell and
  Bloor)
C.T. Oval Phenacetin (Elder)
C.T. Pink (Carr Drug)
C.T. Pink (Caldwell and Bloor)
C.T. Pink (Heyl Physicians Supply)
C.T. Pink (Lampert)
C.T. Pink (Lyons Physician Supply)
C.T. Pink No. 1 CTM (Benet's)
C.T. Red 1-CUD (Caldwell and Bloor)
C.T. Red No. 1-AYJ (Caldwell and Bloor)
C.T. Rose-Pink No. 1-CWT (Durst)
C.T. Round White RX No. 22583 (Elder)
C.T. Special (Dr. Townsend) (Bowman
  Pharm)
C.T. Special Cold Tablets (Elder)
C.T. Tan (S. F. Durst)
C.T. White (Lyons Physician Supply)
C.T. White No. 1-BQR (Caldwell and Bloor)
C.T. White No. 1-BSC (Wendt-Bristol)
C.T. White No. 1-CER (Pan American)
C.T. White No. 1 CEV (Carr Drug)
C.T. White No. 1-CQO (Davis and Sly)
C.T. White No. 1-CUE (Caldwell and Bloor)

C.T. Tan No. 1-DDL (Maceslin)
C.T. Yellow (Caldwell and Bloor)
C.T. Yellow (S. F. Durst)
C.T. Yellow No. 1-ARE (Schuemann)
C.T. Yellow No. 1-BMP (Caldwell and Bloor)
C.T. Yellow No. 1 BNK (Carr Drug)
C.T. Yellow 1CDP (Herman)
C.T. Yellow No. 1 CTB (Harvey)
C.T. Yellow No. 1 CYA (Caldwell and Bloor)
Cal-Sed (Philips Roxane)
Calcidrine Syrup (Abbott)
Calmate Tablets (Henry Schein)
Calmax
Calmiren
Calpental (P. J. Noyes)
Calphodes (Affiliated)
Caltrol (Lanpar)
Cambrised (Cambridge)
  Elixir
  Tablets
Cambrised Jr. Tablets (Cambridge)
Camphen DHC Tablets (Liden Labs)
Canquil-400 Tablets (Canfield)
Cap-O-Sed (Croyden-Browne)
Cap-O-Tran (Croyden-Browne)
Carbadex (Stanford)
  Capsules
  Tablets
Carboxyphen
Carbrital (Parke-Davis)
  Capsules
  Elixir
Carbrital Half Strength (Parke-Davis)
Carbropent (Blue Line)
Cardia Sedative Compound (Wendt-Bristol)
Cardinals (Lafayette)
Carnusen (Queen City)
Carodone (various)
Carodone Jr. (various)
Carrbutabarb (various)
  Elixir
  Tablets 16 mg.
  Tablets 32 mg.
  Tablets 97 mg.
Carrmine Syrup (Century)
Cav-Caps (Kare)
Cedital (Franklin)
Cekophen (Veltex)
  Capsules 49 mg.
  Capsules 97 mg.
Cellamine (Echos)
Cel-O-Rex No. 1 (C. S. Ruckstuhl)

Celludrine (Gotham)
Cellumine Tablets (Ferndale)
Celmol Liquid (various)
Celu-Len (Len Tag)
Cenamal Capsules (Central)
Centra-Sed (Southern)
Centra Sed Plus (Southern)
Cephalgia (Crest)
  Capsules
  Tablets
Cephebs with Dovers Tablets (Lusher)
Cerased Liquid (Pharmak)
Ceretol-B (Barre)
Certigan VC with Codeine (Certified)
Certigan with Codeine (Certified)
Certussin with Codeine (Certified)
Cetro-Cirose (Ives)
Cervo with Morphine (E. W. Huen)
Char-Hal (Halsom)
Char-Ken Tablets (Approved)
Charbel (Delavau)
Charbell (Sonnenberg)
Charbelphen (Modern)
Charbophen (Tricounty)
Charcoal w/ Bellophen Tablets No. 2775 (Richlyn)
Chardonna Tablets (Rorer)
Charloid (Wesley)
Charlynn (Lynn)
Charspast (Truxton)
Cheracol (Upjohn)
Cheradine Cof Liquid (Modern Drugs)
Cheradyne Liquid (Archer-Taylor)
Cherahist Jr. (Ketchum)
Cheralate (Rondex Labs)
Cher and Codeine Liquid (Delavau)
Cherekoff Liquid (Ads Labs)
Cherex Liquid (R. Daniels)
Cheri Hance (Hance)
Cherijen Liquid (Jenkins Labs)
Cherikoff (Purepac)
Cherola Kolex (various)
Cheropine with Codeine (Certified)
Cherosed Liquid (Mallard)
Cheround with Morphine Syrup (Superior)
Cherralex Codeine Liquid (National Pharm)
Cherralex/Dionin Liquid (National Pharm)
Cherrepel with Codeine (Wynn Labs)
Cherripine w/ Codeine (Moore Kirk)
Cherripine w/ Morphine Sulfate (Moore Kirk)
Cherritus and Codeine (Vita Fore)
Cherry Cough Syrup with Codeine (Ladco)

Cherrydel Cough Syrup (Pennex Products)
Cherrymaster No. 3 (Drugmaster)
Chinicol Adult (Rondex Labs)
Chlor (various)
  Capsules 243 mg.
  Capsules 486 mg.
  Vials
Chloral
Chlorhexadol
Chlor Mal No. 3 Liquid (Modern Drugs)
Chlor-A-Drine Elixir (Lusher)
Chlor-Mag-Pent (Curt Labs.)
Chlorpheniramine with SPC, H.S. = 1 (Rich-
  lyn)
Chlorphenyl B Capsules (Darby)
Chlorphenyl B Tabs (Darby)
Chlor-Stron (Edom)
  Liquid
  Tablets
Chloral Betaine
Chloral Bromide Compound (Davis and Sly)
Chloral Hydrate
  Capsules 250 mg.
  Capsules 500 mg.
  Crystals
  Suppositories
  Syrup
  Tablets
Chloral Hydrate and Hyoscine (Durst)
Chloral Hydrate-Betaine Adduct
Chloral-Ten (Mid-Atlantic)
Chlorde Tablets (various)
Chlor-Trimeton Expectorant w/ Codeine
  (Schering)
Cidicol (Upjohn)
Citra (Boyle and Co.)
  Syrup
Citra Forte (Boyle and Co.)
  Capsules
  Syrup
Citradine (Moore Kirk)
Citro-Codea (First Texas)
Citro-Keene-AC (E. W. Huen)
Citropam No. 2 (Jenkins Labs)
Citrose Liquid (Naman)
Clinicol Jr. (Rondex Labs)
Co-Entero Tablets (Coast)
Co-Xan Elixir (Central)
Cobenzil (Abbott)
Cocil w/ Codeine (Rondex Labs)
Cocila with Codeine Liquid (Denison Labs)
Cocila w/ Dionin (Denison Labs)
Cocilar with Morphine Sulfate (Moore Kirk)

Cocilco with Codeine Syrup (Pennex Pro-
  ducts)
Cocilco with Dionin Syrup (Pennex Prod.)
Cocillana and Codeine Syrup (Pharmak)
Cocillana Compound Syrup (various)
Cocillana Compound Syrup w/ Dionin (vari-
  ous)
Cocillana/Codeine No. 1 (National Pharm)
Cocillana/Dionin Liquid (National Pharm)
Cocillco with Codeine (Burrough Bros.)
Cocillin and Codeine (Vita Fore)
Cocillona/Codeine Liquid (Ads Labs)
Codadyne
Codagesic Capsules (Defco)
Coda-Phed with Codeine (Robinson Labs)
Codachlor (Wynn Labs)
Codahist Syrup (Burrough Bros)
Codalan Tablets (Lannett)
  No. 1
  No. 2
  No. 3
Codalex (Mallard)
Codamasal Capsules (Defco)
Codamide Tabs (Cambridge)
Codapec Liquid (Life)
Codasa Capsules I (Stayner)
Codasa Capsules II (Stayner)
Codasa Forte Capsules (Stayner)
Codasa Tablets (Stayner)
Codaspro No. 1 Tablets
Codaspro No. 2 Tablets
Codatuss (Moore Kirk)
Codatuss C (Moore Kirk)
Codecol with Codeine (Wynn Labs)
Codeine Compound Syrup (Denison Labs)
Codel Syrup (Elder)
Codempiral (B.W. & Co..)
  Capsules No. 2
  Capsules No. 3
Codenil (Wynn Labs)
Codesal (Tilden-Yates)
  Tablets No. 1
  Tablets No. 2
Codexin (Arco)
Codexin-T (Arco)
Codilene (Hance)
Codimal DH Syrup (Central)
Codimal PH (Central)
Coditrate (Central)
  Syrup
  Tablets
Codone Tablets (Lemmon)
Codrene C Liquid (R. Daniels)

Codsal
Coem No. 2
Co-Estrovite No. 2 (Robinson)
Cofamine No. 1 (Physicians Drug and Supply)
Cofamine No. 2 (Physicians Drug and Supply)
Cofamine No. 3 (Physicians Drug and Supply)
Colamide No. 3 Tablets (Morton)
Colana with Dionin (Hance)
Cold Capsules (Lafayette)
Cold Tablets =3 (Darby)
Cold Tablets No. 5852 (Savoy)
Coldate Tablets (Massengill)
Cole-Inei (Pharmacole)
Colfant Tablets (Jenkins Labs)
Collancc w/ Codeine (Claflin)
Colrex Compound (Rowell)
  Capsules
  Syrup
  Tablets
Col-Trim (Columbia)
Comad (Bush)
Combisede Elixir (Sherry)
Combital (Rand)
Combituss Syrup (Table Rock)
Combogel-B (Comboceuticals)
Comfex (Bush)
Comfort Tabs (Park)
Complagesic Tablets (Coast)
Compobarb Capsules (Vitarine)
  Forte
  Regular
Cona-Forte No. 2 Liquid (Crystal)
Continex Liquid (National Pharm)
Continucaps (Davis and Sly)
Contramal No. 2 (Purdue-Frederick)
Contramal No. 3 (Purdue-Frederick)
Control-15 (W. E. Boody)
Control-30 (W. E. Boody)
Contussis Syrup Green (Merrell)
Copac Tabs (Towne, Paulsen)
Copavin (Lilly)
  Capsules
  Tablets
Copavin Compound Elixir (Lilly)
Copecoryl Liquid (Na-Spra)
Cophenate (Wynn Labs)
Cor-Caps (United Research)
Cordets, Single Strength, Gray (Toledo)
Cordets, Single Strength, Pink (Toledo)
Cordets, Single Strength, White (Toledo)
Cordets No. 1, Single Strength, Gray (Cord)

Cordets No. 2, Single Strength, Natural-White (Cord)
Cordets No. 3, Single Strength, Pink (Cord)
Cordets No. 1, Double Strength, Gray (Cord)
Cordets No. 2, Double Strength, White (Cord)
Cordets No. 3, Double Strength, Pink (Cord)
Corenil Tablets (McNeil)
Corexin Forte (U.S. Ethicals)
Coricidin/Codeine (Schering)
  Tablets 16 mg.
  Tablets 32 mg.
Corel (Moffet)
Coriforte (Schering)
Corodan w/ Codeine (R. Daniels)
Corparex Meta-Kaps (Sutliff and Case)
Cor-Tabs (United Research)
Cosadein (Parke-Davis)
Cosanussin with Morphine (P. J. Noyes)
Cosanyl (Parke-Davis)
Coscriptin/Codeine
Cosedate Liquid (Pharmak)
Cosiline with Dionin (Wynn Pharmaceuticals)
Cotussis (National Drug)
Cough Syrup No. 3 (E. W. Huen)
Cough Syrup No. 3216 (Savoy)
Cough Syrup No. 3222 (Savoy)
Cough Syrup No. 7 (E. W. Huen)
Cough Syrup w/ Codeine (Bates)
Cough-Eaze (Foy)
Covon No. 1
Covon No. 2
Covon No. 3
Crestanil (Crest)
  Tablets 200 mg.
  Tablets 400 mg.
Crupic Tablets (Jenkins Labs)
Cumbercidin Forte Capsules (Cumberland)
Cyclex (M.S. and D.)
Cyclopal (Upjohn)
Cyclopen (Massengill)
Cycotin (Reed and Carnrick)
Cycotran
Cydril with Toluidin Tablets (S. J. Tutag)
Cydril-TX (S. J. Tutag)
Cypron

Dakamin (Ferrill and Schank)
Danstat (Oxford)
D.F.C. Dophenco (Blue Line)
Darbeda (Darby)
Darbeda-T (Darby)

D-A-S-T Capsules (Caldwell and Bloor)
D-A-S-T-A-L Capsules (Caldwell and Bloor)
D-A-S-T-E-N Capsules (Caldwell and Bloor)
D-O-X Tablets (Davis and Sly)
D-Tab No. 3 (Direct)
D-9-Desophen (Starr)
Dadex (Mar)
Dalatussin Liquid (Life)
Dalby Carminative (Dunwody)
Damason-P (Mason)
  Capsules
  Tablets
Damason/Codeine Tablets (Mason)
D-Amitrene (Normand)
Dantal (Daniels)
  Tablets 16 mg.
  Tablets 32 mg.
Daro (Fellows Testagar)
  Capsules
  Capsules Jr.
  Tablets
Dasa-C (Lynn)
Dasin-CS (Massengill)
Dasin (Massengill)
  Capsules
  Tablets
Daspan Tablets (Naman)
Dat (Blaine)
Dat Comp. (Blaine)
Davis Sedative Cough Syrup (Pharmak)
Davit Capsules (PRL)
Daysed (New England)
De Algianil (De Leon)
De-Amo Timed Capsules (Spartan)
Deamsu Capsules (Hanlon)
Deba
Decabamate (M.S. and D.)
Deeglans (Westerfield)
De-Em Timed Capsules (Spartan)
Deewee Carminative (Dunwody)
Deewee's Mixture (Drug Developments)
Delacom Gradules T.D. (Schuemann-Jones)
Del-Caps (Organd)
Delaphen Capsules (Naman)
Deledex Capsules (Lynn)
Delobese Injectable (Delco)
Delvinal Capsules (M.S. and D.)
Delvinal-Asperin (M.S. and D.)
Delvinal-Diethylstilbestrol (M.S. and D.)
Demido Capsules (Wendt-Bristol)
Demotal Tablets (Philadelphia)
Deoxie (Foy)
  Injection
  Tablets

Deprol (Wallace)
Derfule Pink (Cole)
Desa-Bamate
Desahist AT Syrup (various)
Destab (Marsin Medical Supply)
Descolate Syrup (Vita Fore)
Descolate/Codeine (Vita Fore)
Desephine Tablets (Studebaker)
Deseroid No. 3 (Harvey)
Desital Tablets (Caldwell and Bloor)
Desital No. 2 Tablets (Caldwell and Bloor)
Desobarb (various)
Desobarb 1/2 Strength (Tilden-Yates)
Desodrin (various)
Desoid PB (Schlicksup)
Desoids (Philips Roxane)
Desonine Tablets (Jabert)
Desophen (Starr)
  Capsules No. 1
  Capsules No. 3
Desoroids Tablets (Tracy)
Desothins No. 1 (Haberle)
Desothins No. 2 (Haberle)
Desothins No. 3 (Haberle)
Desothins Forte No. 1 (Haberle)
Desothins Forte No. 2 (Haberle)
Desothins Forte No. 3 (Haberle)
Desoxaloid (Halsom)
Desoxo-5 (Sutliff and Case)
Desoxohab No. 1 (Haberle)
Desoxohab No. 2 (Haberle)
Desoxohab No. 3 (Haberle)
Desoxyephedrine and Thyroid Tablets,
  No. 1 (Wendt-Bristol)
Desoxyephedrine and Thyroid Tablets,
  No. 2 (Wendt-Bristol)
Desoxyephedrine and Thyroid (Wendt-
  Bristol)
Despasmol Tablet (Luly-Thomas)
Destab (Marsin Medical Supply)
De-Stat (Schlick)
Desympatin A (Vitamin Specialties)
Desympatin B (Vitamin Specialties)
Desympatin C (Vitamin Specialties)
Detonal Tablets (Thompson)
Dewux (Halsom)
Dexacap (Marsin Medical Supply)
Dexalate Injection (various)
Dexamar No. 1 (Marsin Medical Supply)
Dexamar No. 2 (Marsin Medical Supply)
Dexamar No. 3 (Marsin Medical Supply)
Dexambar Improved (General Medical
  Supply)
Dexaphen (Moffet)

Dex-Cell-Ate (Westerfield)
Dex-O-Phet Tablets (Laurel)
Dexam (Mayrand)
Dex-Sal (Richlyn)
Dexesul Compound No. 1 (Garde)
Dexesul No. 2 (Garde)
Dexesul No. 3 (Garde)
Dex-Obesity (Garden)
Dex-Tri-Mer (Spencer-Mead)
Dextro-Amphetamine Compound (Cord)
Dextro-Amphetamine Compound (Toledo)
Dextroamphetamine Sulfate Compound:
    15/3 (Shaw)
Dextro O.B. Compound (Lustgarten)
Dextrosal (Fellows-Testagar)
Dextro Teen-Caps (Rugby)
Dextro Teen-Tabs =1 (Rugby)
Dextro Teen-Tabs =2 (Rugby)
Dextro Teen-Tabs =3 (Rugby)
Dextro Trim (Richlyn) Dys
DFA Anamine (Paul B. Elder)
Dia-Quel (Certified Labs)
Diabusmul Suspension (Drug Master)
Diacap Unicelles (Hiss)
Diaceto/Codeine (Archer-Taylor)
    Capsules 16 mg.
    Capsules 32 mg.
    Tablets 16 mg.
    Tablets 32 mg.
Diadem Liquid (National Pharm)
Diadol (various)
    Tablets 32 mg.
    Tablets 97 mg.
Dial (Ciba)
Dialog with Codeine No. 2 (Ciba)
Dialog with Codeine No. 3 (Ciba)
Diamet (Lynn)
Diampha (Direct)
Diamulsin Liquid (Vale)
Dianil and Paregoric (Chase)
Diapect with Paregoric (Rondex Labs)
Diarol with Paregoric (Manhattan Drug)
    No. 1
    No. 2
Diascaphen Tablets (Caldwell and Bloor)
Diatal C.T. (Prof. Drug Service)
Diaval (Moore Kirk)
Dicitradine (Moore Kirk)
Dicodamor (Moore Kirk)
Dicode Liquid (Schlicksup)
Dicodethal Elixir (Lannett)
Dicodid (Knoll)
    Powder

Tablets
Dicodrine Syrup (Tilden-Yates)
Dicomal Syrup (Naman)
Dicomin Special (R. Daniels)
Dicoril Syrup (Lemmon)
Dicosil (S. J. Tutag)
Dietabs, Series A, No. 1 (Key)
Dietabs, Series A, No. 2 (Key)
Dietabs, Series A, No. 3 (Key)
Dietaid (Medco Supply)
Dietaid No. 1 (Medco Supply)
Dietaid No. 2 (Medco Supply)
Dietaid No. 3 (Medco Supply)
Dietcap (Blaine)
Di-Tal (Academy)
Di-Trol (Bellevue Surgical Supply)
Di-Trol T (Bellevue Surgical Supply)
Digeratone (Direct)
Dihistacod (Moore Kirk)
Dihistine DH Liquid (National Pharm)
Dihydrocodeinone Syrup (Linden Labs)
Dimetane Expectorant-DC (Robins)
Dimethylose C.T. (Veltex)
Diofed Syrup (Vale)
Diofedrin (Vale) (Durst)
Dipental Tablets (Haug)
Diphenhydramine Compound Expectorant
    (various)
Diphenoloid (Direct)
Diphylets-T (Tutag)
Dobeline S.C. Tablets (Archer-Taylor)
Docam Tablets (Delavau)
Docaps (Lafayette)
Docodrine Syrup (Tilden-Yates)
Docosil (Cord)
Doffs-Wt-Heavy (Dofs)
Doffs-Wt-Light (Dofs)
Dohiston Tablets (Delavau)
Doloal (various)
Donnagesic Extentabs No. 1 (Robins)
Donnagesic Extentabs No. 2 (Robins)
Donnagel-PG (Robins)
Dorico
Dorico Soluble
Doriden (Ciba)
    Capsules
    Tablets 125 mg.
    Tablets 250 mg.
    Tablets 500 mg.
Doriden-Sed
Dorodol-Dex (Buffington's)
Dormased Tablets (Crest)
Dormitol Compound (various)

Dosal Cold Capsules (Standard)
Dosarbital (Bowman)
Double D-Tab No. 1 (Direct)
Double D-Tab No. 2 (Direct)
Double D-Tab No. 3 (Direct)
Dov. Tablets (Delavau)
Dovacet Capsules (Vale)
Dovacin (E. W. Huen)
Dovahist (High)
Dovalgen (various)
Dovamor (Moore Kirk)
  Capsules
  Tablets
Dovamor Jr. (Moore Kirk)
  Capsules
  Tablets
Dovaphen (Jenkins Labs)
Dovaphen Jr. Tablets (Jenkins Labs)
Dovaspirin Capsules (various)
Dovaval (Moore Kirk)
Dover Capsules (High)
Doveram Capsules (Elder)
Doverdale Capsules (Ferndale)
Doveret Tablets (High)
Doverin Capsules (High)
Doverlyn (Davis and Sly)
  Capsules
  Tablets
  Tablets, Children's
Dovernon Capsules (Tutag)
Dovets Tablets (J.W.S. Delavau)
Dovium Capsules (Hance)
Dovogic Jr. Tablets (Auburn Labs)
Dovogic S/C Blue (Auburn Labs)
Dovogic S/C Red (Auburn Labs)
Dovogic Tablets (Auburn Labs)
Dovosal Tablets (Bowman)
Doxytal Elixir (Sherry)
Drex (Boyle) Powder
Drocogesic No. 3 Tablets (Century)
Drodeine (Dow)
Drotamine Sulfate (Bush)
D.T.A. (Schlicksup)
D-Tab (Direct)
D-Tab No. 1 (Direct)
D-Tab No. 2 (Direct)
D-Tab No. 3 (Direct)
Dys-Tabs (E. K. Cook)
Ducevim (Bernhoft) Capsules
Duenite (Superior) Ampules
Duobarb No. 2 (Vita Fore)
Duobarb No. 3 (Vita Fore)
Duobarbital (Generix)

Duobarbital Cap (Richlyn)
Duobarbital 1 Capsules (Tracy)
Duobarbital 2 Capsules (Tracy)
Duobarbital 1 1/2 (Wolins)
Duobarbital 3 (Wolins)
Duobarbital 3 Gr. (Jan)
Duobarbital-HS (A.B.A.)
Duobrophen (Massengill)
Duocaps (Flatbush)
Duodex (Misemer)
Duodon (Kirkman)
Duoson 3 Gr. (H. Sonnenberg)
Duotal Capsules (Approved)
Duotal (Morton)
Dura-B-Sules Capsules (Tully)
Duradorm (Lincoln)
Duraduosules Capsules (Tully)
Durenosules Capsules (Tully)
Durfule Slosol (Cole)
Dusotal (G. F. Harvey)
  Capsules 97 mg.
  Capsules 195 mg.
Dys-Ban Capsules (Northwest)
Dysenaid (Jenkins Labs)
Dysmengesic (Walden)

Eazette (Freeport)
E.C. Green No. 4-AJE (Schuemann)
E.C. Green No. 4-AJT (Airhart)
Edrisal (Smith, Kline and French)
Ekrised Tablets (Mallard)
Elasate (Dunhall)
Eldecon with Codeine (P. B. Elder)
Elibese Capsules (Pisgah)
Elixsed (Chicago)
Elpagen/Codeine
Elpanal (Lemmon)
Elpandryl Capsules (Elder)
Emebarb-TM (Elder)
Emeracol Syrup (Upjohn)
Emesert No. 1 Suppository (Arnar-Stone)
Emesert No. 2 Suppository (Arnar-Stone)
Emesert No. 3 Suppository (Arnar-Stone)
Emesert No. 1 (Storck)
Emesert No. 2 (Storck)
Emesert No. 3 (Storck)
Empirin Compound No. 1 (B.W. & Co.)
Empirin Compound with Codeine No. 2
  (B.W. & Co.)
Empirin Compound with Codeine No. 3
  (B.W. & Co.)
Empirin Compound with Codeine No. 4
  (B.W. & Co.)

Emprazil-C Tablets 1/4 gr. (Burroughs Wellcome)
En-Chlor (Ulmer)
  250 mg.
  500 mg.
Endotussin-C (Endo)
Endotussin NN Pediatric Syrup (Endo)
Endotussin NN Syrup (Endo)
Ental Elixir (Allison)
Ental Tablets (Allison)
  16 mg.
  32 mg.
Enzobarb (K. & M.)
Ephedrine and Amytal (Lilly)
Ephedrine and Nembutal 50 (Abbott)
Ephedrine/Nembutal (Abbott) Capsules
Ephedrine and Phenobarbital Sodium (Massengill)
Ephedrine and Phenobarbital Tablets (various)
Ephedrine and Seconal (Lilly)
Ephedrine Sulfate w/ Sodium Secobarbital (Davis-Edwards)
Ephedrol (Lilly) w/ Codeine
Ephedrotal Solu-Caps (Sutliff and Case)
Equagesic (Wyeth) Tablets
Equalysen (Wyeth) Tablets
Equanil (Wyeth)
  Suspension
  Tablets 200 mg.
  Tablets 400 mg.
  Wyseals 400 mg.
  Tablets Veterinary 400 mg.
Equanil LA (Wyeth) Capsules 400 mg.
Equi-Thesin Injection (Jensen-Salsbery)
Erasen (Davis-Edwards)
Eskabarb (S.K. & F.)
  Spansule 65 mg.
  Spansule 97 mg.
Eskaphen-B (S.K. & F.)
  Elixir
  Tablets
Esperon (Table Rock)
Estracorp (Sutliff and Case)
Ethalyl (Premo)
Ethalyl Sodium (Premo)
Ethaminal
Ethchlorvynol
Ethinamate
Ethobral (Wyeth)
  Capsules 65 mg.
  Capsules 130 mg.
Euphased (Schenley)
Euphased-5 (Schenley)

Euphenex (Westerfield)
Euphenex, Jr. (Westerfield)
Eurodex-Plus (Euron)
Euthanasia (Arnold)
Evipal (Winthrop)
Evipal Sodium (Winthrop)
Ev-Ren (Zimmers)
Evronal Sodium (Evron)
Ex-O-Bese (Wabash)
Expansatol Elixir Butabarbitol (Merit)
Expectacod (Auburn)
Expectamor (Auburn)
Expectorant Codel Syrup (P. B. Elder)

Facaps (H. A. Pell)
Fatal Injection Veterinary (Syracuse Pharmacal)
Febridyne No. 2
Febridyne No. 3
Feleen =1 (Jeffrey Fell)
Feleen = 2 (Jeffrey Fell)
Feleen =3 (Jeffrey Fell)
Fello-Sed Elixir (Fellows, Testagar)
Felsules (Fellows-Testagar)
  Capsules 3 3/4 gr.
  Capsules 7 1/2 gr.
  Capsules 15 gr.
Fenadin w/ Codeine (Burroughs Bros.)
  Capsules 16 mg.
  Capsules 32 mg.
  Tablets 16 mg.
  Tablets 32 mg.
Fenbane (Walker)
Fenbro (Cole)
Fenbutal Tablets (Tutag)
Fenobex (Strasenburgh)
Fenta (Lusher)
Feridexate (U.S. Standard)
Feta Capsules (Misemer)
Fetabarb No. 1 (Misemer)
Fetabarb No. 2 (Misemer)
Fetacomp No. 1 (Physicians Drug Supply)
Fetacomp No. 2 (Physicians Drug Supply)
Fetacomp No. 3 (Physicians Drug Supply)
Fetasulf No. 1 (Physicians Drug Supply)
Fetasulf No. 2 (Physicians Drug Supply)
Fetasulf No. 3 (Physicians Drug Supply)
Fiorinal (Sandoz)
  Capsules
  Tablets
Fiorinal with Codeine Capsules No. 1 (Sandoz)
Fiorinal with Codeine No. 2 (Sandoz)
Fiorinal with Codeine No. 3 (Sandoz)

Flatutive Childtabs (Garde)
Floramine (Lemmon)
Floranerval Tablets (Roger)
Floraphen-SCT (Prof. Drug Service)
Florased (Caldwell and Bloor)
Floratal (Sherman)
Flornal Capsules (North American)
Forbutol (Plymouth)
For-Dyne/Codeine
    Rmasal and Camphor
Formula =1 Light Green Square (Bariatric)
Formula =1 Orange Square (Bariatric)
Formula =4 Brown Oval (Bariatric)
Formula No. 3 and Formula No. 4 (Cumberland)
Formula No. 1 and Formula No. 5 (Cumberland)
Formula No. 13 (Spencer-Mead)
Formula No. 14 (Spencer-Mead)
Formula No. 15 (Spencer-Mead)
Formula No. 16 (Spencer-Mead)
Formula No. 17 (Spencer-Mead)
Formula No. 30 (Bariatric)
Formula No. 31 (Bariatric)
Formula No. 80 (Bariatric)
Formula No. 81 (Bariatric)
Formula No. 107 (Bariatric)
Formula No. 108 (Bariatric)
Formula No. 109 (Bariatric)
Forpane Capsules (Bates Labs)
Four Green Liquid (Mallard)
Four Red Liquid (Mallard)
4-25 Suppositories (Langer Labs)
Fox-Nux (Foy)
Fre-Tense Tablets (Westerfield)
Fre-Tense Tablets (Kendall)

G-3 Tabs (Palmedico)
    Capsules
Gabail (Fougera)
Galapose Capsules (Galen-Allison)
Galliadine (Astor)
Ganone (Endo)
Gemonil (Abbott)
Genedex-5 Tablets (General)
Genegesic Cap. (General)
Geralert (Nysco)
Gerapenta (Schlicksup)
Geriatonic (Kraft)
Geri-Flav (Direct)
Gerilets (Abbott)
Gerisal Tab. (Geriatric)
Glamour Time Caps (Halsey)
Glamour Set No. 1 (Halsey)

Glamour Set No. 2 (Halsey)
Glamour Set No. 3 (Halsey)
Glutethimide
Glyceryl AC Guaiacolate (Wynn Labs)
Glyco-Pruni with Codeine (First Texas)
Godfrey Cordial (R. G. Dunwody)
Gothotabs-CR (Gotham)
Grey Obesity No. 1 (Byrne)
Guaiacodeine Adult (P. B. Elder)
Guaiacodeine Jr. Syrup (P. B. Elder)
Guaiatrate Syrup with Codeine (Bowman)
Guaiatuss AC Liquid (National Pharm)
Guianate (Wendt-Bristol)
Guiosan with Morphine Acetate (Vale)
Gyaphen (Durst)

Habgesic (Haberle)
Hakritan (Lemmon)
Halabar Tablets (Carnrick)
Halital Injection (Jensen-Salsbery)
Hal-Obese (Halsom)
Haltran (Haller)
H-A-M (Blair)
H-A-M C T (Blair)
Hamtussin with Codeine (Certified)
Harmonyl-N (Abbott)
Harmonyl-N Half Strength (Abbott)
Harvey Dever (High)
Harvodyne/Codeine
Hasacode C.T. 1/4 gr. (Arnar-Stone)
Hasacode Strong 1/2 gr. (Arnar-Stone)
Haxsen (Haack)
Headache and Neuralgia Capsulets (Standard)
Hebaral
Hebaral Sodium
Henbro Elixir (Bowman)
Henofor Elixir (Bowman)
Henotal (Bowman)
    Elixir
Heprodyne Tablets (Westerfield)
Hexemal
Hexemal Calcium
Hexethal
Hexethal Sodium
    Hexett
Hexanastab
Hexenal
Hexobarbital
Hexobarbital Sodium
Hexshortal (Sabra)
Heyl Hy-Lets (Heyl Physicians Supply)
H.F. Doveram Rx No. 24163 (Elder)
H.F. Doveram Rx No. 24214 (Elder)

H.F. Doveram Rx No. 24434 (Elder)
Hi-Cof (Linden)
Hi-Potency Thin Grey, 10 mg. (Henry Schein)
Hi-Potency Thin Pink, 10 mg. (Henry Schein)
Hisdrin (Massengill)
Histachlor with S.P.C. Forte (Lustgarten)
Hista-Cof Liquid (Linden)
Histacof with Codeine (Ladco)
Histadeine Cough Syrup (Pennex Products)
Hista-Derfule (Cole)
Histadyl E.C. Syrup (Lilly)
Histajen (Jenkins Labs)
    Liquid
    Tablets
Histalme (Meyer)
Histalme Duracap (Meyer)
Histam No. 2 Liquid (P. B. Elder)
Histamak Liquid (Pharmak)
Histapco (Apco Labs.)
Histaphed (Rondex Labs)
Histapro No. 32 (Drug Master)
Histapro No. 65 (Drug Master)
Histatussin with Codeine (Ketchum)
Histexpel with Codeine (Ketchum)
Holbamate
Homaphine (C.D. Smith)
Homex (C. O. Truxton)
Hourdex (Delta)
Hoursed Capsules (Delta)
Hovizyme (Ayerst)
H-P-A (Paine, Elder)
H.S. Capsules Clear No. 2-ALD (Caldwell and Bloor)
H.S. Capsules Clear No. 2-AKA (Hiss)
H.S. Cap (Luke)
H.S. Capsules Yellow No. 2-AKJ (Pan American)
H.S. Need Capsules (Hanlon)
Hybar Tablets (Jenkins)
Hycodan Syrup (Endo)
Hycodan Tabs (Endo)
Hycohist Liquid (Endo)
Hycomine Syrup (Endo)
    Syrup Ped.
    Compound Tablets
Hydradine (Auburn Labs)
Hydra-Hal (Halsom)
Hydral Capsules (Person and Covey)
Hydrosoxy (Prof. Drug Service)
Hyobarb (Haberle)
Hyobarb (Indianapolis)
Hyonal (Durst)

Hyophen Tablets (Kendall)
Hyophen Tablets (Westerfield)
Hyophen-BB Tablets (Kendall)
Hyophen-BB Tablets (Westerfield)
Hyoscyamus-Phenobarbital (Davis and Sly)
Hyoscyamus-Phenobarbital Tablets (Tilden-Yates)
Hyo-Sed (Bowman)
Hypasen (Queen City)
Hyper-Sed (Sutliff and Case)
Hyphenal (Blaine)
Hypivals (Physicians Supply)
Hypnettes (Fleming)
    Suppos. 16 mg.
    Suppos. 8 mg.
Hypnodram Computabs (Dram)
Hypnofer
Hypnogene
Hypno-Sed (Jenkins)
Hypocal (Benton)
Hypronate (Franklin)
Hyptran Tablet (Wampole)
Hy-Quad-Phed Tablets (High)
Hysophen (Halsom)
Hyssen-AC (Canright)
Hytrobarb (Dalen-Kaemp)
Hy-Val-Flora w/ Phenobarb

Iacol and Codeine Syrup (W. B. Boyer)
Idenal Tablets (Interstate)
Inazar (Indianapolis)
Indorex (Pasadena)
Indorex No. 1 and No. 2 (Pasadena)
Indorex-C (Pasadena)
Indybese 15 (Indianapolis)
Indybese 30 (Indianapolis)
Infadorm Drops (Reid-Provident)
Infaease Elixir (Tri-State)
Insolat (Denab)
    Tablets 15 mg.
    Tablets 30 mg.
Iodizem Compound Syrup (Zemmer)
I-Pac (Spencer-Mead)
Ipral
Ipral Calcium (Squibb)
    Tablets 130 mg.
Ipral Sodium (Squibb)
Ipsatol-C (Davies, Rose-Hoyt)
Isobarb (U.S. Standard)
Isobarb-APC Tablets (Richlyn)
Isobutal (Henry Schein)
Isobute-APC (Columbia)
Isoclor Expectorant (Arnar-Stone)
Isollyl (Rugby)

Isomnital Tablets (Buffington)
Isonal (Roussell)
Isosed Tablets (Nysco)
Isothal (U.S. Standard)
  Tablets 30 mg.
  Tablets 100 mg.

Jantussin with Codeine (Bates)
Jaydex Tablets (Mid-Atlantic)
Jelobese, Single Strength Gray, =1 (Lit Drug)
Jelobese, Single Strength White, =2 (Lit Drug)
Jelobese, Single Strength Pink, =3 (Lit Drug)
Jensenex (Jenkins)
Juniors Phenobarbital (P. J. Noyes)
Jurasule Jr. (Storck)
Jurasule Sr. (Storck)

K plus P plus Paregoric (Chase)
Kalicyanate (St. Louis)
Kalory (Tyler)
Kalory-Plus (Tyler)
Kamagel Liquid (Towne Paulsen)
Kaobarb (Bernhoft)
Kaodene Liquid (Pfeiffer)
  Kaodene No. 2
Kaogoric (Hance)
Kaolin plus Pectin with Paregoric (Supreme)
Koaparic (Blue Line)
Kaophen (Vale)
Katy Special Formula No. 5 (Katy)
Katy Special Formula No. 7 (Katy)
Katy Special Formula No. 12 (Katy)
Katy Special Formula No. 15 (Katy)
Kelav (Halsom)
Kemithal
Kenital (Kendall)
Kenpectin P (Ormont Drug and Chemical)
Kessobamate (McKesson)
Kessodrate (McKesson)
  250 mg.
  500 mg.
Kessolana Liquid (McKesson)
Kiddikoff (Cord)
Kirkobee (Moore Kirk)
Klort (Lemmon)
Kni-Tal (Knight)
  Tablet 65 mg.
  Tablet 97 mg.
Knised Tablets (Knight)
K-N-S (King) Elixir
K-O Injection Veterinary (A. J. Buck)

Kobac Tablets (Zemmer)
Kodoven (Drug Master)
Kodrene with Codeine (Ads Labs)
Kolana Compound with Codeine (R. Daniels)
Kolana Compound with Codeine (Purepac)
Kolephrin (Pfeiffer)
Koparin with Paregoric (McKesson)
Kopectolin with Paregoric (National Pharm)
KPB with Opium (Cole)
K-Peck with Codeine (Ketchum)
Kraftgesic (Kraft)
Kraftphenamide (Kraft)
Kraftpress (Kraft)
Kraftstat (Kraft)
Kused Capsule (Kremers-Urban)
Kylobee Tablets (Kyle)

Laevobese (Kay)
Laevobese No. 1 (Haberle)
Laevobese No. 2 (Haberle)
Laevobese No. 3 (Haberle)
Larten
Latrodol w/ Phenobarbital (Physicians Products)
Lavabo (Superior)
Lavadex (Jabert)
Lavodrine Chroncaps (Cenci)
Lead and Opium Lotion
Lead and Opium Wash
Lee-Sed (Rucker)
Lemidyne with Codeine Tablets (Lemmon)
Lemo-FP Tablets (Pisgah)
Lemobese Tablets (Pisgah)
Lepetown
Leptagesic (Bowman)
Lestense (Sherry)
Lethol Injection (Pitman-Moore)
Levatrol (Pasadena)
  Capsules 15 mg.
  Tablets 5 mg.
Levo-Ducevim (Bernhoft)
Levo-Trisules (Wilfred)
Linoxsol (S. F. Durst)
Lipogen Trisules (Wilfred)
Lipogen-S Trisules (Wilfred)
Liquid No. 6-AAP (Stuart)
Liquid No. 6-AEG (Wendt-Bristol)
Liquid No. 6-AGM (Wendt-Bristol)
Liquid No. 6-AMT (Davis and Sly)
Liquid No. 6-ANU (Lyons)
Liquid No. 6-BAT (Durst)
Liquital EM. S. and D. N.
List No. 1601 C.T. (Kirkman)

Lixophen (Massengill) Elixir
Lomotil (Searle)
  Liquid
  Tablets
Lora (Wallace)
Lorinal (Arnar-Stone)
Loryl (Kremers-Urban)
Lotusate (Winthrop)
  Caplet 30 mg.
  Caplet 50 mg.
  Caplet 120 mg.
Loubarb (Louisons)
Lowate Tablets (Key)
Lowebarb-CTR (Lowe)
Lull Tablets (Foy)
Lull-S Tablets (Foy)
Lumiflora (Bluffingtons)
Luminal (Winthrop)
  Elixir
  Ovoids 16 mg.
  Ovoids 32 mg.
  Ovoids 100 mg.
Luminal Sodium (Winthrop)
  Powd. Ampul 130 mg.
  Powd. Ampul 320 mg.
Luminal Sodium in Propylene Glycol Injection (Winthrop)
  Soln. Ampul 130 mg.
  Soln. Ampul 160 mg.
  Soln. Ampul 320 mg.
Luxsul Capsules (Luly)
Lycodyne (Wynn Labs)
Lycoral (Fellows)
Lycoral (Fellows-Testagar)
Lyn-TD Capsules (Lynwood)
Lynnbuserp (Lynn)
Lynnkol Tablets (J.W.S. Delavau)
Lynnocell Tablets (Lynn)
Lynnsed (Lynn)
Lynntrims Gradual =47 Release Capsules (Lynn)
Lynntrims with Dextro =1 Tablets (Lynn)
Lynntrims with Dextro =2 Tablets (Lynn)
Lynntrims-High Potency =1 Tablets (Lynn)
Lynntrims-High Potency =2 Tablets (Lynn)
Lynntrims No. 1 Tablets (Lynn)
Lynntrims No. 2 Tablets (Lynn)
Lyn-T.D. Caps No. 1 (Lynwood)
Lytogen (Wilco)

M-A Barb (Medical Arts)
M-Buta (Misemer)
M-Buta L.A. (Misemer)
M-Sed Liquid (Misemer)

M-Tablets (Winning-Peplau)
Mabutone (Reed and Carnrick)
Magnox (Bowman)
Mall-etts No. 1 (Mallard)
Mall-etts No. 2 (Mallard)
Mall-etts No. 3 (Mallard)
Mallo-B (Mallard)
Malobrom Sodium Elixir (Loyes)
Manhattan Special Formula Cough Syrup (Nyal Co.)
Mannecaps (T.D.) (Kenneth A. Manne)
Mannetabs No. 1 (Kenneth A. Manne)
Mannetabs No. 2 (Kenneth A. Manne)
Mannetabs No. 3 (Kenneth A. Manne)
Mantrim (Kenneth A. Manne)
MO Caps (Blaine)
Margane (Northrup)
Margesic Tablets (Teemar)
Marlibar X-L (Lexington)
Marlibar-B Tablets (Lexington)
Marlibar-LA Capsules (Lexington)
Marlibeph (Lexington)
Marpex (North American)
Masobarb No. 1 and 2 (Mason)
Masopent Capsules (Mason)
Mauve (Superior)
Maxefed 2.5 (Noyes)
Maxefed 5 (Noyes)
Mebaral (Winthrop)
  Tablets 1/2 gr.
  Tablets 3/4 gr.
  Tablets 1 1/2 gr.
  Tablets 3 gr.
Mebroin (Winthrop)
Mebusal-C (Ethical Specialties)
Mebutal (Medco)
Medarsed (Medar)
  Elixir
  Tablets 1/4 gr.
  Tablets 1/2 gr.
Medcohist 1/4 gr. (Palmedico)
Medcohist/Codeine
Mediatric Cap Tab, Liq. (Ayerst)
Medi-Barb (Spencer-Mead)
Medicobie Regular Strength No. 1 (Medical Supply)
Medicobie Regular Strength No. 2 (Medical Supply)
Medicobie Regular Strength No. 3 (Medical Supply)
Medinal (Warner)
Medique Anti Pain Pill (Pharmak)
Medique Pain Relief Cappette (Bates Labs)
Medituss with Codeine (Manhattan)

Meditussin Syrup (Palmedico)
Medomin (Geigy)
Melbert's Cough Syrup (Ads Labs)
Melbert's Cough Syrup (Purepac)
Melfiat Unicelles =1 (Hiss)
Melfiat Unicelles =2 (Hiss)
Meneferoid (Physicians Drug Supply)
Meneferoid No. 1 (Physicians Drug Supply)
Meneferoid No. 2 (Garde)
Menobese-T.D. (Remsen)
Mentabal (Walker)
Mepavlon
Mephabarb Elixir (Mayrand)
Mephamosin (Oxford)
Mephelex (Garde)
Mephenamide (Lynn)
Mephenesin w/ Pentobarbital MLT-TD
    (Nysco)
Mephesal (various)
Mephobarb Injection, Veterinary (Kay)
Mephobarbital (various)
    Tablets 1/4 gr.
    Tablets 1/2 gr.
    Tablets 1 1/2 gr.
Mepho-Dex (Rowell)
Mephonyl Tablets (Lynn)
Meposed
Meprin
Meprindon
Meprobamate (various)
    Tablets 200 mg.
    Tablets 400 mg.
Meproban
Meprocompren
Meprocon CMC
Meprol
Meproleaf
Meprolone (M.S. & D.)
Meprosin
Meprospan-200 (Wallace)
Meprospan-400 (Wallace)
Meprotabs (Wallace)
Meprotan
Meptran (Reid-Provident)
Mercodinone Tablets (Merrell)
Mercodol (Merrell)
Mercodol with Decapryn Succinate (Merrell)
Meth-OD Tablets (Trimen)
Methabese (Paramount Surgical Supply)
Metha-Bese (Roder)
Metha-Bese T (Roder)
Methachlor Tablets (Jabert)
Methacil Liquid (Jenkins Labs)
Methaloid (S. J. Tutag)

Methamphetamine Compound (Shaw)
Methaplex Liquid (Caldwell and Bloor)
Metharbital
Methefed (Mid-Atlantic)
Methent-TD (Interstate)
Methio-Bismadene Liquid (Weeks and Leo)
Methitural Sodium
Methobese-T (Paramount)
Methohexital
Methohexital Sodium
Methoserp Tablets (Nysco)
Methostat (J.W.S. Delavau)
Methyprylon
Metrosed (Metro-Med)
    Capsules
    Tablets
Mey-Bese (Meyers)
Meycoff Syrup (P. B. Elder)
Migesic (Thea-Medic)
Milatran Tablets (Milan)
Mill-A-Sed (E. S. Miller)
Miltown (Wallace)
    Ampule 400 mg.
    Tablets 200 mg.
    Tablets 400 mg.
Minabar (Minette)
Minibese Nyscaps (Nysco)
Minispan (Rugby)
Minto-Chlor (Vale)
Minukol (Elder)
Monacet Compound/Codeine
Monacet Compound with Codeine 1/30 gr.
    (Rexall)
Monacet Compound with Codeine 1/4 gr.
    (Rexall)
Monacet Compound with Codeine 1/2 gr.
    (Rexall)
Monacet Compound with Codeine 1 gr.
    (Rexall)
Monodorm
Monsyl (Arcum)
Morbam
Morphus Syrup (Caldwell and Bloor)
Multibarb (Cole)
Multibarb-MLT (Hartford)
Muslax (Cole)
Mylodorm
Myocars Cap. (Phila. Caps. Co.)
Myosin (Caldwell and Bloor)
Myotal Injection, Veterinary (Warren-Teed)
Myothesia Injection, Veterinary (Massengill)
Myrobie =1 (Meyer)
Myrobie =2 (Meyer)
Myrobie =3 (Meyer

Na-Pent Injection (Mayrand)
Nalline (Merck)
   Injection 0.2 mg./cc. Ampule
   Injection 5 mg./cc. Ampule
   Injection Vial 10 cc.
Nalorphine
Nalorphine Hydrobromide
Nap-Tabs (Santa)
Napaphen w/ Chloral Hydrate Syrup (Vitamix)
Napental (Massengill)
Napental Injection, Veterinary (Massengill)
Narkine Syrup (Tilden-Yates)
Nascobarb Ovalets (Mayrand)
Nascobarb-100 (Mayrand)
Naus-A-Tories (Table Rock)
Nebralin Tablets (Dorsey)
Nembu-Donna 1/2 (Abbott)
Nembu-Gesic (Abbott)
Nembu-Serpin (Abbott)
Nembu-Serpin Half Strength (Abbott)
Nembudeine Tablets 1/4 gr. (Abbott)
Nembudeine Tablets 1/2 gr. (Abbott)
Nembudeine Tablets 1 gr. (Abbott)
Nembudeine/Codeine
   Filmtab 1/4
   Filmtab 1/2
   Filmtab 1
Nembutal and Belladonna No. 1 (Abbott)
Nembutal (Abbott) Elixir Gradumet 100 mg.
Nembutal Calcium (Abbott)
Nembutal Sodium (Abbott)
   Capsules 50 mg.
   Capsules 100 mg.
   Suppositories 30 mg.
   Suppositories 60 mg.
   Suppositories 120 mg.
   Suppositories 200 mg.
Neo-Amproid (Remsen)
Neo-Be-Cal (Nysco)
Neo-Codenyl M Liquid (Westerfield)
   Tablets
Neo-Ducevim Tablets (Bernhoft)
Neo-Migrainoid (Moore Kirk)
Neoparbel (Central)
Neo-Pectin (Manhattan)
Neo-Sedaphen (Smith Miller and Patch)
Neo-Slowten (Smith Miller and Patch)
Neo-Tritabs Anphetacomp =1 (Eastern Research)
Neo-Tritabs Anphetacomp =2 (Eastern Research)

Neo-Tritabs Anphetacomp =3 (Eastern Research)
Neobese =1 (Nysco)
Neobese =2 (Nysco)
Neobese =3 (Nysco)
Neocylate/Codeine
Neodyne Tablets (Studebaker)
Neonal (Abbott)
Neotuss-PT (Westerfield)
Neotuss with Codeine (Westerfield)
Neotussin Liquid (Lusher Labs)
Neraval (Schering)
Nervonus
Neulin (Walker)
Neuramate
Neuramin (Evron)
Neurinase (Fougera)
   Solution
   Tablets
Neurobarb
Neuronidia Elixir (Schieffelin)
Neurophen Elixir (Naman)
Neuroval Elixir (Vale)
Neutrased (Mallard)
Nevrotose No. 2 (Vale)
Nevrotose No. 3 (Vale)
New Pen Codeine Liquid (Purepac)
New-Pen Codeine Liquid (Ads Labs)
Ni-Tabs (Bowman)
Nicobalic Tablets (Lynn)
Nicobarb (Modern)
Nicodex Tablets (Stanford)
Nicotal No. 1 (Hart)
Nicotal No. 2 (Hart)
Nicotal-G (Hart)
   Elixir
   Tablets
Nidar (Armour)
Nika Caps (Lemmon)
Nilorex (A.V.P.)
Nilox (Direct)
Nilox-R Cap. (Direct)
Nipirin (Massengill)
Nitensar (Armour)
Nitrobar (McNeil)
Nobese Half Strength (Tilden-Yates)
Nobese Full Strength (Tilden-Yates)
Noctec (Squibb)
   Capsules 250 mg.
   Capsules 500 mg.
   Syrup
Noludar Hoffmann-Laroche

Tablets 50 mg.
Tablets 200 mg.
Noludar 300
Noratuss Syrup (P. B. Elder)
Norexin (Smith-Dorsey)
Nortussin with Codeine (P. B. Elder)
Novacin D.H. Liquid (Bates)
Novahistine-DH (Dow)
Novahistine Expectorant (Dow)
Novatuss (Ketchum)
Nullicof with Codeine (Noyes)
Numal (United Chemical)
Nurocam Tablets (Westerfield)
Nurodol (Buffington)
Nurokardiac Tablets (Rorer)
Nuxaphen (Durst)
Nuxi-Barb (Hazleton)
Nuxogen Tablets (Studebaker)
Nyomin-BA (Elder)

Oasil
O.B. Formula No. 15A (Kalmar)
O.B.L. Lozenges (Len Tag)
O.B. Tablets Purple (Henry Sonnenberg)
Obaloss L-T (Beverly Medical Supply)
O.B. Comp (Henry Schein)
O-B Comp No. 1 (Lustgarten)
O-B Comp No. 2 (Lustgarten)
O-B Comp No. 3 (Lustgarten)
O-B Comp No. 1 Hi-Potency (Lustgarten)
O-B Comp No. 22 Hi-Potency (Lustgarten)
O-B Comp No. 3 Hi-Potency (Lustgarten)
O-B Comp No. 1 Morning-Grey (Henry Schein)
O-B Comp No. 1 Morning-Red (Henry Schein)
O-B Comp No. 1 Hi-Potency, Morning Brown (Henry Schein)
O-B Comp No. 2 Noon-Natural (Henry Schein)
O-B Comp No. 2 Hi-Potency, Noon-Clear (Henry Schein)
O-B Comp No. 3 Evening-Green (Henry Schein)
O-B Comp No. 3 Hi-Potency, Evening Pink (Henry Schein)
O-B13 Tablets (Wolins)
O-B15 Tablets (Wolins)
O-B8 Tablets (Wolins)
O-B-E, Double Strength No. 1 (Kay)
O-B-E, Double Strength No. 2 (Kay)

O-B-E, Double Strength No. 3 (Kay)
OBE =1 E.C. Tablet (Queen City)
OBE = 1 C.T. Tablet (Queen City)
OBE =2 C.T. Tablet (Queen City)
OBE =2 E.C. Tablet (Queen City)
OBE =3 C.T. Green Tablet (Queen City)
OBE =3 E.C. Tablet (Queen City)
Obecaps 15 T.D. (Jabert)
Obecaps-Jrs-7 1/2 (Jabert)
Obecord T.D. (Cord)
Obedex G (Cabell)
O-Bee Capsules (Superior)
Obees (Bryant)
Obelones Tablets (Nejo)
Obe-Lyn (Lynwood)
Obelynn G.R. (Lynn)
Obemak =1 (Jabert)
Obemak =2 (Jabert)
Obemak =3 (Jabert)
Obemak Fortis =1 (Jabert)
Obemak Fortis =2 (Jabert)
Obemak Fortis =3 (Jabert)
Obesa-Mead (Spencer-Mead)
Obesa-Mead T (Spencer-Mead)
Obesavit (S. F. Durst)
Obese Caps S.A. (American Tablet and Capsule)
Obese T.D. (Physicians Supply)
Obesity (Jabert)
Obesity No. 3 (Standex)
Obesity Caps (Garden)
Obesity Comb. No. 1 (Spartan)
Obesity Combination Set =1 (Plymouth)
Obesity Combination Set No. 2 (Spartan)
Obesity Combination Set =2 (Plymouth)
Obesity Comb. No. 3 (Spartan)
Obesity Combination Set =3 (Plymouth)
Obesity Compound (Plymouth)
Obestat (Lemmon)
Obestat TY-Med (Lemmon)
Obestina (Vincent Christina)
Obetabs (Bentex)
Obets-T =5 (F. and S. Surgical)
Obex (Greens)
Obex Half Strength (Greens)
Obex-Tabs =1 Grey (Greens)
Obex-Tabs =2 White (Greens)
Obex-Tabs =3 Pink (Greens)
Obex-Tabs H.P. =1 Grey (Greens)
Obex-Tabs H.P. =2 White (Greens)
Obex-Tabs H.P. =3 Pink (Greens)
Obi-Caps Formula No. 1 (National)

Obi-Caps Formula No. 2 (National)
Obi-Caps Formula No. 3 (National)
Obital (Caldwell and Bloor)
Obital No. 2 (Caldwell and Bloor)
O-B-Len (Len-Tag)
Obozet Capsules (Cenci)
Obrex (Caldwell and Bloor)
O.B.X. (Henry Schein)
Off-Tabs (Kare)
  Nised (Delta)
  Tablets 1/4 gr.
  Tablets 1/2 gr.
  Tablets 1 1/2 gr.
Opasal (P. B. Elder)
Orbital (Organd)
Ori-Hist Capsules (Lafayette)
Orioles Capsules (Lafayette)
Ortal Sodium (Parke-Davis)
Ova-Bese (Harvey)
Oveen (Warren-Teed)
  Green
  Yellow
Ovofen Capsules (Warren-Teed)
Oxabar (Durst)
Oxydessin Tablets (Conal)

P-26,881 Tablets (Standard)
P-27,413 Tablets (Standard)
P-29,649 (Standard)
P-30,231 Capsules (Standard)
P-30,617 (Standard)
P-30,700 (Standard)
P. and B. (Schlicksup) Elixir
P. and H. No. 1 (Halsom)
P. and H. No. 2 (Halsom)
P. and H. No. 1 (Moffet)
P. and H. No. 2 (Moffet)
P.C. Chocolate No. 9-AAQ (Davis and Sly)
P.D.A. Pain Tablets (Morton)
PF 5264 (Superior)
P.F. No. 109 (Table Rock)
P.F. No. 175 (Table Rock)
P.F. No. 364 (Table Rock)
P.F. No. 708 (Table Rock)
P.F. No. 287 Elixir (Winston)
P.F. No. 1103 (Winston)
P.F. No. 1263 (Winston)
Pabazol with Codeine (Rexall)
Pabirin/Codeine
P-A-C Compound/Codeine

  Capsules 32 mg.
  Tablets 16 mg.
  Tablets 32 mg.
  Tablets 65 mg.
P-A-C w/ Cyclopal (Upjohn) Tablets
Pain-Tabs (Tracy)
Painex Tablets (Ketchum)
Palagren (Kendall)
Palagren Liquid (Westerfield)
Palapent (Bristol)
Palgesic (Pan American)
  Capsules
  Tablets
Pambromal (Whittier)
Pamine-PB Drops (Upjohn)
Panbutal (Pan American)
  Capsules
  Elixir
  Tablets
Panediol
Pannuxital (Airhart)
Papaverine HCl (Various)
  Ampoules
  Ampoules
  Powder
  Tablets 32 mg.
  Tablets 65 mg.
  Tablets 97 mg.
  Tablets 195 mg.
Papaverine HCl (Towne Paulsen) TD Capsules
Para Hycodan Tablets (Endo)
Parabarb-3 Capsules (Paramed)
Parabin Tablets (J.W.S. Delavau)
Paradexsets No. 1 (Paramount Surgical Supply)
Paradexsets No. 2 (Paramount Surgical Supply)
Paradol (Medics) Tablets
Parafon/Codeine (McNeil) Tablets
Paral (Fellows) Ampules
Paral Capsules (Fellows-Testagar)
Paraldehyde (various)
  Ampules
  Liquid
Paree Bupec (National Pharm)
Parepectolin (Rorer) Liquid
Paregoric (various)
Pasa-Flora (Indianapolis)
Pascotal List No. 384 (Bowman) Tablets
Pascotal List No. 385 (Bowman) Tablets
Pasibar (Lima) Tablets
Pasijen Tablets (Jenkins)

Passi-Barb (Smith Miller and Patch) Tablets
Passibarbital (C. D. Smith)
Passi-Dyne Tablets (Tri-State)
Passilynn (Lynn)
Passimil (Superior) Tablets
Passiphen (McNeil) Tablets
Passital (Moffet)
Passitilla (Stuart, Elder)
Passobar (Arrow)
Pavadon No. 3 (Coastal)
PB Tablets (Cenci)
PB-30 (Schlicksup)
PBR/12 Capsules (Scott-Allison)
Pecterol with Morphine Syrup (P. J. Noyes)
Pectogoric (Bates Labs)
Pedasol Liquid (E. W. Huen)
Pedestal Capsules (Len Tag)
Pediacof (Winthrop) Syrup
Pedules No. 7 Tabs (Superior)
Pellbarb (Kirkman)
Pell-Sed Tablets (H. A. Pell)
Pembrin (Novocol)
Pembule (Novocol)
Pen Bisma Paregoric (Purepac)
Pen Bisma with Paregoric (Ads Labs)
Pendex Tempo-Kaps (Penn)
Pentacine (Walker)
Pental (Malinkrodt)
    Capsules 49 mg.
    Capsules 97 mg.
Pental (Van Pelt and Brown)
Pentasom Tablets (Archer-Taylor)
    Capsules 50 mg.
    Capsules 100 mg.
Pentobarbital Acid (various)
Pentobarbital Sodium (various)
    Capsules 49 mg.
    Capsules 97 mg.
    Powder
    Tablets 32 mg.
    Tablets 97 mg.
Pentobarbital-Asperin (Davis and Sly)
Pentobarbital-Asperin Capsules (Bush)
Pentobarbital-Asperin Capsules (Tilden-
    Yates)
Pentobarb-Caps (Wesley)
Pentobarbitol (Webb)
Pento-Del (Boyle) Capsules
Pentodyne (Tri-State)
Pentolen Capsules (Len Tag)
Pentolixir (Maceslin)
Pento-Meph Injection (Foy)
Pentoneed Capsules (Hanlon)

Pento-Pheno-Barb (Harvey)
Pentosal Capsules (Normand)
Pentotabs 1 1/2 (Prof. Drug Service)
Pentothal Sodium (Abbott)
    Rectal Susp.
Pepsibarb Tablets (Tilden-Yates)
Pepsin Nux and Pheno (Dalen-Kaemp)
Peralga (Warner-Chilcott)
Perased Liquid (Jenkins Labs)
Percogesic-C (Endo) Tablets
Perequil
Perical D.C. (Cord)
Perichlor (Ives-Cameron)
Peridyne (Queen City)
Perquietil
Pertranquil
Pex with Paregoric (Robert Daniels) Liquid
Phac (Cole) Tablets
Phanodorn (Winthrop)
    Tablets 195 mg.
Pharb Liquid (Cole)
Pharma-Hist Syrup (P. B. Elder)
Pharmatussin with Codeine (P. B. Elder)
Phazyme w/ Phenobarbital (Reed and Carn-
    rick)
Phedracol Liquid (Mallard)
Phedrahist Capsules (Lafayette)
Phelantin (Parke-Davis)
Phenabee Liquid (Veltex)
Phenacetyl/Codeine
Phenadex (Detroit First Aid)
Phenamine C (P. B. Elder)
Phenaphen with Codeine No. 2 (Robins)
    Capsules
Phenaphen with Codeine No. 3 (Robins)
    Capsules
Phenaphen with Codeine No. 4 (Robins)
    Capsules
Phenaserp No. 1 (Bernhoft)
    Tablets No. 2
    Tablets No. 3
Phenatuss (Rondex Labs)
Phenedrine (MacAllister)
Phenergan Expectorant with Codeine
    (Wyeth)
    Troches w/ Codeine
Phenergan VC Expectorant (Wyeth)
Phenital Sodium Capsules (Archer-Taylor)
Pheno-Amus (Bowman)
Phenobane Tablets Veterinary (Syracuse
    Pharmacal)
Phenobarb and Bromide Effervescent (B.W.
    & Co.)

Phenobarbital (various)
Ampules
Capsules 100 mg.
Elixir
Powder
Tablets 8 mg.
Tablets 15 mg.
Tablets 30 mg.
Tablets 65 mg.
Tablets 100 mg.
Tablets
Phenobarbital Calcium
Phenobarbital and Aspirin (Direct)
Phenobarbital and Aspirin (Medical Arts)
Phenobarbital and Belladonna (various)
Tablets
Phenobarbital and Bromides (Medical Arts)
Phenobarbital and Bromides Elixir (Moore Kirk)
Phenobarbital and Bromides Elixir (Philips Roxane)
Phenobarbital and Bromides Elixir (Tilden-Yates)
Phenobarbital and Ephedrine Sulfate (Direct)
Phenobarbital and Hyoscyamus (Zimmers)
Phenobarbital and Hyoscyamus No. 1 (Zimmers)
Phenobarbital and Hyoscyamus 1/4 (Superior)
Phenobarbital and Hyoscyamus 1/2 (Superior)
Phenobarbital 1/4 gr w/ Extract Hyoscyamus 1/8 gr (Queen City)
Phenobarbital 1/4 and P.E. Hyoscyamus 1/4 (Medco)
Phenobarbital and Hyoscyamus Formula No. 2 (Medical Arts)
Phenobarbital 1/4 and Hyoscyamus 1/4 (Caldwell and Bloor)
Phenobarbital-Hyoscyamus Tablets (Westerfield)
Phenobarbital Hyoscyamus Comp. P.F. No. 1576 (Maceslin)
Phenobarbital and Passiflora Compound (Blaine)
Phenobarbital Hyoscyamus and Passiflora (Briar)
Phenobarbital Hyoscyamus and Passiflora Comp. (Med. Arts)
Phenobarbital w/ Sodium Bromide Elixir (Zemmer)
Phenobarbital, Sodium Citrate, Potassium Iodide (Blaine)

Phenobarbital Sodium (various)
Ampules
Powder
Phenobarbital Sodium in Propylene Glycol (Endo, Rorer)
Phenobarbital Stronger Elixir (Sutliff and Case)
Phenobarbitol (Webb)
Pheno-Bell Tablets (Starr)
Phenobella (Ferndale) Tablets
Pheno-Bepadol (Ives)
Pheno-Brom (St. Louis)
Phen-O-Brom (Tri-State)
Phenobrom (Schuemann)
Phenobromal (Amco)
Phenobromide (Central)
Pheno-Bromide (Halsom)
Phenobromidine Elixir (Tilden-Yates)
Phenocaps (Jabert)
Phenocaps Fortis (Jabert)
Phenocyamus (Cole)
Pheno-Dex Capsules (S. J. Tutag)
Phenodonna No. 2 (Modern)
Phenodyne with Codeine No. 2 (Blue Line)
Phenodyne with Codeine No. 3 (Blue Line)
Phenoflora (Philips Roxane) Tablets
Pheno-Nux (Vale)
Pheno-Nux and Pepsin (Wesley)
Phenosate Elixir (Bryant)
Phenosedophen Tablets (Studebaker)
Phenotropine (Moffet)
Phenoturic (Ethical)
Phenroid Capsules = 1 T.D. (Starr)
Phensal/Codeine
Phenylhist (Drug Master)
Phenylin Liquid (Life)
Phetabar (Moore Kirk)
Phetabarb Delacaps (Sig)
Phetamide (Moffet)
Phob (Brewer)
Phy-Somol (Physicians Supply)
Pine Tar with Codeine (Robinson Labs)
Pink Obesity No. 3 (Byrne)
Placidyl (Abbott)
Capsules 100 mg.
Capsules 200 mg.
Capsules 500 mg.
Capsules 750 mg.
Plexamine Liquid (Naman)
PMP (Schlicksup)
Capsules
Expectorant
Syrup
Tablets, Chewable

Tablets, Compound
Tablets, Jr.
Poly Barb Capsules (Arnell)
Polycodilene (Hance)
Polygesic (Arnar-Stone)
Pomadex (Standex)
Pomadex-15 (Standex)
Pomatran (Standex)
Potocal Syrup (Zemmer)
Pre-OB Tablets (Rasman)
Pre-Tense Tab. (Phila. Caps. Co.)
Prednal Tablets (Nysco)
Prelital (PRL)
Preslyn (Wynn Labs)
Private Formula Liquid No. 6-AZJ (C&B) (C.M. Bundy)
Private Formula Liquid No. 6-BFG Jenkins (Bundy)
Private Formula Liquid No. 6-BHG (Horton) (C.M. Bundy)
Private Formula 1 DGG (Jenkins)
Private Formula 1 CJV (Medical Arts Pharmacy)
Private Formula H.S. Capsules Blue-Yellow No. 2 ACU (Wendt-Bristol)
Private Formula H.S. Capsule Clear No. 2 AKF (Hiss)
Private Formula H.S. Capsule Red/Clr No. 2-ANT (Cornersburg)
Private Formula H.S. Capsule Red Clear No. 2-ANL (C.A. Mell)
Private Formula H.S. Capsule Yellow-Blue No. 2-AOT (Corners)
Private Formula Liquid 6-ADW (W.B.) (C.M. Bundy)
Private Formula Liquid 6-AXN (C.M. Bundy Co.)
Private Formula No. 1-BEQ (Heyl Physician Supply)
Private Formula No. 1-BOH Tablets (W.B.) (C.M. Bundy)
Private Formula No. 1 BRH (Lyons Physician Supply)
Private Formula No. 1-BUL Tablets (D&S) (C.M. Bundy)
Private Formula No. 1-CMD Tablets (Raymers) (C.M. Bundy)
Private Formula No. 1-DET (Harvey)
Private Formula No. 1-DFP Jenkins (Bundy)
Private Formula No. 1-DGZ (Caldwell and Bloor)
Private Formula No. 1-DHO (Maceslin)
Private Formula No. 1-DIO (Jenkins)
Private Formula No. 1-DJL (Schlick)

Private Formula No. 1-DJT Tablets (Jenkins)
Private Formula No. 1-DLG Tab. (C.M. Bundy) (Dr. John Kraai)
Private Formula No. 1-DNC (Lynwood)
Private Formula No. 1-13425 Tablets (S.J.) (C.M. Bundy)
Private Formula No. 1-14555 Tablets (C&B) (C.M. Bundy)
Private Formula No. 1-14979 Tablets (C&B) (C.M. Bundy)
Private Formula No. 2-AIN Bellevue (Bundy)
Private Formula No. 2-AKB Tablets (Lampert) (C.M. Bundy)
Private Formula No. 2-APM Caps. (Cornersburg Pharmacy)
Private Formula No. 2-AQB Tablets (C&B) (C.M. Bundy)
Private Formula No. 3 AEL (Lyons Physician Supply)
Private Formula No. 3-AGT Tab. (Boericke and Tafel)
Private Formula No. 3-BCN (Jenkins)
Private Formula No. 3-BCT Tablets (Jenkins) (C.M. Bundy)
Private Formula No. 3-BDQ (Lafayette)
Private Formula No. 3-BDW Tab. (Lynwood)
Private Formula No. 3-BDY Tab. (Jenkins)
Private Formula No. 3-BEM Tablets (Hobson) (C.M. Bundy)
Private Formula No. 6-AXN Liquid (C.M. Bundy)
Private Formula No. 7-BFM (Syrup Sedacel) (Jenkins)
Private Formula No. 163 (Table Rock)
Private Formula No. 1432, C.T. Blue (Table Rock)
Private Formula No. 1433 Tablets (Superior)
Private Formula No. 1533 (Table Rock)
Private Formula No. 1775 Cap. (Table Rock)
Private Formula No. 1777 Cap. (Table Rock) (Bell Pharmacal)
Private Formula No. 22397 Dover (Elder)
Private Formula No. 222 Liquid (W.B. Boyer)
Private Formula No. 4220 Tablets (Superior)
Private Formula No. 4226 Tablets (Superior)
Private Formula No. 4263 Tablets (Superior)

Private Formula No. 4329 Tablets (Superior)
Private Formula No. 4330 Tablets (Superior)
Private Formula No. 4399 Tablets (Superior)
Private Formula No. 4420 Tablets (Superior)
Private Formula No. 4484 Tablets (Superior)
Private Formula No. 4493 Tablets (Superior)
Private Formula No. 4499 Tablets (Superior)
Private Formula No. 4727 Tablets (Superior)
Private Formula No. 4970 Tablets (Superior)
Private Formula No. 4993 Tablets (Superior)
Private Formula No. 4995 Tablets (Superior)
Private Formula No. 5388 (Superior)
Private Formula No. 5425 (Superior)
Private Formula No. 8997 (First Texas)
Private Formula No. 9-AAD Tablets (Harvey) (C.M. Bundy)
Private Formula No. 9-AAM (Jenkins)
Private Formula No. 910 Tablets (Superior)
Private Formula No. 1992 Tablets (Superior)
Private Formula No. 2-AOE Tablets (Jenkins) (C.M. Bundy)
Private Formula No. 4832 Tablets (Superior)
Private Formula S.C. Green No. 3-AQL (Davis and Sly)
Private Formula S.C. Green No. 3 AXE (Caldwell and Bloor)
Private Formula S.C. Orange No. 3-BBO (Schlick)
Private Formula Tablets 1-DOD (Hobson) (C.M. Bundy Co.)
Probamin
Probamyl
Probar (Allan)
Probarbital
Probarbital Calcium
Probarbital Sodium
Probate
Procalmidol
Prodyne No. 3 with 1/2 gr. Codeine (Strong Cobb Arner)

Profundal
Promate (Truett)
Promethazine VC with Codeine Liquid (National Pharm)
Promethazine with Codeine Liquid (National Pharm)
Prominal
Propallylonal
Prophen Expectorant (Drug Master)
Prophen No. 37 (Drug Master)
Prophen No. 76 (Drug Master)
Proponal
Prorenata Tablets (Palmedico)
Prorenata Tabs with 1 gr. Codeine (Palmedico)
Protran
Proval No. 3 (various)
Prozine (Wyeth)
  Capsules, Half Strength
  Capsules
Prunatol (First Texas)
Prunicodeine (Lilly)
P.T.Z. (various)
Pulsabarb (Physicians Supply)
Pulsaphen List No. 113 and 114 (Wesley)
Pulsobarb (Dalen-Kaemp)
P-V-Tussin Syrup (Reid-Provident)
Pyne-Tarco with Codeine (Robinson Labs)
Pyra-Phed Syrup (various)
Pyracal and Codeine (Vita Fore)
Pyracodeine RX No. 22950 Liquid (P. B. Elder)
Pyradeine Liquid (Life)
Pyrahist Jr. with Codeine (R. Daniels)
Pyramid (Barre)
Pyranel Capsules (Burrough Bros.)
Pyratuss and Codeine (Vita Fore)
Pyrihist with Codeine (R. Daniels)
Pyriladex (Caldwell and Bloor)
Pyrroxate/Codeine (Upjohn)

Q Caps (Testagar) Capsules
Quabese T.D. (Quaker City)
Quabese H.P., T.D. (Quaker City)
Quacharbell (Quaker City)
Quad Histamine (Lynwood)
Quad-Set Tablets (Kenyon)
Quadra-Bar Tablets (Columbus)
Quadra-Barb (Moffet)
Quadra-Sed (Smith Miller and Patch) Liquid
Quadsed Capsules (Lynn)
Quahistasin Capsules (J.W.S. Delavau)
Quakerdex Capsules (Quaker City)

Quaname
Quanil
Quartal Tablets (Tully)
Quasedate (Quaker City)
Quasin Capsules (J.W.S. Delavau)
Quasin Jr. Tablets (J.W.S. Delavau)
Queen-Caps T.D. (Wolins)
Qui-A-Zone (Walker) Tablets
Quiebar (Nevin)
  Elixir
  Spantabs
  Tablets
  AC-Capsules
Quiedrate Capsules (Luly)
Quiess (Durst) Tablets
Quietuss AC (Rondex Labs)
Quilate
Quintal (Penn) Elixir

R-3 Gray (Winning-Peplau)
R-3 Pink (Winning-Peplau)
R-3 Yellow (Winning-Peplau)
Rac Cough Syrup (Plymouth)
Raldrate Syrup (Jones and Vaughan)
Ram-B-Phen (Northwest)
Ratiodrine (Metro-Med) Tablets
Raudilan-PB Tablets (Lannett)
Rectal Ointment (Hance)
Rectodyne Ointment (Massengill Co.)
  Suppository
Rectules (Fellows) Suppos.
  Ten-Grain
  Twelve-Grain
Redcomp, Half Strength (Interstate Drug
  Exchange)
Redex-Caps (Tri-State)
Redexcel (Central)
Redocomp, Full Strength (Interstate Drug
  Exchange)
Reducap (Morton)
Reducaps (Werner)
Reducer 5 mg. No. 1 Gray (C.M. Bundy)
Reducer 5 mg. No. 2 White (C.M. Bundy)
Reducer 5 mg. No. 3 Pink (C.M. Bundy)
Reducer 10 mg. No. 2 White (C.M. Bundy)
Reducer 10 mg. No. 3 Pink (C.M. Bundy)
Reducets No. 1 (Virtal)
Reducets No. 2 (Virtal)
Reducets No. 3 (Virtal)
Reducincaps T.D. (Spartan)
Reducing-Caps, No. 1 (Davis-Edwards)
Reducing-Caps, No. 2 (Davis-Edwards)
Reducing-Caps, No. 3 Pink (Davis-Edwards)

Reducing Tabs 5 mg. No. 1 Grey (Davis-
  Edwards)
Reducing Tabs 5 mg. No. 2 White (Davis-
  Edwards)
Reducing Tabs 5 mg. No. 3 Pink (Davis-
  Edwards)
Reducing Tabs 10 mg. No. 1 (Davis-
  Edwards)
Reducing Tabs 10 mg. No. 1 Grey (Davis-
  Edwards)
Reducing Tabs 10 mg. No. 1 Red (Davis-
  Edwards)
Reducing Tabs 10 mg. No. 1 White (Davis-
  Edwards
Reducing Tabs 10 mg. No. 2 White (Davis-
  Edwards)
Reducing Tabs 10 mg. No. 2 (Davis-
  Edwards)
Reducing Tabs 10 mg. No. 3 (Davis-
  Edwards)
Reducing Tabs 10 mg. No. 3 Pink (Davis-
  Edwards)
Reducing Tabs 15 mg. No. 1 White (Davis-
  Edwards)
Reducing Tabs 15 mg. No. 1 Red (Davis-
  Edwards)
Reducing Tabs 15 mg. No. 2 Gray (Davis-
  Edwards)
Reducing Tablets No. 1, Regular Strength
  (Classic)
Reducing Tablets No. 2, Regular Strength
  (Classic)
Reducing Tablets No. 3, Regular Strength
  (Classic)
Reducing Tablet with Phenobarbital
  (Bucher Clinic)
Reducotabs No. 1 Regular-Gray (Philadel-
  phia)
Reducotabs No. 2 Regular-Natural
  (Philadelphia)
Reducotabs No. 3 Regular-Pink (Philadel-
  phia)
Reducotabs No. 1 Hi-Potency-Gray
  (Philadelphia)
Reducotabs No. 2 Hi-Potency-Natural
  (Philadelphia)
Reducotabs No. 3 Hi-Potency-Pink
  (Philadelphia)
Redutab (Morton)
Redutabs No. 1 (Allan)
Redutabs No. 2 (Allan)
Redutabs No. 3 (Allan)
Regumen (U.S. Ethicals)

Relaxan (Pitman-Moore)
Relaxinal (Success Chemical)
Releas-Obese (Vanguard)
Release Tabs T.D. (M.W. Fisher)
Release Tabs H T.D. (M.W. Fisher)
Reme (Caldwell and Bloor)
Renbu Tablets (Wren)
Reniphen (Winston) Tablets
Reniphen No. 2 (Winston) Tabs
Reostral
Reoxyn Injection (Pasadena)
Reposans (Physicians Prod.)
Resedex (Cenci)
Reserbutal (Lustgarten)
Reserbutal No. 2 (Lustgarten)
Reserpal (Garde)
Reserpine and Phenobarbital (Direct)
Reserpine w/ Mebaral (Winthrop) Tablets
Reserpodex Tablets (Teemar)
Resitab 1/2 (Arnell)
Resital Elixir (Arnell)
Respazem (Zemmer) Tablet
    Tablet No. 2
Respi-Sed (Conal)
Respi-Sed (Linden)
Restenil
Restinal Tablets (Sanford)
Restophen Tablets (Noyes)
Restophen Half-Strength (Noyes)
Resydess Tablets (Conal)
Retabs Tablets (Caldwell and Bloor)
Reycodel (Reyman) Tablets
Rhiningesic/Codeine
Rhinodex Tablets (Stanford)
Rid-A-Pain Tablets (Pfeiffer)
Ridupois Improved Tablets (Elder)
Robahist (Ruby)
Robamate (Robinson)
    Tablets 200 mg.
    Tablets 400 mg.
Robarb Tab. (Rocky Mt. Pharmacal)
    Tablets 16 mg.
    Tablets 32 mg.
    Tablets 65 mg.
Robillana with Dionin (Robinson Lab)
Robitussin A-C (Robins) Syrup
Rochlorate Capsules (Robinson)
Ro-Dex (Rowell)
Rola Methazine Expectorant with Codeine
    (Robinson Labs)
Ro-Thin =1 (Robinson)
Ro-Thin =2 (Robinson)
Ro-Thin =3 (Robinson)
Rotran (Rocky Mountain) Tabs

Rotrim (Rocky Mountain)
Rotrim =2 (Rocky Mountain)
Roxyn (Rocky Mountain) Tabs
R-S-Tabs (Kare)
Rubarsin (Rupp and Bowman)
Ruck-Sed (Rucker) Liquid
    Tablets
Ru-Tuss (E. W. Huen)
RX 800 (Kirkman)
RX 861 (Kirkman)
RX 871 (Kirkman)
RX 875 (Kirkman)
RX 975 (Kirkman)
RX 4088 (Zemmer)
RX No. 822 (Kirkman)
RX No. 988 (Kirkman)
RX No. 989 (Kirkman)
RX No. 4148 (Zemmer)
RX No. 4156 (Zemmer)
RX No. 4176 (Zemmer)
RYD C Liquid (R. Daniels)
RYD-C Liquid (Ormont)

S. No. 5 Tablets (Starr)
S.B.P. (Lemmon) Tablets
S.C. Blue No. 3-AXF (Harvey)
S.C. Blue No. 3-BAF (Durst)
S.C. Cream No. 3-AJP (Fox)
S.C. Gray No. 3-APY (Davis and Sly)
S.C. Gray No. 3-ATC (Caldwell and Bloor)
S.C. Green No. 3-AVR (Raymer)
S.C. Green No. 3-AYL (J. Allan Shaw)
S.C. Green No. 3-14826 (Caldwell and
    Bloor)
S.C. Lavender No. 3-BBH (Maceslin)
S.C. Pink (Caldwell and Bloor)
S.C. Pink No. 3-AVJ (Raymer)
S.C. Pink No. 3-13310 (Scheumann)
S.C. Purple No. 3-ATG (Sherwood)
S.C. Purple No. 3-AXV (Caldwell and Bloor)
S.C. Red No. 3-AXO (Lampert)
S.C. Red No. 3-AYE (Durst)
S.C. T. Passitilla Yellow (Stuart)
S.C. Violet No. 3-AZW (Caldwell and Bloor)
S.C. White No. 3-ASB (Physicians Supply)
S-F-D-1 (Riders)
S-H-Tabs Tablets (Southern States Phar-
    macal)
So-Mel
S-T Forte Syrup (Scott-Tussin)
S-T-Barb (Scott-Tussin) Capsules T.D.
S-T-Desex-15 (Scott-Tussin) Capsules T.D.
S-T-Pephedex (Scott-Tussin) Capsules T.D.

S-T-Secobarb (Scott-Tussin) Capsules T.D.
Sal-Codeia Bell (Hollings-Smith)
   Tablets
Sal-Meph Improved (Fisher)
Saladex (Wesley)
Salatin Tablets 1/4 gr. (Ferndale)
Salatin Tablets 1/2 gr.
Sali-Dex Tabs (United Research)
Sali-Dex (Lustgarten)
Salimeph-C w/ Codeine 1/8 gr. Tablets
   (Kremers-Urban)
Salipral (Kenyon)
Salipral (Lustgarten)
Salipral (Wynn)
Salisil w/ Phenobarbital (Elder)
Salitrin (James S. Airhart)
Salol and Bismuth Compound (Vale)
Sandoptal (Sandoz)
Santalgesic Tablets (Santa)
Santaminic Syrup (Santa)
Schlickative (Schlicksup)
Schlickinol 100 Capsules (Schlicksup)
Scophenesin (Nelson-Boyer)
Seal-Tabs T.D. 15 (Jabert)
Sebadar Tablets (Klug)
Sebephen (Haag)
Sebutal (Tilden-Yates)
Sec-Am-Bital Capsules (Columbia)
   Capsules 1 1/2 gr.
   Capsules 3 gr.
Secamine Stankaps (Standex)
Secolen Capsules (Len Tag)
Secolynn Sodium Capsules (Lynn)
Seco-Perles (Caldwell and Bloor)
Seco-Pro 1 1/2 (Prof. Drug Service)
Seco-8 R Cap. (Fleming)
Secobar Capsules (Naman)
Secobarbital
Secobarbital Elixir (Lannett)
Secobarbital Capsules (H.L. Moore) 97 mg.
Secobarbital Sodium Powder
   Capsules 49 mg.
   Capsules 97 mg.
   Elixir
   Inj. 50 mg./cc.
   Sterile Powder 100 mg.
Secocaps (Hiss)
Secodrin (Premo) Tablets
Secodrin Encore (Hart)
Secomob Capsules (Allen)
Seconal (Lilly) Elixir
Seconal Sodium (Lilly)
   Ampules 0.25 gm.
   Ampules 50 mg./cc.

   Enseals 97 mg.
   Inj. 50 mg./cc.
   Inj. 100 mg./2 cc.
   Powder
   Pulvules 32 mg.
   Pulvules 49 mg.
   Pulvules 97 mg.
   Suppos. 32 mg.
   Suppos. 65 mg.
   Suppos. 130 mg.
   Suppos. 195 mg.
Seconeed Capsules (Hanlon)
Seconesin (Crookes-Barnes)
Secotress (Wampole)
Sectal (St. Louis)
Sectal Capsules (United)
Sed-A-Nat (National) Tablets
Sed-A-Ped Liquid (Steven)
Sed-A-Plex Tablets (Austin)
Sed-O-Et (Drug Products) Tablets
Seda-Bute (Cole)
Seda-Symtol Temsules (Veltex)
   No. 1
   No. 2
Sedabamate Tablets (Mallard)
Sedabarb No. 2 Tablets (Tilden-Yates)
Sedacaps (Dumas-Wilson)
Sedacil (Maceslin)
Sedades (Marin Medical Supply)
Sedadrops (Walker)
Sedafax (Eastern Research)
Sedaflora (Philips Roxane) Tablets
Sedagesic (Kay) Tablets
Sedalgesic Inserts (Table Rock)
Sedalixir (Walker)
Sedalones Tablets (Nejo)
Sedalyn (Lynwood)
Sedamine (Boody)
Sedamine-1 (Modern)
Sedamorph (J.W.S. Delavau)
Sedapav (Moore Kirk) Tablets
Sedaphen (Smith Miller and Patch) Liquid
Sedaplex (Walker)
Sedapro-TD (Prof. Drug Service)
Sedaserp (Dooner) Tablets
Sedaserpin (Oxford)
Sedatal (Medco)
Sedatal Cap. (Caldwell and Bloor)
Sedative Compound with Codeine Liquid
   (National Pharm)
Sedative No. 1 (Lampert)
Sedative No. 2164 (Borneman)
Sedative No. 6 (Philips Roxane)

Sedative with Codeine (National Pharm)
Sedavin (Wendt-Bristol)
Sedavol (Wendt-Bristol)
Sedazil
Sedelixir (Maceslin)
Sedeval
Sedex (Nysco)
Sedex Nyscaps (Cumberland)
Sedinyl (Smith Miller and Patch)
Sedital (Halsom)
Sedital (United Research)
Sedital Tablets (Wolins)
Sedital Tablets No. 4614 (Richlyn)
Sednotic
Sedo-Bee Tablets (Southern)
Sedobarb (Whittier)
    Tablet No. 1
    Tablet No. 2
Sedogel (Medical Arts)
Sedoral Liquid (Mallard)
Sedotane (Wendt-Bristol)
Sedoval Tablets (Westerfield)
Sedovas (Massengill)
Sedpane (Freeport)
Sendex Delay-Caps (American)
Senodin Syrup (Squibb)
Senostim Liquid and Tablets (Lynn)
Ser-Doma (Haag) Tablets
Serbuta (Freeport)
Seril
Sernyl (Parke-Davis)
Sernylan (Parke-Davis)
Serpabarb Tablets (Misemer)
Serp-Ex-5 Tablets (Scott-Tussin)
Sertal (Medical Arts)
Sertec-M Tablets (Arnell)
Sertec-M w/Codeine Capsules (Arnell)
Setaflem (Rupp and Bowman)
Setared (Rupp and Bowman)
Setran
Sevital (Academy)
Sevocol (Wendt-Bristol)
Sherobese (Sherry)
Sherry-Bese (Sherry)
Silano with Dionin (Ads Labs) (Purepac)
Silbar (Haack) Tablets
Sima Capsules (Superior)
Sima Dult Tablets (Superior)
Sima Pediatric Tablets (Superior)
Sinexen Timekaps (Caldwell and Bloor)
Sinotuss and Codeine (Vita Fore)
Sinutabs/Codeine (Warner-Chilcott)
    Tablets

Sistol Elixir (Studebaker)
    Tablets
Slentab No. 1 (Moore Kirk)
Slentab No. 2 (Moore Kirk)
Slentab No. 3 (Moore Kirk)
Slimzen Forte (Zemmer)
Slim T.D. (W. F. Baker)
Slim-Tabs No. 1 Morning Gray (Wesley)
Slim-Tabs No. 1 Hi-Potency Morning Gray
    (Wesley)
Slim-Tabs No. 2 Noon Natural (Wesley)
Slim-Tabs No. 2 Hi-Potency Noon White
    (Wesley)
Slim-Tabs No. 3 Evening-Pink (Wesley)
Slim-Tabs No. 3 Hi-Potency Evening-Pink
    (Wesley)
Slimetts (Wesley)
Slim-Zem =1 (Zemmer)
Slim-Zem =2 (Zemmer)
Slim-Zem =3 (Zemmer)
Socumb Injection, Veterinary (Syracuse
    Pharmacal)
Sodacitrol/Codeine Liquid (Davis and Sly)
Sodital (Arnar-Stone)
Sodium Phenobarbital w/Sodium Bromide
    Soln. (Durst)
Soduben (Arcum) Elixir
    Tablets
Solfo-Serpine (Poythress)
    Capsules
    Tablets
Solfoton (Poythress)
    Capsules
    Tablets
Solfoton S/C (Polythress)Tablet
Solsed (Jackson-Mitchell)
Solu-Barb (Fellows Testagar)
    Tablets
    Pediatric Tablet.
Soma Compound with Codeine (Wallace)
    Tablets
Somatal (Person and Covey)
Sombitol (Wesley) Liquid
Sombrul (Columbus)
Sombucaps (Riker)
Sombulex (Riker) Tablets
Sominal-Phenobarb (Davis and Sly)
Sominol Phenobarbital (Tilden-Yates)
Sominal-PB (Flint-Eaton)
Somlethal Injection Veterinary (Syracuse
    Pharmacal)
Somlyn Tablets (Davis and Sly)
Somlyn-Phenobarbital (Davis and Sly) Tab-

lets
Somnalar Tablets (Lardon)
Somnalert (Warren-Teed)
Somnesin Injection, Veterinary (Central)
Somni-Sed (Tutag)
Somnofen Parenteral (Wesley)
Somnopentyl (Pitman-Moore)
Somnos (M S & D)
  Capsule 500 mg.
  Elixir
Somonal Capsules (Croyden-Browne)
Somorsed (Philips Roxane)
  Capsules
Somtrol (Philips Roxane)
Sonazar (Tutag) Tablets
Sondrate Elixir (Kenyon)
Sonnenberg Oblets (Sonnenberg)
Sopena-MRT (Thompson)
Sopento (St. Louis)
Sp. Cough Syrup for Keese Chem. (Strong Cobb.Arner)
Spa (Darby)
Spabelin No. 2 (Arcum) Tablets
Spancap No. 3 (North American)
Spancab No. 3, Half Strength (North American
Spantab No. 3 (North American)
Spasmal (Franklin)
Spasmanol (Bluffingtons) Tablets
Spas-Meth-Barb (American Tablet and Capsule)
Spasmosed (Lustgarten)
Spasmosed (Zimmers)
S.P.C. (P. J. Noyes)
SPC with Codeine (Bates)
SPC with Codeine (R. Daniels)
SPC with Codeine Tablets (Ketchum)
SPC with Codeine Tablets (Standard)
SPC/Codeine (Linden Labs)
  16 mg.
  32 mg.
Special Formula Amogel (Bates Labs)
Special Formula 711 Tab (Detroit First Aid)
Special Formula C.S. (Manhattan)
Special Formula Capsules (Hasley)
Special Formula L-77 (Lentag)
Special Formula L-88 (Lentag)
Special Formula No. 1 (Table Rock)
Special Formula = 3 (Davis-Edwards)
Special Formula No. 20 (Drug Master)
Special Formula No. 25 (Drug Master)
Special Formula No. 32 (Drug Master)
Special Formula No. 33 (Drug Master)

Special Formula No. 53 (Penn State)
Special Formula No. 58 (Drug Master)
Special Formula No. 59 (Drug Master)
Special Formula No. 63 (Drug Master)
Special Formula No. 64 Tabs (Drug Master)
Special Formula No. 109 (U.S. Hospital Supply)
Special Formula =203 (Davis-Edwards)
Special Formula No. 1228 (Table Rock)
Special Formula No. 1248 (Archer-Taylor)
Special Formula No. 1313 (Vale)
Special Formula No. 1381 (Archer-Taylor)
Special Formula No. 1392 (Archer-Taylor)
Special Formula No. 1432 (Archer-Taylor)
Special Formula No. 1449 (Archer-Taylor)
Special Formula No. 1805 1-BJV (Wendt-Bristol)
Special Formula No. 4283 (Ferndale)
Special Formula No. 17750 (Upjohn)
Special Formula No. T-60 (Schlicksup)
Special Formula Rx T-211 (Schlicksup)
Special Formula 1-BRV (Blaine)
Special Formula Verdahist Expectorant (Bates)
Special Formula White No. 1 (Supreme)
Special Formula Grey No. 2 (Supreme)
Special Formula Pink No. 3 (Supreme)
Special Nonau F (Wendt-Bristol)
Special Obesity Formula No. 3 (Garden)
Special Obesity Capsule No. 401 (Rugby)
Special Obesity Capsules No. 441 (Rugby)
Special Obesity Capsules No. 451 (Rugby)
Special Obesity Capsules No. 501 (Rugby)
Special Obesity Capsules No. 551 (Rugby)
Special Obesity Formula =40 (Paramount Surgical Supply)
Special Obesity Formula =44 (Paramount Surgical Supply)
Special Obesity Formula =45 (Paramount Surgical Supply)
Special Obesity Formula =50 (Paramount Surgical Supply)
Special Obesity Formula =55 (Paramount Surgical Supply)
Special Reducing Formula Caps (Wayne)
Special RX (Davis and Sly)
Special RX 2247 (Spabelin No. 2) (APC, Arcum)
Special RX 2295 (APC, McKesson)
Special RX No. 6389 (Moore Kirk)
Special RX No. 10305 (Dr. McCrea)
Special RX No. 10313 (Dr. Keller) (Bowman)
Special RX No. 22458 (Elder)

Standex Forte (Standex)
Stannitol No. 3 (Standex)
Stato (Cumberland)
Stental (Robins) Extentabs
Stokes Expectorant (various)
Sulfonal
Sulfondiethylmethane
Sulfonethylmethane
Sulfonmethane
Su-Tuss (Lusher)
Su-Tuss Liquid (Superior)
Sulphet Tab. (Kay Pharmacy)
Sulphet-AB Ovules No. 3 (Vita Elixir)
Sunchol Tablets (P. J. Noyes)
Sureno Capsules (Superior)
Surital Sodium (Parke-Davis)
Sybotan (Massengill) Tablets
Synacetyl (Airhart)
Synalgos-DC Capsules (Ives)
Synorex (Schilling)
Syrajen Liquid (Jenkins)
Syrcodate (Blue Line) Syrup
Syrcohist (Blue Line)
   Expect.
   Syrup
Syridyl AF Liquid (Southern Drug)
Syrtane Jr. C.S. (Vitarine)
Syrup Cheround with Codeine (Superior)

T-23 (Bell
T-32 (Bell)
T-33 (Bell)
T-35 (Bell)
T-36 (Bell)
T-37 (Bell)
T-38 (Bell)
T-40 (Bell)
T-41 (Bell)
T-45 (Bell)
T-50 (Bell)
T-55 (Bell)
T-101 (Bell)
T-110 (Bell)
T-115 (Bell)
T 126 (George N. Bell)
T 130 (George N. Bell)
T 132 (George N. Bell)
T 140 (George N. Bell)
T-332 (St. Louis)
T-829 (Bush)
T-A Tabs No. 1 (Bush)
T-A Tabs No. 2 (St. Louis Physicians Supply)

T-A Tabs No. 3 (St. Louis Physicians Supply)
Tablet No. 1-BKK (Caldwell and Bloor)
Tablet No. 1-BND (Caldwell and Bloor)
Tablet No. 1-BRI (Lyons)
Tablet No. 1-BRQ (Davis and Sly)
Tablet No. 1-BVO (Davis and Sly)
Tablet No. 1-BZC (Caldwell and Bloor)
Tablet No. 1-13450 (Davis and Sly)
Tablet No. 3-AGC (Heyl)
Tablet No. 3-AJA (Sherwood)
Tablet No. 3-ASJ (Davis and Sly)
Tablet No. 3-ASK (Davis and Sly)
Tablet No. 312717 (Lyons)
Tablet No. 4-AIH (Caldwell and Bloor)
Tablet No. 4-AJE (Schuemann-Jones)
Tabs No. 1 (Caldwell and Bloor)
Tabs No. 2 (Caldwell and Bloor)
Tabs No. 3 (Caldwell and Bloor)
Tad-Caps (Kare)
Taf/Tabs-T T.D. (Federal)
Tanorex (Laser)
T.D. Capsules 10 (St. Louis)
T.D. Capsules 15 (St. Louis)
T.D. Caps 15-3 (Detroit Pharmacal)
T.D. Capsules 15-100 (Bush)
T.D. Green and White Thyroid Compound
   (Shaw)
T.H. Capsules (Saron)
T.M. 10 and 15 (TMCO)
T.M. 10-60 (TMCO)
T.M. 10-60 Capsules Special (TMCO)
T.M. 15-100 (TMCO)
T.M. 15-100 Capsules Special (TMCO)
T.V.D. Formula (Adams)
T-Barb (Tennessee)
T-D Capsules A (Wendt-Bristol)
T-D-Caps O (Wendt-Bristol)
Takabarb No. 1 (Cenci)
Takabarb No. 2 (Cenci)
T-D Capsules 10 (Wendt-Bristol)
T-D Capsules 15 (Wendt-Bristol)
T-O-W Tablets (Kenyon)
Talalf Tablets (Tully)
Talamo (Merrell)
Talesco (Merrell)
Tamate
Talpento (Merrell)
Talpheno (Merrell)
   Inject.
   Elixir
   Tablets 15 mg.
   Tablets 30 mg.

Tablets 100 mg.
Tangene Cough Syrup (Na-Spra)
Tatol Tablets (Craig)
Taxite Capsules (Lancer)
Tecodan
Tee-Dees Capsules (Pasadena)
Tee-Dees w/ Amobarbital (Pasadena)
Teedex-LC Capsules (Teemar)
Teedexal Tablets (Teemar)
Teek Cough Syrup with Codeine (Norwich)
Teen Caps 15 mg. (Rugby)
Teen Tabs 10 mg. (Rugby)
Teen Tabs =1 (Darby)
Teen Tabs 10 mg. No. 2 White (Darby)
Teen Tabs = 2 15 mg. (Darby)
Teen Tabs =2 (Darby)
Teen Tabs 10 mg. No. 3 Pink (Rugby)
Teen Tabs =3 (Darby)
Tega-Atric (Ortega)
Tega-Tussin (W. Huen)
Tega-Zol (Ortega)
Tega-Zol Elixir (Ortega)
Tempo-Dex Tablets (Rasman)
Tempo-Dex 15 (Buffalo)
Tempophene (Tutag)
Tempophene-H (Tutag)
Tempotraid Liquid (Smith, Miller and Patch)
Temsert No. 2 (Arnar-Stone)
Ten-Shun (Haberle)
Tense-Less (Medical Service)
Tensel (Foy)
Tensenal (Foy)
Tension Aid (Lit)
Tenstan (Standex)
Tenstat S.R. (St. Louis Physicians Supply)
Teolaxin (Paul Maney)
Teragen (S.F. Durst)
Terhydrol with Codeine Liquid
Terhydrol with Morphine (Neisler Labs)
Terp Cough Tabs (United Research)
Terpacof Liquid (Jenkins Lab)
Terpan (Wynn)
Terpi-Chlor (Richlyn)
Terpi-Kal Tablets (Approved)
Terpicol (Garde)
Terpin Hydrate and Codeine Elixir
Terpin Hydrate Wafers with Codeine (W. T. Thompson)
Terpin-Hy-Chlor (Darby)
Terpinodeine (Moore Kirk)
Terponium (Medco)

Terpyamous (Lustgarten)
Tetrahydrophenobarbital
Tetronal
Thalmased (Kenyon)
Thencodin with Dionin Liquid (National Pharm)
Thenital (Ascher)
Theolaxin Ph. Unoday 748 (Paul Maney)
Theratone (Day-Baldwin)
Theratone-B (Day-Baldwin)
Thesant (Norden)
Thiabarb (various)
Thiamine-P (Vitamix)
Thiamital-CT (Standex)
Thiamylal Sodium
Thin-Tabs No. 1 Yellow (Henry Schein)
Thin-Tabs No. 2 Green (Henry Schein)
Thin-Tabs No. 3 Orange (Henry Schein)
Thin-Tabs, Pink (Henry Schein)
Thin-Tabs, White (Henry Schein)
Thin-Tabs 5 mg. Grey (Henry Schein)
Thiodex (North American)
Thiogenal
Thiopental
Thiopental Sodium
Thiopentone Sodium
Thora-Dex No. 1 and 2 (Smith, Kline and French)
Thoryza Capsules (Warren-Teed)
Threamine with Codeine Liquid (National Pharm)
Three Bromides Syrup (various)
Thy Obese T.M. (TMCO)
Thy-Obese No. 3 Jr. (TMCO)
Thy-O-Caps (Bush)
Thy-O-Caps, Jr. (St. Louis Physicians Supply)
Thycochen with Codeine Liquid (Wisconsin Pharm)
Thypet (Kraft)
Thyramo (Darby)
Thyrex (Prof. Drug Service)
Thyrobarb T.R. (Harvey)
Thyrodex (Marin Medical Supply)
Thyrophen, F.S. No. 1 (Premo)
Thyrophen, F.S. No. 2 (Premo)
Thyrophen, F.S. No. 3 (Premo)
Thyrophen, H.S. No. 1 (Premo)
Thyrophen, H.S. No. 2 (Premo)
Thyrophen, H.S. No 3 (Premo)
Thyro-Spandex No. 2 (Bock)
Thyro-Spandex No. 3 (Bock)

Thyroquad (Medical Specialties)
Tilyards Mixture (National Pharm)
Timecaps 10 and 15 (Jabert)
Timely Delstat Tablet (Queen City)
Timely Obe Capsules (Queen City)
Timo-Tabs No. 2 (Superior)
Timo-Caps No. 2 (Superior)
Tio-Pentemal
TMCO Sodium Pentobarbital (TMCO)
Capsules 49 mg.
Suspension
T.O.B. Caps (Zimmers)
Tobaral Forte (Ascher)
Tobie Tablet =1 Double Strength
(Fellows-Testagar)
Tobie Tablet =2 Double Strength
(Fellows-Testagar)
Tobie Tablet =3 Double Strength
(Fellows-Testagar)
Tobie Tablet = 1 Regular Strength
(Fellows-Testagar)
Tobie Tablet =2 Regular Strength
(Fellows-Testagar)
Tobie Tablet =3 Regular Strength
(Fellows-Testagar)
Tolamine Tablets (Clark and Clark)
Tolaphen-Phenobarb (Invenex)
Tolbuzem (Zemmer)
Tolsamide w/ Phenobarbital (Cenci)
Tolserol/Codeine
Tolsom No. 2 (Superior)
Tolu-Sed (First Texas)
Tolumint DHC (P. J. Noyes)
Tonedom (Edom)
Toni Barbital (TMCO)
Toni Secobarbital (TMCO)
Toni-Tran (TMCO)
Tonodex Tablets (Key)
Toxital Injection (Jensen-Salsbury)
Tran-B (Byrne)
Tranbusol (Southern)
Trangic Tablets (Kenyon)
Tranizer (Wabash)
Trankuilan
Tranlisant
Tranquil (Detroit)
Tranquilan
Tranquilans (Noyes)
Tranquilax
Tranquiline
Transen (Gateway)
Transibarb (Breon)
Trantab (Plymouth)
Tred-Caps (Santa)

Trenket-Tabs (Lustgarten)
Tresodex (Midwest)
Tri Comph (Tricounty Surgical Supply)
Tri Peptum/Paregoric (Ads Labs)
Tri-Barbs (High)
Tri-Caps No. 1 (Vita-Fore)
Tri-Caps No. 2 (Vita-Fore)
Tri-Caps No. 3 (Vita-Fore)
Tri-Caps P.A. (Vita-Fore)
Tri-Dex (Testagar)
Tri-Dextro (Kenyon)
Tri-Peptum Paregoric (Purepac)
Tri-Phetamine Capsules (Wayne)
Tri-Thyram' (Tricounty Surgical Supply)
Triaminic Expectorant DH (Dorsey)
Triaxin (Mayrand)
Tablets 16 mg.
Tablets 32 mg.
Tablets 97 mg.
Tribromatal Tablets (Parker)
Trico-Tabs No. 1 '5' (Vita-Fore)
Trico-Tabs No. 1 '10' (Vita-Fore)
Trico-Tabs No. 2 '5' (Vita-Fore)
Trico-Tabs No. 2 '10' (Vita-Fore)
Trico-Tabs No. 3 '1' (Vita-Fore)
Trico-Tabs No. 3 '5' (Vita-Fore)
Tricodene Liquid (Pfeiffer)
Tricodene No. 2 Liquid (Pfeiffer)
Tricopec (Tricounty Surgical Supply)
Tricostat (Tricounty Surgical Supply)
Triforms with Thyroid, Blue (Conwell)
Triforms with Thyroid, Green (Conwell)
Triforms with Thyroid, Orange (Conwell)
Trigesic/Codeine
Triko No. 1 (Bryant)
Triko No. 2 (Bryant)
Triko No. 3 (Bryant)
Triko T.D. (Bryant)
Trimbak (Reyman)
Trim Caps =1 5 mg. H.S. =4 Grey (Richlyn)
Trim Caps =2 5 mg. H.S. =4 Clear (Richlyn)
Trim Caps =3 5 mg. H.S. =4 Pink (Richlyn)
Trim Caps =1 10 mg. H.S. =1 Grey (Rich-
lyn)
Trim Caps =2 10 mg. H.S. =1 Clear (Rich-
lyn)
Trim Caps =3 10 mg. H.S. =1 Pink (Richlyn)
Trim Capsules =1 Regular (United Re-
search)
Trim Capsules =2 Regular (United Re-
search)
Trim Capsules =3 Regular (United Re-
search)
Trimcap No. 1 Timedcaps (Robinson)

Trimcap No. 2 Timedcaps (Robinson)
Tri-Mer (Richlyn)
Trim Tabs =1 5 mg. Grey (Richlyn)
Trim Tabs =2 5 mg. Natural (Richlyn)
Trim Tabs =3 5 mg. Pink (Richlyn)
Trim Tabs = 1 10 mg. Grey (Richlyn)
Trim Tabs =2 10 mg. Natural (Richlyn)
Trim Tabs =3 10 mg. Pink (Richlyn)
Trim Tablets =1 (United Research)
Trim Tablets =1 High Potency (United Research)
Trim Tablets =2 Regular (United Research)
Trim Tablets =2 Regular-Sugar Coated (United Research)
Trim Tablets =2 High Potency (United Research)
Trim Tablets =2 High Potency-Sugar Coated (United Research)
Trim Tablets =3 Regular (United Research)
Trim Tablets =3 Regular-Sugar Coated (United Research)
Trim Tablets =3 High Potency (United Research)
Trim Tablets =3 High Potency-Sugar Coated (United Research)
Trim Tab (Franklin)
Trim Tabs =1 (J.W. S. Delavau)
Trim-Tabs 1 (Franklin)
Trim-Tabs =2 (J.W.S. Delavau)
Trim-Tabs 2 (Franklin)
Trim-Tabs =3 (J.W.S. Delavau)
Trim-Tabs 3 (Franklin)
Trimer-Caps T.D. (Spencer-Mead)
Trinotic (Testagar)
Trio (Rondex)
Trio No. 1 (Rondex)
Trio No. 2 (Rondex)
Trio No. 3 (Rondex)
Tri-Ob No. 1 (Superior)
Tri-Ob No. 2 (Superior)
Tri-Ob No. 3 (Superior)
Triocap (Evron)
Triofate Tablets (Hiss)
Trional
Trip-Notic (Ortega)
Triphenatol (Tri-State)
  Tablets 16 mg.
  Tablets 32 mg.
  Tablets 65 mg.
  Tablets 97 mg.
Triple-Barb (Moore Kirk)
Triple Obesity (Halsom)
Triple Obesity No. 1, Grey (Drugmaster)
Triple Obesity No. 2, White (Drugmaster)

Triple Obesity No. 3, Pink (Drugmaster)
Trisobarb Tablets (Cenci)
Trisobarb w/ Belladonna (Cenci)
Tri-Tabs No. 1 '5' (Vita-Fore)
Tri-Tabs No. 1 '10' (Vita-Fore)
Tri-Tabs No. 2 '5' (Vita-Fore)
Tri-Tabs No. 2 '10' (Vita-Fore)
Tri-Tabs No. 3 '5' (Vita-Fore)
Tri-Tabs No. 3 '10' (Vita-Fore)
Tritabs Amphetacomp, Green (Eastern Research)
Tritabs Amphetacomp, Yellow (Eastern Research)
Tritabs Amphetacomp, Pink (Eastern Research)
Trital (Testagar)
Tri-Trim Tabs MLT =1 (Richlyn)
Tri-Trim Tabs MLT =2 (Richlyn)
Tri-Trim Tabs MLT =3 (Richlyn)
Tritussin Cough Syrup (Towne, Paulsen)
Trivased Tablets (Wesley)
Tro-Pam (Amco)
Trycoval Liquid (National Pharm)
TS-192 (Calvin Scott)
TSB (Calvin Scott)
TSG Croup Syrup (P. B. Elder)
TXB (Calvin Scott)
Tuinal (Lilly)
  Capsules 49 mg.
  Capsules 97 mg.
  Capsules 194 mg.
Tussaminic
Tussanil DH (various)
Tussar-SF (Armour)
Tussar-2 (Armour)
Tussarol-CC (Burrough Bros)
Tusseez No. 18 Cough Syrup (Sutliff and Case)
Tussend Liquid (Dow)
Tussend Tablets (Dow)
Tussihab (Haberle)
Tussi-Organidin (Wampole)
Tussionex (Strasenburgh)
  Capsules
  Suspension
  Tablets
Tussirex with Codeine Syrup (Scott-Tussin)
Tussomyl Syrup (P. B. Elder)
Tusstrol (Reid-Provident)
Twendex-PB (Allison)
Twin-Barb (Ascher)
Twin-Barb Improved (Ascher)
Twinital 1 1/2 (TMCO)
Twistussin Syrup (McNeil)

Two-Bar (Key)
Two-Bar-HS Tablets (Key)
Two-Barb (Key)
Two-Barbital Capsules (Supreme)
Tylenol with Codeine No. 1 (McNeil)
Tylenol with Codeine No. 2 (McNeil)
Tylenol with Codeine No. 3 (McNeil)
Tylenol with Codeine No. 4 (McNeil)

Una-Nike (Physicians Supply)
Uni-Bese (United Research)
Uni-Bese =2 (United Research)
Uni-Bese-T =3 (United Research)
Unibese-T (United Research)
Uni-Butamph-Dex (United Research)
Unicel Tablets (United)
Uni-Dextro-B (United Research)
Uni-Haponal TDC (United Research)
Uni-Test Barbital Buffer Catalog Nos. 8093,
    8094, 8096
Uni-Test Barbital Buffer (Vaughn)
    Catalog No. 8093
    Catalog No. 8094
    Catalog No. 8096
Uni-Trim (United Research)
Urbil

V-13 (Starr)
V-27 (Starr)
Valamin (Schering)
Valana with Codeine Sulfate (Vale)
Valaspas (Moore Kirk)
Valeripass (Standex)
Valmid (Lilly)
Valora (Superior)
Valtobarb (Valentine)
Valtuss Syrup (Vale)
Vanaphen (various)
    Elixir
    Tablets
Vee-Gera basic (Schlicksup)
Vee-Gera Basic (DAS 2.5 mg) Tablets
    (Schlicksup)
Vellada Tablets (Testagar)
Veraflex (Neisler)
Veralzem No. 2 (Zemmer)

Verbital Elixir (Burroughs Bros.)
Verdex Capsules (Lynn)
Verolettin
Vertavis-Phen (Neisler)
Vertens (Wabash)
Veruphen No. 2 (Zemmer)
Viage (Kenneth A. Manne)
Viatric (various)
Vio-Dexose Chewables (Rowell)
Vio-Lectal (Rowell)
Viobamate (Rowell)
    Tablets 200 mg.
    Tablets 400 mg.
Virtal-B Tablets (Virtal)
Vita-Dex Elixir (Vita-Fore)
Vita-Phen Elixir (Vita-Fore)
Vita-Sed Tablets (Klug)
Vito-Bese P.A. (Vita-Fore)

W-10 (Wolins)
Waitplex 1/2 (Schlicksup)
Waitplex (Schlicksup)
Wans No. 1 (Webster)
Wans No. 2 (Webster)
Watrol Liquid (U.S. Vitamin)
Waytrol Graduals (Federal)
Wefeta Capsules (Webb)
Wendased (Wendt-Bristol)
Wescoid-B (Wesley)
Wescophen-S (Wesley)
Weytabs No. 1, 2, & 3 (Vale)
Win-Codin Tablets (Winthrop)
Wiscollana with Codeine Liquid (Wisconsin
    Pharm)
Wolgraine (Wolins)
Wolstat (Wolins)
Wolstat-T (Wolins)

X-Ameen Capsules (Xttrium)
Y-Tussin (E. W. Huen)
Yelophen Tablets (Durst)
Zem Histine with Codeine Syrup (Zemmer)
Zeni-Bese (Zenith)
Zeni-Bese T (Zenith)
Zeni-Bese T-15 (Zenith)
Zenobese 15 Capsules (Zenith)
Zo-Tussin (E. W. Huen)

Catalog

If you are interested in a list of fine Paperback
books, covering a wide range of subjects
and interests, send your name and address,
requesting your free catalog, to:

McGraw-Hill Paperbacks
1221 Avenue of Americas
New York, N.Y. 10020